THE WARDENS: MANAGING A LATE MEDIEVAL HOSPITAL

BROWNE'S HOSPITAL, STAMFORD 1495-1518

edited by Alan Rogers
and members of the Stamford Survey Group

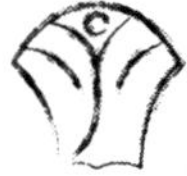

Published by the Stamford and District Local History Society,
with support from and in association with the Lincoln Record Society
and Abramis Academic Publishing

Cover illustrations:
(a) Bedehouse Farm, North Luffenham, Rutland, acquired by William Browne and passed to the Hospital (photo: Nick Hill); (b) Audit Room (formerly Gildhall of Gild of All Saints), Browne's Hospital (photo: Nick Hill); (c) extract from Hospital Account Book from MS. Rawl. B. 352, The Bodleian Libraries, University of Oxford (with permission)

Published 2013 by abramis academic publishing

www.abramis.co.uk

ISBN 978 1 84549 599 2

Printed and bound in the United Kingdom

abramis is an imprint of arima publishing.

arima publishing
ASK House, Northgate Avenue
Bury St Edmunds, Suffolk IP32 6BB
t: (+44) 01284 700321

www.abramis.co.uk

CONTENTS

LIST OF IMAGES

FOREWORD

Bodleian Library Rawlinson MS. B. 352 is an account book from Browne's Hospital, Stamford, covering the years 1495 to 1518. Its existence has been known for many years, and the first two and a half pages were published in *Antiquaries Journal* in 1966. But the riches contained in the rest of the volume have not been tapped.

The current edition is the result of many years of work by a large number of people. It was begun in the late 1960s by Canon J Paul Hoskins, former rector of St John's and then of St Mary's church, Stamford, and confrater of Browne's Hospital 1952-1958, jointly with Dr Alan Rogers, University of Nottingham Resident Tutor in south Lincolnshire. The University of Nottingham funded a microfilm of the volume. On Canon Hoskins' death, the work was taken up by several members of the Stamford Survey Group, notably Mrs Winifred Bowman and latterly Ann Matthews, who between them completed the first transcript of the volume. Ann and other members of the Group have been involved in further work on the glossary. But the editing of the volume in its present format and the Introduction have both been my work.

We are all very grateful to a large number of people who have assisted this work over many years. They are too many to be listed in full, but the following need particular acknowledgement: Dr Bruce Barker-Benfield and the staff of the Bodleian Library; the staff of Lincoln Archives Office (LAO); Nick Hill of English Heritage; Dr James Ross (then) of the National Archives; Dr Nicholas Amor; Dr Nicholas Bennett of Lincoln Record Society; the trustees and residents of Browne's Hospital, especially Pam Sharp and David Goodison; the staff of the Town Hall, Stamford; the former staff of the (now defunct) Stamford Museum and their successors at the Stamford Public Library. Andy Hall of Cambridge provided the map.

The Lincoln Record Society made a substantial grant to the Stamford and District Local History Society to enable this publication to appear in a timely fashion; and our publisher of several of our volumes, abramis academic publishers, Bury St Edmunds, have once again done us proud in the difficult work of producing a volume which represents as far as possible the complicated formatting of the original volume. To them all, we are very grateful.

But I would like, if I may, to dedicate this volume to the memory of Canon Paul Hoskins, whose enthusiasm for both Browne's Hospital and his adopted town of Stamford sparked off this production. This is the last of the published volumes in this project on medieval Stamford which the Stamford Survey Group commenced many years ago; future texts will appear on the society's website.

Alan Rogers
September 2013

INTRODUCTION:
THE WARDENS - MANAGING THE HOSPITAL AND ITS ESTATES

(*Note: the numbers in brackets refer to folio numbers in the text of the account book, not to page numbers*[1])

If we are to judge by the story told in this account book, the life of a warden of a late medieval almshouse must have been hell. The troubles of Mr Harding in Barchester make his life look like a bed of roses compared with what successive wardens of Browne's Hospital, Stamford, experienced in the late fifteenth and early sixteenth century. These wardens may not of course have been typical for this period, but their lives were real enough.

The problems seem to have been caused by three factors. First was a chronic shortage of money which, as time went on, forced successive wardens into a variety of strategies. Secondly, there was William Browne's inheritance. Browne endowed the Hospital with an estate and an estate management system which, while Browne with his staff and personality could manage it, the warden was completely inexperienced and ill-equipped to deal with; and the resulting difficulties of arrears of rents and distraints and repairs to properties drained the energies of the warden. But thirdly, in 1506 the then warden (probably prompted by a predecessor) found himself launched on an injudicious dispute with the gild of All Saints, Stamford, which took up a great deal of time and financial resources and caused him to resign.

THE PRE-WARDEN DAYS

To understand the situation, we need to survey briefly the early history of the Hospital. William Browne, a wealthy wool merchant, and his wife Margaret founded it in 1475 as Clement Hospital, a gild hall for the parish gild of All Saints of which Browne was Alderman for life, combined with an almshouse for ten poor men and two women attendants. The Brownes managed the institution. Prior to their deaths in 1489, they endowed it with a portfolio of estates, rural and urban, and they incorporated the Hospital in the names of the warden and confrater[2]. They appointed the staff of whom John Coton (warden) and William

---

[1] The folio numbers in brackets are indicative only, not a full list; for more comprehensive references to the subjects mentioned, consult the index. Some of the quotations used in this Introduction have been modernised to make them more easily understood; the text below will show the original.

[2] Initially, rather than appoint long-term trustees, the Brownes intended to incorporate the warden, confrater and all ten bedesmen and two bedeswomen; but in the end it was only the warden and confrater who had the responsibility of incorporation. See Nick Hill and Alan

Hawkyns (confrater) came from the earlier Hospital, in that office by at least July 1488 and probably earlier[3].

On the death of William and Margaret Browne, Margaret's brother Thomas Stokes[4], formerly vicar of All Saints in the Market, Stamford, continued the foundation. He drew up statutes, arranged for the (re-)dedication of the chapel and paid all the costs from the estates; the warden did nothing.

> *I have reserved to myself* [he wrote] *during my life over the said Almshouse, the Warden and Confrater of the same and their successors, and also over the profits, revenues, or possessions, or what things soever are bestowed or hereafter to be bestowed upon the same Warden, Confrater or their successors, a full power and absolute authority of further ordering*[5]

Like Browne, he ruled the Hospital. This is indicated in the first account which is described as

> *the first accompt' off thys almos hows aftyr the deth off Mastyr thomas stok fownder of the seyd hows* (fol 2)

Stokes died in October 1495, and the warden John Coton took over: as John Taylor his successor, quoting the statutes, reported (with some exaggeration),

> *After whose death the said John Coton actively executed his said office, namely warden in this almshouse, to pay, receive, administer, preside over, correct what needed to be corrected and did such other things that belong to his office in this almshouse from the feast of the Nativity of Our Lord in the said year* (1v)

The patronage

William Browne clearly saw himself as patron of the Hospital in a personal capacity rather than as Alderman of the gild. He had built the Hospital in the grounds of his own house and (when the time came) he endowed it from his own family estates. It was his personal fiefdom; hence the change in title from Clement Hospital to *'the Hospital of William Browne of Stamford for ever'*.

Rogers 2012 *Gild, Hospital and Alderman: new light on the foundation of Browne's Hospital, Stamford 1475-95* Bury St Edmunds: abramis academic publishers

[3] Coton and Hawkyns were named as feoffees by Browne in the Hospital estates in July 1488, Lincolnshire Archives Office (LAO), Browne's Hospital archives (BHS) 7/12/24; for more complete details of this deed, see Alan Rogers 2012 *People and Property in Medieval Stamford* abramis, pp 293-4. It is probable that Hawkyns was not confrater from 1475, since Hawkyns did not die until 1517, and that would imply 42 years at the Hospital; as it was, from 1488 (or earlier) to 1517 was 29 years or more.

[4] For Thomas Stokes, see Alan Rogers, 2011 Eton's First 'Poor Scholar': Sir William Stokes of Warmington, Northamptonshire (c1425-1485) and his family in the fifteenth century, *Northants Past and Present* 64 pp 5-21

[5] H P Wright 1890 *The Story of the Domus Dei of Stamford: the Hospital of William Browne* London: Parker, pp 29-30; see Appendix III.

On Browne's death, the patronage came to Thomas Stokes, while the Aldermanry of the gild came to Browne's young grandson and heir William Elmes, a lawyer. The two worked closely together, for Elmes (at least for a time) lived in Browne's house next door to the Hospital as well as on his manor of Wolfhouse (now Woolfox), Rutland. In his statutes (see Appendix III), Stokes provided that on his death, the patronage would descend to William Elmes (by name) and then to the dean of Stamford and the vicar of All Saints jointly. If that were not possible, then "the heirs of the said William Browne" shall become patron "for that time only"; in the event that the heirs were not able to act, the patronage would descend to the Alderman of the borough and the abbot of Crowland, then to the bishop of Lincoln; "and so forward *ad infinitum*".

After the death of Coton in 1497, Elmes, as patron, appointed John Taylor as warden and then William Sharpe as Taylor's successor in 1504. After the death of Elmes in 1504, the vicar of All Saints acted as patron. The dean of Stamford (an office which moved around among the parish clergy of the town) joined with the vicar in the annual audit of the Hospital's accounts, but the vicar was clearly in charge.

The vicarage of All Saints was in the patronage of the nuns of St Michael, Stamford, but it would seem that William Browne had considerable influence. Browne's early home stood next door to the vicarage. John Holliday, vicar for nearly fifty years, 1419-68, was a feoffee (trustee) and associate of Browne. On his death in 1468, the nuns appointed Browne's brother-in-law, Thomas Stokes, as vicar, and when Stokes resigned in 1479 to go to his living of Easton-on-the-Hill, he obtained from the nuns the next presentation and appointed Henry Wykes who stayed until his death. Wykes was a member of the wealthy family of Burley[6] by Stamford and again a very close associate and trustee of Browne. Wykes appointed Robert Sheppey, another protégé of Stokes, as warden after the departure of Sharpe in 1507. Wykes died in 1508 and was succeeded by Thomas Morrand as vicar of All Saints church and patron of the Hospital.

After the death of William Elmes, few residual links remained between the Hospital and the Elmes family. William and Margaret Browne's daughter Elizabeth, by now widow of John Elmes esq[7] of Lilford and mother of William Elmes, survived as a widow until 1511, and she and her second son John both left substantial legacies to the Hospital. The Hospital continued to draw supplies from the Elmes' manor of Wolfhouse; and the warden on one of his travels stayed at the Elmes' manor of Swinstead, Lincs[8]. The accounts speak of 'my

[6] Now Burghley

[7] Not 'Sir' John Elmes as in other accounts; he was never knighted. The error comes from the late seventeenth century pedigree printed in *Visitations of Northamptonshire, 1564 and 1618*, edited W.C. Metcalfe, London 1887, p 18; the pedigree is inaccurate.

[8] If Hoggerston (which is not otherwise identified) is Oakington in Cambridgeshire, then the wardens stayed at another Elmes' manor on several occasions. See Appendix V

lady' when referring to Elizabeth Elmes (70v, 73). But it is very unlikely that she had any real influence on the fortunes of the house during her lifetime; she lived mainly at Henley on Thames or at Lilford, Northants.

THE WARDENS

After the death of Stokes in October 1495, the day-to-day management of the Hospital and its estates fell onto the warden - and apparently onto the warden alone. The confrater for almost the whole of this period (1495-1518), William Hawkyns, is notable by his almost complete absence from the pages of this account book. In early 1497 when Coton died, Hawkyns did not pick up the warden's duties; it was Wykes who paid the weekly stipend to the bedesmen and women. The confrater did not succeed to the office of warden on the death of the warden. Hawkyns did go to North Witham with William Elmes at Christmas 1495 in place of Coton (who may have been ill), and he is named once or twice as being present at the annual audit of the warden, but apart from that, his activities remained outside the orbit of this account. The burden - and burden it clearly was - fell on the warden, with some support from the vicar of All Saints.

Who then were the wardens who found themselves suddenly carrying such onerous duties of estate management as these accounts show?

Of **John Coton (Warden to 1497),** we know little. He is referred to as 'the first warden' of the Hospital[9]; and since he was in the Hospital by 1488, it is probable that he was warden of Clement Hospital, the predecessor of Browne's Hospital. He was one of William Browne's connection; he and Hawkyns were feoffees for William Browne in 1488, and both witnessed Margaret Browne's will in 1489. He was confirmed in office by Stokes in December 1494 and took over his responsibilities a year later when Stokes died. There was some confusion immediately after the death of Stokes (October 1495) but in December 1495, Robert Beomond, William Browne's agent who also worked for Thomas Stokes, made payments to the warden from the estates so that the warden could pay the bedesmen and women at the statutory rate of 7d per week. Coton took over from January 1496. Optimistically, he raised the weekly rate to 8d which persisted until he died just over a year later, on 10 January 1497. The next warden, Taylor, kept this increase going for six months but reversed it in August 1497 (8).

William Elmes, patron, appointed **John Taylor (Warden 1497 to 1504)** as successor to Coton. Taylor is the key figure throughout the whole of this account book, for he was involved with Hospital affairs before becoming warden

[9] It is clear that Thomas Stokes and successive wardens regarded the re-foundation and re-naming of the Hospital in 1494 as the foundation of Browne's Hospital, and Thomas Stokes as its founder; for this, see Hill and Rogers *Gild, Hospital and Alderman*

and continued to pull the strings after he resigned; indeed, as we shall see, he initiated the book. His appointment was somewhat unusual in two respects; he was a relatively young man, and he was and continued to be an academic at Oxford University.

It must have been his prior links with William Browne which caused his appointment in 1497. John Taylor had been personal chaplain to William Browne (we know Browne had a chapel in his house next to the Hospital[10]). In July 1488, with Coton, he had been named as a trustee in the Hospital estates. On the death of William Browne in 1489, Taylor proceeded to Oxford, probably supported by the Browne estate, now in the hands of feoffees but effectively in the hands of Thomas Stokes. Taylor remained close to the Browne family; in 1499, he was feoffee for Elizabeth Elmes[11].

He was admitted to Oriel College in 1489-90 and took his MA in that same year. He continued at Oxford, quickly becoming junior treasurer (1491-2) and senior treasurer (1493-4) of the college. The support of Thomas Stokes for his Oxford career is indicated by the provision in Stokes' will (1494):

> *Item I will that C li* [£100] *be delyvered into the keping of sir Henry Wykes and maister Thomas Hykam for the exhibicion of ij prests that is to say maistre John Taylour scolar of Oxford and sir Robert Shipley, the said maistre Taylour to have his stipend to Oxford by cause of his Lernyng there viij marcs by yere.*

So that after Stokes' death in October 1495, Taylor continued to receive support for his studies in Oxford. But in February 1497, a month after Coton died, Taylor was installed as warden of Browne's Hospital; and (despite a prohibition in the statutes against the warden having any other preferment) for most of his time as warden, he combined an active academic career with the wardenship of the almshouse - senior treasurer of Oriel 1498-1501, principal of St Mary Hall from 1499 until September 1502, and dean of Oriel for part of the year 1501-2. He was a bookish man - almost certainly owner of the English translation of the *Speculum Inclusorum* which he gave to the Hospital[12], and the recipient of a book from a fellow Oriel scholar in 1500 while he was warden in Stamford.

It seems he only became full-time warden in Stamford in 1502 when he left Oxford[13]; he then engaged energetically in the administration of the Hospital and

---

[10] The will of Margaret Browne in 1489 mentions a 'chamber over the chapel', see Alan Rogers 2008 Some kinship wills of the late fifteenth century from Stamford, Rutland and the surrounding area, *Rutland Record* 28 pp 285-6

[11] Devon Record Office, Simcoe M/T/13/6,7

[12] Rogers, Wills pp 290-1; Alan Rogers, The Ownership of *The Myrour Of Recluses* (British Library Harl Ms 2372) in the late fifteenth century, *The Library* (forthcoming).

[13] Emden A B 1957 *Biographical Register of the University of Oxford to 1500* Oxford iii p 1851; there was a second John Taylor who held Northmoor, Oxford, with licence for absence for purposes of studying (Margaret Bowker 1968 *Secular Clergy of the diocese of Lincoln 1495 to 1520*

its estates. He dismissed the estate bailiff, taking part of the bailiff's fee for himself (43v-44), and chose his own assistants. He cancelled at least one major tenancy (43v). But this did not last long: in January 1504, he resigned the wardenship to take up the somewhat more remunerative[14] and less stressful position of vicar of St Martin's parish church in Stamford, from where he continued to be closely involved in the affairs of the almshouse until he died in 1517/8[15].

The coincidence of Taylor leaving the Hospital in February 1504 and Elmes dying in March 1504 cannot be ignored. Elmes had been ill for some years ("with the sweating sickness", see fol 10) and on occasion the vicar of All Saints had had to act on his behalf. It would have been known that on the death of Elmes, the next Alderman of the gild would be Christopher Browne, the senior surviving member of the Browne family; and there had already (1502) been trouble between Taylor and Christopher over some of the Hospital estates in Lincolnshire. And it cannot be doubted but that the gild had already raised questions about the role of the gild in the management of the Hospital, probably at the time of the appointment of Taylor. Taylor may have wished to relocate himself to avoid the trouble which he saw would clearly follow. But this must remain as speculation.

William Elmes lived long enough to appoint Taylor's successor, **William Sharpe (Warden 1504 to 1508)** before Elmes himself died in March 1504. Sharpe too seems to have been a scholar; one William Sharpe graduated at Cambridge University in 1499, and in 1514, Master William Sharpe was reprimanded for being non-resident from his benefice of Careby, Lincs, perhaps for the purposes of studying[16]. The exact date of his appointment to Browne's Hospital early in 1504 is not certain, since the accounts for his first two and half years are missing. Similarly, the date of his '*departyng*' (of which he speaks in his final account, folio 65) is equally uncertain. But since he bore the brunt of the law suit between the Hospital and the gild, being summoned to London twice in a few months, and since he left immediately after his London court appearances, he may have

---

Cambridge University Press p 206) and from 1510 the benefice of Frome Selwood in Somerset, until his death about 1524; the Stamford John Taylor died in 1517 (see note 15 below). Emden *Oxford* confuses the two Taylors. I am certain that our man was the Oxford fellow of Oriel because of Thomas Stokes' legacy to support his studies at Oxford.

[14] The wardenship paid £6 13s 4d p.a, the vicar of St Martin's church received about £8, see John S Hartley and Alan Rogers 1974 *Religious Foundations of Medieval Stamford* Stamford Survey Group p 32

[15] On 18 January 1518, Richard Hardy was instituted to the vicarage of St Martin's church, Stamford, on the death of Master John Taillour, Bishop Atwater's register, LAO, Register 25, fol 17v; I owe this reference and other help to Dr Nicholas Bennett. Hardy remained there until his death about 1526, H E Salter 1913 *Clerical subsidy in the diocese of Lincoln 1526*, Oxford Historical Society vol 63 p 61

[16] J Venn *Alumni Cantabrigiensis to 1751* (4 vols 1922-27) sub nom; A B Emden *Biographical Register of the University of Cambridge to 1500* (1963) p 511; Bowker *Secular Clergy* pp 133, 196

departed with some bitterness between himself and Taylor. Taylor clearly remained active in relation to the Hospital, acting as deputy for the vicar of All Saints in the annual audit of the accounts of the wardens (83, 89v). Sharpe is next seen in 1511 when he was instituted as rector of Careby, a rich benefice in south Lincolnshire; in 1514, he was ordered to pay for repairs to the rectory; in 1526, he was serving the parish by a curate and a parochial chaplain, and he died in office there in 1531[17]. He appears to have been pious – we know he fasted every Wednesday, and his accounts include payments for two images of saints, St Blaise and St Anne; so the active life of the warden may not have been congenial to his nature.

Sharpe seems to have used lawyers for much of the work that Taylor had done. But he departed in a hurry; the final part of his account was written (by Sharpe) in a scrawl and there was a dispute over the wording of the audit. Before he left, he met his successor '*to show him where our debts lay*' (65); and although he held unaccounted-for debts to the almshouse to the tune of £10 4s 2½d for which he was pursued for several years, he was paid handsomely before he left:

> *Md yat the warden ys allowed for hys gret laburs and troblese yat he hath had for hys suet off thys almeshouse* *xxiiijs viijd* (68v)

The hurried nature of his departure almost certainly accounts for the next appointment, made by Henry Wykes. **Robert Sheppey (Warden 1507-1518)** was one of the Browne-Stokes circle. As Robert Shipley, he was named in the will of Stokes (1494, proved 1495) as Thomas Stokes' chantry priest in Easton on the Hill at a stipend of £5 p.a. until the endowment ran out; he may have combined this with the benefice of Duston, Northants (Robert Shipley, vicar 1497-1503)[18]. In 1503, Sheppey became rector of St Paul's church in Stamford (with a stipend of about £4 p.a.), so that his elevation in 1508 to the wardenship at a stipend of over £6 p.a. would have been an advancement. Indeed, he can be seen as acting for Sharpe during the last months of Sharpe's administration; Sheppey went to London on behalf of warden Sharpe, and there were hand-over discussions with Sharpe. But like the other wardens, Sheppey clearly found the task too much; he

---

[17] William Sharpe (or Scharpe) instituted to the rectory of Careby on 20 December 1511 on the presentation of Tattershall College (LAO Register 23 fol 143v); his successor, Nicholas Sclater, was instituted on 1 August 1531, on the death of Master William Sharp (LAO Register 27 fol 50v) (I owe these references to Dr Nicholas Bennett); *An Episcopal Court Book 1514-1520,* ed M Bowker, Lincoln Record Society (LRS) vol 61 (1967) p 6; Salter *Clerical subsidy 1526* p 56; is he also the cantarist in Lincoln cathedral, ibid p 84? He cannot be the William Sharpe of Worcester diocese who went to Oxford in 1505, despite Emden *Oxford*, for the Oxford scholar was not ordained until 1512-13; this Sharpe died in 1534. But our man may be the William Sharpe vicar of Heacham who had a licence for plurality in 1489, *Calendar of Papal Letters 1484-92* p 392.

[18] Rogers, Wills pp 290-1; H I Longden, *Northants and Rutland Clergy from 1500* Northants Record Society (NRS) 1938-52, vol 12 p 155; his resignation from Duston in 1503 supports the identification. Throughout the account book, he signs as Sheppey, not Shipley.

seems to have been ill for much of his term of office, and he failed to complete several of his accounts, others having to stand in for him.

His death in January 1518 caused a crisis. A number of persons rallied round the Hospital - Thomas Morrand vicar of All Saints, Thomas Forster rector of St Michael the Greater and dean of Stamford, Thomas Hykeham rector of St Peter's church, and especially Thomas Williams, a relation of the Wykes family and one of the richest residents[19] of Stamford Baron (the suburb of Stamford south of the river Welland) and seemingly a friend of Taylor who was vicar of that part of the town; Williams was employed by the Hospital in some capacity (125).

We know that Sheppey was replaced in 1518 by **Richard Dykelun**, bachelor of decrees, a member of a very prominent local clerical family. He was son of John Dykelon husbandman of Northborough and brother of John Dykelun vicar of Deeping St Guthlac (1504); he may have attended Cambridge University. But the account book ends with only a fragment of his first account[20].

The accounts

It was the wardens then who compiled the book edited here. Apart from an account of the foundation of the Hospital from 1475 to the time of writing (c1506) which occupies the first three pages, an account which I have called 'the Narrative', it contains the annual accounts of income and expenditure of the wardens in relation to the Hospital for most of the years from 1495 to 1518. In this respect, it is unusual for this region, for there are few comparable accounts of estate management in detail such as this, but one which does provide some similar material is the informal notebook of the almoner of Peterborough abbey,

---

[19] In 1524, apart from his property in the town north of the river, Williams was assessed in Stamford Baron for goods worth £120, the largest sum in that part of the town, The National Archives (TNA) E179/135/315

[20] Northants Record Office (NRO), Fitzwilliam F/M Charter 1458. Earlier, one Richard Dykelun was vicar of East Deeping and Northborough; he was one of the godparents for two of the children of William Fairfax esquire of Deeping Gate in 1447 and 1464, Alan Rogers, 2007 A fifteenth century family Bible from Northamptonshire? *Nottingham Medieval Studies* LI, 2007 pp 167-179; and c1444-5 (the date is uncertain), he was president of a consistory court in Stamford, *Lincoln Diocesan Documents* EETS second series vol 149 pp 115-6 He was a servant of the abbot of Peterborough, NRS vol 16 *Book of Morton 1448-67* pp 30, 43-45, 67, 78, 81, 168; he may also have been Cambridge don and rector of St Edward's church in Cambridge, Emden *Cambridge* sub nom. He was a member of William Browne's circle. John Dykelun was rector of Peakirk nearby in 1467 and similarly a godparent for the Fairfax family; he held a consistory court in 1451, NRS vol. 16 p 43. Our man may be the Dykelun at Cambridge University between 1468 and 1475, Emden *Cambridge* p 202. A Richard Dyklyn was vicar of Boston 1526, Salter *Clerical subsidy 1526* p 59.

William Morton, "a careful and provident manager"[21] for the years 1449 to 1471. While there are differences, as we shall see, there are significant parallels, for the almoner was often engaged in the same kind of activities and making similar purchases in the same region of the country.

We shall discuss below the immediate causes for the creation and format of this account book, but here we can look briefly at each accountant.

Coton clearly kept accounts but not in this book and perhaps not fully, for Taylor, when he wrote the first part of the book, did not just copy up Coton's accounts but created them in this form; indeed, he paid some of Coton's bills. They cover just over one year. **Taylor,** presumably because of the legal nature of the book (see below), presented meticulous accounts, scrupulously justifying every expenditure. **Sharpe's** accounts for his first two and a half years were not available when they needed to be copied up, but he kept a very detailed account of his final year in office during which he went to London twice to attend court. He left in a hurry, and his successor Sheppey may even have made payments for Sharpe. **Sheppey** followed the precedents of earlier wardens for his first couple or so years but as time went on, the accounts became briefer and were sometimes completed by his auditors.

The chief value of these accounts is that they reveal the main problems which faced the successive wardens of Browne's Hospital, Stamford - the declining income, the problems of relating to the tenants, and the large number of disputes which presented themselves to the warden willy nilly, all (apart from one dispute, and that the most significant and most costly) arising from the management of the estates. So that the estates became the primary focus of attention of the warden rather than the Hospital.

THE ESTATES

William Browne seems in the last years of his life to have concentrated more on building up his properties in both urban and rural contexts than on his wool trade, probably with a view to endowing the Hospital which he had founded[22]. In 1488, some six months before he died, he split his estates into two, one part going to his daughter and sole surviving heir, Elizabeth Elmes, and the other part to the Hospital. Both were settled onto feoffees, and in 1494 the leading feoffee of the Hospital part, Thomas Stokes, passed these to the warden and the confrater who in 1495, when Stokes died, became sole owners of the whole estate.

---

[21] *The Book of William Morton* edited by W T Mellows and P I King, Northants Record Society 16 (1954) p xxxv - hereafter *Morton*. Morton engaged in more hands-on estate administration than the wardens, grazing and selling cattle etc.

[22] For Browne, see Alan Rogers 2012 *'Noble Merchant': William Browne (c1410-1489) and Stamford in the fifteenth century* abramis academic, Bury St Edmunds

What then were the estates which were 'dumped' on John Coton after the death of Thomas Stokes?

They consisted on two manors in south Lincolnshire, Swayfield and North Witham. Swayfield seems to have comprised the whole settlement, but in North Witham, there were other landholders, especially Sir Thomas Delalaund who resided there. Each manor had outlying interests in neighbouring villages, and each was burdened with 'chief rents' to neighbouring lords. We do not have surveys of these manors, so the number of tenants is not known; but the properties were extensive. Manor courts were held twice a year in each manor.

There were properties in another twenty parishes, ten in Lincolnshire, three in Rutland and seven in Northamptonshire. The most southerly was Warmington, Margaret Browne's birth village. The most distant estates were some 18 kms (just over ten miles) from Stamford, so "*the circuit of our lands*" (91v) as described by the warden was some 22 miles from north to south and about ten miles from east to west (see map).

In addition, there were sixteen tenements in Stamford itself, several with land in the open fields. There were also some gardens and further lands in all three open fields of the town, East, Middle and West (42v) and in Pinglefield, some closes at Small Bridges (on the road to Uffington), two closes and some meadow in Bredcroft (a suburb of Stamford to the west lying in Rutland), and property in Wothorpe (37v)[23], a small parish to the south west, almost a suburb. Some of these properties were very substantial, especially the Angel on St Mary's Street at the top of St Mary's Hill and the Crane in St Peter's parish.

Increase of estates

The estates did not remain unchanged from Browne's donation. Margaret Browne gave some woodland to the Hospital in 1489[24]. Other land was bought from time to time; presumably with a view to consolidating the estates rather than investment, for the Hospital did not have spare cash for purchases of land. A great amount of time and effort was spent in the early years discussing land with Sir Thomas Delalaund - first, an exchange of property (17v), then the sale of part of the wood of Swynhaw, and finally a grant of two sets of property in North Witham. One was a messuage ("*beside the river*") and 40 acres of land which Delalaund had received from his brother-in-law Sir Maurice Berkeley. The other consisted of three tenements and some land, granted specifically in return

---

[23] In these accounts, the Hospital divided its estates into rural and urban; Wothorpe, south of the river Welland, was frequently among the rural estates but at times among the urban group of properties. Bredcroft paid the subsidy at the urban rate of one tenth, TNA E179/135/24; 179/135/20, but Wothorpe seems to have paid at one fifteenth.

[24] Wright p 71

for the names of himself and his family being added to the Hospital bederoll[25]. A licence of mortmain was obtained from the abbot of Peterborough (22).

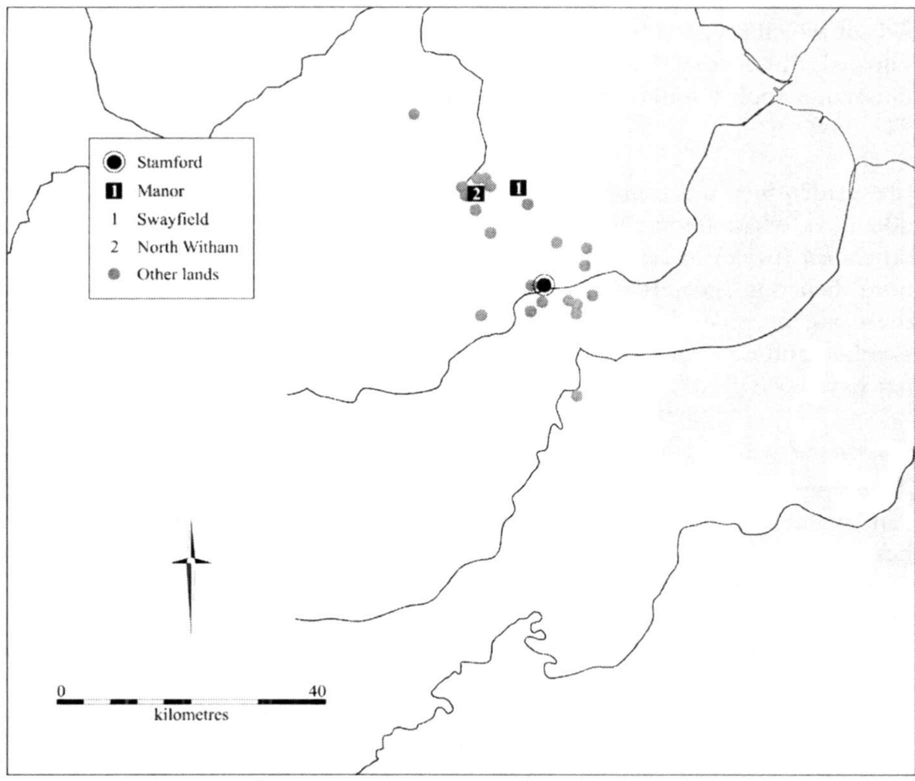

Map of estates of Browne's Hospital as granted by William Browne in 1488

A few other properties were purchased. In 1501-2, a close in Counthorpe was acquired from John Misterton (26, 38). In 1503, the warden opened discussions to purchase 'Eltham thyng' in Carlby from the widow of a tenant:

> *for horshyer to gretham to speke with hyr that was hyksons wyffe off carlby for to bye hyr hows and land in carlby that joynyth opon owr hows xviij day off junii;*

the lands were measured (53), but it was not until 1506-7 that a later warden (Sharpe) could write

> *for makyng ye dede off alic' hykson in hyr wedoo hode viijd*

and all other legalities[26] were completed (43v, 57). Purchases from Sir John Hussey and Christopher Browne and others appear to have been buying out chief rents; one chief rent of 3s p.a. was acquired for 5 marks (£3 6s 8d) (106).

[25] LAO, BHS 7/7/9, 10; see Appendix III

Equally, there were occasional sales, including part of Swynhaw wood in North Witham in which Delalaund was also involved. The wood to be sold was measured (the exact dimensions are given) and once sold, the remainder was hedged, which suggests the sold area was cleared (6). A second part of this wood followed three years later "*to increase the stock*", i.e. to raise cash. But this transaction took a long time and involved a visit to London for some reason (24v, 30v).

The warden then was immersed in paper work - title deeds, leases, contracts and indentures occur frequently. Messengers were sent to various places including Tattershall (twice) to fetch 'evidences'. Paper, parchment and ink were bought; more than one account book was acquired (43v, 56v, 57, 72, 80v, 106, 111). There are no signs here, as with Morton some fifty years earlier, of tallies, inscribed and cut wooden sticks used widely for accounting purposes, but they may have been used[27].

A new rental

The accounts do not give us a detailed breakdown of the tenancies, although the many repairs provide information on a number of the individual tenements on these estates. But a revised rental (92b) drawn up in 1517-8 gives more indication[28]. It is detailed for the Stamford properties with names of tenants and rents due, but the outlying rural estates are indicated more generally by the names of the villages, and several are grouped together. There is evidence here and elsewhere that, apart from Swayfield, which with a nominal yield of £12 18s 6d was always in a class by itself, the Lincolnshire villages were treated as one group under one rent collector; and on a wider scale, the whole estate was regarded as one. For example, building materials needed at Woolsthorpe were prepared at Swayfield (50v). An annual feast was held for all tenants in April on the anniversary of William Browne's death.

The rural economy

The Lincolnshire estates lay on the limestone ridge of south Kesteven; this was good sheep grazing territory and barley land, perhaps indicated by the number of kilns and ovens listed in the accounts. It was heavily forested and was an area of considerable disturbance by local Robin Hood type gangs[29] - which may help to

---

[26] Releases to Hugh Turner of Collyweston and John Barret of Oakham feoffees in the property; John Barret married the widow Alice Hikson. The purchase price was 5 marks (£3 6s 8d) but other costs added 9s to the total price (57).

[27] *Morton* pp xli-iv

[28] The inquisitions post mortem of William and Margaret Browne 1489 and the indenture of enfeoffment drawn up by William Browne in 1488 provide more details, *Calendar of Inquisitions Post Mortem, Henry VII*, vol. 1 pp 476-8 (202, 203), 219 (525), 230 (551); LAO, BHS 7/12/24; Devon R O, Simcoe 1038 M/T/13/6

[29] Rogers *'Noble Merchant'* pp 16-17

account for a number of the alleged 'distraints' which the wardens had to deal with (see below). The Northamptonshire estates lay in part on the gravels of the fen edge and in part (like the Rutland estates) on good clay land suitable for general agriculture.

The prominence which the accounts give to woodland is striking (see e.g. 80v, 102, 125). As we have seen, Margaret Browne gave woodland to the Hospital, and Delalaund's grant comprised substantial areas of woodland. Two parts of Swynhaw woods were carefully measured and marked out (53-54); the remainder was hedged (14, 50v), on one occasion "*to save the spring from the cattle*" (17v), and exploited (92, 114). Some woodland was cleared, and timber for building was regularly cut and trimmed on site for the use of the estate and for sale to others (17v, 50-50v, 53, 54, 101v). Fuel (*kydds*) for the bedesmen and occasionally for the warden and confrater was purchased every year from the Elmes manor of Wolfhouse. Ashes were planted and again sold very regularly on many parts of the estate, the warden on occasion paying for those he used (14v, 17); willows were also planted[30]. Thorns (*thornys*) for hedging, even in Stamford, were bought and brought to the town (27, 50v). The local woodlands were an important part of the Hospital's economy.

Parts of the estates provided stone. The Hospital owned slate (*sklatt*) pits in Wothorpe and Easton on the Hill, and let them out, paying the tenant for the many slates they purchased from their own pits and from Collyweston (3, 6 etc). Building stone came from Clipsham, Wothorpe, Walcot (6, 45v) and from Barnack (47v). For all of these items and for other building materials which the wardens and their agents acquired from the tenants of the Hospital, they paid what appear to be commercial rates. Even for wood from their woodlands, the going prices were paid. The Hospital did not live off its estates but off its rents.

Estate management

How then did the warden, new to this task, manage such a far-flung empire? Rents had to be collected, manor courts held and other manor courts attended, farms leased and re-leased, disputes which involved tenants dealt with, and above all repairs (*reparacions*) done to the tenants' properties. The fact that they were so scattered made them much harder to manage.

The warden of Browne's Hospital had of course the advantage of taking over the management system of William Browne and then of Thomas Stokes; and for a time, two former bailiffs continued in office:

Bartholomew Holmes in Swayfield and North Witham was apparently taken over from the Misterton family, stewards to Ralph lord Cromwell, at a fee of 15s 10d p.a.; but Holmes proved to be incompetent or corrupt (or both). Taylor paid for

---

[30] See *Morton* p xxxv for ashes and willows on the almoner's estates in the same area

a chief rent which Holmes had claimed he had paid and which had been allowed in his audited accounts (8v), and an account for repairs which Holmes said he had paid had to be settled by Taylor later. Holmes was dismissed by Taylor and left Swayfield to die soon after, but 'Jenett Holm the widow' remained as a tenant of the estate in Swayfield (17), and John Holmes his son was engaged with the Hospital for some time.

Robert Beomond was different; a close intimate of Browne and executor of Margaret Browne's will, he was apparently more reliable. Like the young William Elmes, he was called *literatus* (1489). In 1495, after the death of Thomas Stokes, he paid the warden for the bedesmen and women for a period before John Coton the warden took over (4). He was responsible for the Rutland, Northamptonshire and Stamford tenancies (4, 6v) but when Holmes was dismissed, Beomond became *"holl* [whole] *baylyff off the lyflode* [estate] *off thys hows"* (20) at an increase in his annual fee from 26s 8d to 40s (a slight saving to the Hospital). The warden took him round the tenants in south Lincolnshire:

> *Item for horshyer to Ryde with Robard Beomond to gyff hym autorite in hys offyce off baylywyk the xij day off maij* [1498]

But he too was dismissed by Taylor in 1502-3, perhaps for delays in collecting rents and arrears (see 49) or simply to save costs, since Taylor took on much of the work himself. There was clearly trouble compensating him for the ending of his contract, for as late as 1513-14 (107), there was

> *payd to Robt beymond for ... the redemption of hys patentt that he had gevyn owt of owr howse by owr seal vj li xvjs viijd,*

a substantial sum, compared with his annual fee of £2.

Both the bailiffs produced individual accounts which were audited separately; and the particular bills for property repairs were presumably prepared and submitted to the wardens by the bailiffs, to be copied into the warden's annual account. But soon the warden himself took over. Taylor was energetic and hard-headed and highly committed - he early on expressed his feelings when the annual account showed a loss rather than a profit:

> *Hyt aperyth thatt the stok and superplusage off the last accompt and off new Recepts thys yer that schuld haf incresyd the stok is decayed* (14v)

So that, when he arrived full time at the Hospital in 1502, he assumed responsibility from Beomond for the administration of the estate, using tenants and others as his assistants, such as William Baker in Stamford. Arnold Morton, Beomond's deputy in south Lincolnshire, was retained in some capacity, probably that of bailiff of one part of the estate, for which he received an annual fee and a robe (31v, 38, 43v); but in Taylor's last (part) year, Morton was arrested for some misdemeanour:

> *ffor expens' of a man to go to aylton* [Elton] *to spek with arnold morton aftyr he was atachud to know whethyr hyt wer he or natt;*

and the warden went to Swayfield to take possession of his goods (53).

Stewards were appointed to hold the manor courts. Henry Toky of South Witham was steward in North Witham and Swayfield courts from the start (3v, 9, 22-22v) until 1499. Nicholas Trygge, notary and under-steward of the borough of Stamford, held the manor courts 1508-10 (80, 85v). 'Harry' Lacey, also under-steward of the borough, held the manor courts on several occasions (72v, 91v, 117); he drew up the inventory of the goods of the gild after the end of the law suit (1507) and acted as retained counsel to the Hospital (62, 103v, 122). He was paid an annual fee from 1510 to the end of the accounts (1518). Richard Campion received a fee for 'gathering rents' (91v), as did 'master Colston[31]' (117, 125v) who also supervised some *'reparacions'* (property repairs, 119v). Master Thomas Bagott received an indenture for 40 years as rent collector in south Lincolnshire and for supervising repairs in his area (116v, 122v, 92b). But it seems that no-one really replaced Beomond as a general estate manager, and the warden managed as best he could. It is significant that in the later years, an item appeared in the accounts - cost of 'gathering' the rents, amounting in 1514-15 to £2 11s (110v)

Relations with tenants

The warden's relationship with the tenants was not simply one of rent collector; it is clear he had a much closer relationship with many of them. It is true that, on occasion, some tenants were "*put from the land*" (79), and that the warden distrained some of his tenants for overdue rents (17, 27), although these occasions sometimes went wrong:

> *Item I had ij horsys and j kow dystreynd for the rent and cowd nat sell hem to the valew therfor I ask for abatement* [deduction]...*vjd* (6v)

But it was the warden who had to find new tenants, make contracts and leases with them, and help them to settle. As we shall see below when discussing disputes, he shouldered their burdens and acted as surety for them. Some tenants did their own repairs and improvements, being allowed rent reductions for this. The warden sometimes bought supplies from his tenants. There were times when he did not know their names, referring to them by occupations - where the weaver dwells in St Martin's parish, the tailor in Wothorpe, the roper's house, etc. But generally the impression given is of a warden who knew them and was concerned for them, not simply as rent payers.

[31] on occasion, called 'Colson'.

INCOME

No details are provided in the account book of the real income. What is given here is the 'charge', i.e. the nominal income arising from the estates for which the warden or his bailiffs had to account. This nominal income came from rents, profits of trading (tolls etc) and from the manorial courts. The actual income has to be calculated, allowing for deductions and arrears where they are known. There is virtually no other income itemised in these accounts - a very small amount from sales of some hay, old timber, some building equipment no longer used, and some slates and ash wood. There are a few goods left by those Hospital residents who died, as the statutes provided; these seem to have been reserved for the expenses of the chapel (e.g. 123).

William Browne's intention was to endow the Hospital with a usable annual income of 50 marks (£33 6s 8d). It is not clear how this sum was arrived at. The stipends of the warden (10 marks p.a.) and the confrater (8 marks p.a.) would come to £12 p.a.; payment of 7d per week to each of the ten poor men and two poor women would use a further £18 4s - leaving some £3 per year for maintenance of the building and other costs, hardly adequate.

In fact, the estates granted had a *nominal* value of some £62 p.a., but its actual income was considerably lower. What is indicated in these accounts is only a formal figure - what it *ought* to yield before any deductions. The figure for 'the charge' remained steady at some £62 p.a. (table 1 in Appendix I). In other words, this is what the bailiffs (at first) and the warden in the later years had to account for; if they had not received this sum, they had to give reasons for it.

Deductions at source: There were several ways in which this 'charge' was diminished. First, there were what the accounts called **'decays'** - that is, property empty, or where rents for some reason had not been paid. With these were the **'abatements'** or *'debatements'*, occasions when the rents were reduced by agreement - where property had been burned down or damaged by "the great water" (floods) or where the tenant had paid for repairs and been allowed this sum in their rent. Only a few details of such deductions are recorded but they indicate a more general approach to rent reduction. These figures varied from year to year; and some were carried over:

> *Item John Joyner the tenant axeth allowance for vj yer every yer ijs whych he seyth m[aster] thomas stok promysyd hym to abate off the* Rent *off xxs* (26v)
>
> *Item john lytster hath abate off x acres arabyll for v yers passyd* (31)

The combined decays and abatements increased substantially from £3 in the early years to a high point of £18, remaining stubbornly at £14-15 for several years, out of a charge of £62 p.a..

Thirdly, most of the properties had against them rent charges (**chief rents)** due to the king or other lords, payments for properties belonging to other manors, ranging from £2 10s 4d due from the manor of Swayfield to lord Grey of Codnor's manor of Corby (Lincolnshire), part of the Castle Bytham estate, down to ½d due each year to the earl of Westmorland from Barham. These were of course more fixed and hovered around £6 per year - until 1513-14 when the chief rent of Swayfield to Corby manor (a major bone of contention, which ran on for many years) was rescinded permanently, apparently by being bought out from lord Grey's estate feoffees; the total of chief rents then settled at some £3 p.a. Associated with these were charges for attendances at other manor and hundred courts (**suits and amercements**). These were more variable but amounted to only a few shillings each year. The chief rents and courts would bring the warden into contact with the officers of a number of noblemen and women of a status higher than he would normally have expected to encounter.

All of these were deducted at source, so the annual income of some £62 to the Hospital was reduced. Table 2 (Appendix I) indicates these deductions from the annual income, showing a yield which fell from £54 in the first year of the warden's administration to a low point of £37 in 1510-11, and it settled at about £40 p.a. for the latter half of this period.

So William Browne's aim of providing the Hospital with a *usable* annual income of some £33 (50 marks) p.a. was to be achieved by giving estates worth a *nominal* rental of £62 p.a. But even if we allow for all the inconsistencies and errors in the accounting, the decline of the disposable income to the warden is very clear; by 1515, he had lost some 20% of his real annual income.

The surplus: As tables 1 and 2 show (Appendix I), the only other substantial item recorded in the accounts is the *superplusage* from the previous account. But this is not the excess of income over expenditure, it is not surplus cash in hand. Rather, it comprises all the debts and arrears for which the warden and the officers would have to account when they did come in (if ever). Taylor wrote in 1500:

> *Summa superplusagij off the Rents thys yer* [year] *to the incresyng off the stok thatt was dekayd and gon in arrerag' byfor* *xij li xiiijs iijd qa*

In other words, £12 14s 3¼d was in that year the total of the unaccounted sums, the arrears to be added to the running total.

Each year, the loss grew; by 1501-2, arrears amounted to over £45, more than half the total nominal annual income from the whole estate; so that (nominally) Taylor was due to account the next year for some £108. It would seem that the estate was haemorrhaging at least 10% of its income every year Most of these arrears remained on the accounts of the bailiffs. The losses of Bartholomew Holmes were written off but those of Robert Beomond were pursued after he was dismissed; they were listed by Taylor each year in his annual audit. When Sharpe left in a hurry, he too had substantial sums unaccounted for, and they continued to be listed for several years. This situation appears to have been too much for Sheppey to cope with, and on his death in 1517, a new, more realistic rental was drawn up.

The nature of the accounts

This book then is what it says on the tin - a book of accounts. There is no balance sheet, no overall statement of the position of the Hospital funds at any one time. This is not a day book - we have few signs of the loans the wardens had to take out to cover day-to-day expenses or the unpaid bills on the warden's desk, no idea (except once) of the cash that remained in the chest in the counting house. For this was, on the face of it, a cash economy - payments to tradesmen and to the bedesmen were recorded as having been made in cash on the due date; there is no sign here of any promissory notes, although on occasion, a tenant was reimbursed for work done by a remission of rent (33v).

But we do have to be careful here - for the record may hide the detailed bargaining which must have gone on. How far credit was allowed in the market for food and nails, for example, is uncertain, but in view of the shortage of cash the wardens experienced, I feel certain that many varied arrangements would have been made. The more informal record of William Morton at nearby Peterborough abbey is revealing: "Morton ... buys his own supplies (mainly spices, wine, building materials such as sticks, bricks, lime, nails) on credit from suppliers who are often the same people who buy from him on credit. At regular intervals these mutual debts are set off against each other and net balances are either settled in cash or carried over for another term". Much the same may well have taken place in Stamford markets - different kinds of agreements would probably have been made but are hidden from view in these accounts[32].

What then we have in this book are two unequal items - a statement of actual sums paid out by the warden in any one year up to the moment of the audit, matched against a *nominal* statement of income in part received and in part still due to the warden - unpaid rents, sums in the hands of former bailiffs or former wardens. The annual audit shows that much of this remained in the hands of the bailiffs and of course the tenants; in 1501, Robert Beomond was said at the time of his dismissal to be in arrears by £13 13s 2¾d for 15 Henry VII [1499-1500] and by £22 2s 3¼d for 16 Henry VII [1500-01] (34v, 35v) - at more than £35, a whole year's actual income.

The arrears of rents were clearly a great worry. The warden himself went round "*asking for rent*" (17). The accounts frequently mention debts due to the Hospital and sued for (64v, 65, 83, 85v, 101 etc). Sharpe left with large unaccounted-for sums accumulated during at least two of his three years. The difficulties the warden had in 'gathering rents' show the increasing debt burden. In 1510-11, the

---

32 *Morton* p xxxv.

warden reported that the tenants ran away when the rent collector came; the warden asked for

> *Allowanc' for geyderyng ye rent in stanford and in other plac' and for makkyng good ye rent when they rwn awey with ye rent afor owr rekunyng* (91v)

In 1512-13, the warden had to make allowances to the tenants, as he said, a penny here, there two pence, by agreement, and for making good the missing rents:

> *Item a lowyd for gederyng ye rent in stawnford and in other placs and owerseyng of reparacions and for their expenses and rewards as in gyffyng ageyn somtym jd sumtym ijd by agreement and for makkyng good ye rent' of yem that are not there* [i.e. absent] (98)

(the same phrase is used in 1516-17, 122). The difficulties of collecting rents from a scattered estate which was apparently over-rated clearly became acute: in 1517-18 when Sheppey died, the new rental resulted in an assessment of some £44 p.a. instead of £62 p.a.

Additional income? It is possible that there were additional sources of income not listed in these accounts. In August 1498, Sir Thomas Delalaund leased a messuage and 40 acres of land in North Witham to John Taylor warden and William Hawkyns confrater; and in December he quitclaimed these properties. At about the same time, in return for being added to the Hospital bederoll, he gave three other properties in the same village to "*the Almoshouse called Brouneis Halmoshouse in Stamford*" to the value of 18s p.a.; the money was to increase the stipend of the warden by 4s p.a., the confrater by 3s p.a., and the remainder (11s p.a.) was to go to the twelve bedesfolk[33]. Legacies were left to the almshouse on occasion. In 1504, William Elmes' granted *to the Warden of the almis house at Staunford xs and to his brother vjs viijd and to every pour man and woman and* [sic] *the same house xijd*; and in 1511 Elizabeth Elmes wrote

> *I geve and bequeth unto the ij preests in my fathers almeshouse in Stamford to every of theym xs. And every of theym to saye a trentall of seynt gregory with massez dirige and other observaunces. Also I geve and bequeth to every of the poore men and women beyng in the said almeshouse ijs*[34]

There are however no signs of any of these additional payments in the account book.

Cash flow: There was clearly a problem with cash flow. Prior to the death of Thomas Stokes in October 1495, the warden did not handle the Hospital funds - everything was done by William and Margaret Browne and then by Thomas Stokes, assisted by William Elmes. In the first few months after Stokes' death,

---

[33] LAO, BHS 7/7/10; Appendix III; the account in Wright pp 55-60, 493-5 is inaccurate at times.

[34] See Rogers, Wills pp 293-4

Coton was short of cash, and Elmes (as patron of the Hospital) ordered Henry Wykes vicar of All Saints to give the warden various sums amounting to £20 (later the gild claimed these sums came from the gild's coffers). When Coton died in January 1497 and Taylor took over, he found only 14s 8d in the chest, enough for two weeks' stipends of the almsmen and women. When Taylor left in January 1504, he drew up his accounts for the part of the year for which he had been in office. He had not received money from his agents and only £5 8s 3½d direct from the tenants, and it appears he had had to turn to some other clergy to receive sums of £6 and 3s 4d (apparently loans since they were secured by indentures). This explains why the warden himself went round some of the tenants asking for rents.

Shortage of money is clear. Although the almsmen had received the statutory payments of 7d per week under Thomas Stokes, Coton, when he took over in January 1496, started off paying the bedesmen at 8d per week, but Taylor quickly reduced that during his first year as warden. And soon the warden resorted to keeping some of the bedesmen places vacant and reducing the female assistance down to one person instead of two, which seems to reflect cost cutting to accommodate the lower income. Because of the large arrears carried over from year to year, it is impossible to know what the exact disposable income available to the warden was at any time, but he must have been living from hand to mouth.

The contrast between the situation the wardens found themselves in and the situation under Thomas Stokes (and presumably William Browne) may be hinted at in an unusual surviving account, the *parcelles* of the New Tavern cited below. On the dorse of that bill are some calculations which are hard to interpret but which draw a distinction between *'Rem'* (what remains in hand) and *Superplus'* (what is outstanding). However we interpret the figures, they are in a different world from that of the wardens - remnants of over £300 against arrears of £131[35]. The wardens had much less at their disposal than Stokes had.

EXPENDITURE

But they still had to spend – and the costs they faced were unlikely to have been much lower than those faced by Stokes.

The expenditure is set out in the table in Appendix I under its various headings as listed in these accounts - the bedesmen, the costs of holding courts, casual costs, purchases of stock, and building repairs. The totals in the tables are as often as possible those given in the account book. Once again, they include some

[35] It is possible these figures relate to the whole of the Browne estate, not just to that part which came to the Hospital. In December 1494, the Hospital chest had £119 11s 11d when Stokes launched the Hospital, LAO, BHS 1/2

nominal rather than real items; for example, Taylor in 1501-2 wrote that his expenditure matched his charge to the very half-pence. They must then be taken as simply giving an indication of the problems facing the wardens - not only how to raise the money owing to the Hospital but also how to keep rising costs in hand. Taylor clearly tried in 1498 to rein back on expenditure but costs rose inexorably to a peak in 1502. When Sharpe took over, costs again rose significantly in all sectors of the accounts - except the bedesmen and women.

THE BEDESMEN AND BEDESWOMEN

The first and primary charge on the income was of course the payments to the bedesmen and women and to the warden and confrater; these always come first in the expenditure. Payment was normally on a Friday (15, 53) but at times it varied.

The recorded payments to the bedesmen and women week by week provide us with a kind of register of attendance. The Hospital had its full complement of ten men and two women in December 1495 when the accounts start, but the book does not give us their names. There is however a list of names from December 1498, and by using the departures and admissions in the account book, a more detailed register can be constructed (see Appendix II). There is a gap from January 1504 to October 1506, so some admissions in these years and the dates of the departures of some of those enrolled before 1504 are not known. In the later years, not all the admissions and departures are recorded by name, but they can be traced in the sums paid to the inmates. For example, in September 1509, payments were made for 11 inmates, but in the next month, payments were for ten inmates, although the name of the departing bedesman is not recorded (78, 84).

Numbers of inmates: The potential roll was twelve, ten men and two women. From December 1495 until July 1500, total numbers did not fall below 10, and even then only for very short times - vacancies were usually filled in a month or two. But even under Taylor, numbers began to fall substantially, to 8-9 and once to 7 (i.e. only five men) for four months (October 1500 - February 1501). When he left (January 1504), there were only nine inmates, eight men and one woman.

After the first few years, then, places in the Hospital were often left vacant. The sums paid to the paupers reveal this clearly. Omitting the years for which there is no data or only partial data and the year 1496-7 when for most of the year the stipend was paid at 8d per week instead of 7d per week, the annual totals paid for the poor men and women show a steady decline.

1497-8	Taylor	17. 17. 0
1498-9	Taylor	17. 1. 3
1499-1500	Taylor	17. 14. 8
1500-1	Taylor	12. 7. 11
1501-2	Taylor	16. 1. 5
1502-3	Taylor	16. 9. 2
1506-7	Sharpe	14. 11. 1
1507-8	Sheppey	16. 17. 2
1508-9	Sheppey	16. 10. 9
1509-10	Sheppey	13. 3. 0
1510-11	Sheppey	12. 2. 8
1511-12	Sheppey	12. 3. 6
1512-13	Sheppey	11. 13. 0
1513-14	Sheppey	9. 19. 11
1514-15	Sheppey	10. 9. 5
1515-16	Sheppey	13. 10. 1
1516-17	Sheppey	13. 13. 2

There were increasing gaps between the times of departure and filling those vacancies. For two years, from August 1507 to October 1509, the Hospital was full apart from one woman, but after January 1510 to the end of these accounts (September 1517), the total number rose above nine only once (from July 1516 to February 1517). In May 1512, the numbers dropped to 7 and for the next three years (until August 1515), apart from two months, there were only 6-7 inmates. In other words, there were only 5-6 bedesmen, half the complement.

There are also signs that the increasing burden of work on the warden impacted on his relations with his charges. Taylor clearly knew them well; he used them often for the work of the Hospital – to run errands, for example, to South Luffenham to fetch court rolls, to Tattershall for 'evidences' or to Grantham (30v, 38), to accompany him on some of his visits (43v), and to fetch and carry (17) - and he paid for their costs. Sheppey did not keep careful records of admissions and departures, at least in these accounts (he or the vicar of All Saints may have had a separate register of admissions) and he referred to some of them by surname only rather than by full name, but the paucity of records may be due to his being unwell. On the other hand, Sharpe and Sheppey used the bedesmen more frequently for building work: for daubing a wall, for bringing in timber, for carrying building materials etc. For help with some of the many tasks, he gave them *mete* and *drynk* (64v, 74v, 87v, 88v, etc). Later, when Sheppey was apparently incapacitated, they were involved more often and were paid for their work:

> *Item to ye bedmen for helpyng in wyntter and now in sommer abowte ye wal making I gaf yem to drynk* *vd* (88v)
>
> *Item gyffyne to ye bedmen at sertyn tymys whey the[y] haf doyne for well of ye hows* *vjd* (108v)

Some bedesmen were clearly independent; "*two of ye more discreet paupers of ye said house John Parkyn and John Calays*" were included in the audit team in 1510 (89v, 95v) as required in the statutes, and they were used several times as messengers (72v, 80v) or to supervise or support some of the reparation work (81v, 82, 100v):

> *Item for gaderyng of ye same sond and for doyng mony other thyngs yat has don gud to ye hows to calys and perkyn* *viijd*

On the other hand, there was an issue with discipline on occasion. One of the bedesmen (Bulkeley, July 1498) was expelled on the grounds of being 'intractable', and another (Arnold, May 1512) was also expelled. In 1507-8, the warden withheld 3s 2d from the weekly sums due to the bedesmen for 'corrections'; in the following year, this sum was 4s, and in 1509-10, 2s 8d.

In the early years, one of the bedesmen, Bentley, was given licence to be absent three times, but on the last occasion in 1499, he did not return, the warden having been reliably informed that he had died. Other licences for absence were granted (24v, 25v).

The length of stay varied greatly. Some died within weeks of entering the almshouse; others survived for 7-8 years. One or two years was an average stay. Not all departures were due to death. Several left, presumably, like the attendant Margaret, to stay with relatives. There is no record of anyone being removed on the grounds of disease, as the statutes stipulate.

Little can be said of the choice of candidates for welfare. Thomas Bentley, tenant, became a bedesman and seems to have been privileged. Phylyp may be related to the elite family of that name and to tenants. John Holand was succeeded by Robert Holand, Henry Walch by Thomas Walch. The families of the tradesmen used by the Hospital may occasionally be represented among the bedesmen. Thomas Andrew, William Bacon and Robert Hall bedesmen may be related to tradesmen who supplied the Hospital; Lynley may have been a tenant from North Witham. The issue of whether the gild members had any claim to priority is one for which there is no evidence either way.

OTHER DISBURSEMENTS

What I have called disbursements are listed more or less under standardised headings - annual charges, cost of holding our courts, payments for suits in other courts and amercements, casual costs, the *'stoor'* [store] and *'reparacions'*. From time to time these categories become confused, so that it is not possible to enumerate comparative costs under these headings with assurance that in each case the same items are covered. To ease comparison, the totals in the account book are given (see tables in Appendix I: there are a number of inaccurate calculations in the book).

Annual charges: Each year, the warden paid a pension of 6s 8d from the Angel Inn to the rector of St Michael's church, Stamford, a settlement which William Browne made very reluctantly in the last few months of his life to settle a claim by the rector for church fees, since the chapel of the Hospital lay in the parish of St Michael and not in the parish of All Saints. Secondly, fuel (specified as 1000[36] kydds or faggots) for the Hospital was collected each year, for which they paid some 5s 10d, a figure which rose slightly in the later years to 6s and once to 7s; carriage cost 8s or 10s. Sharpe included under the heading of annual charges the cost of the founder's celebration (which does not appear in earlier accounts) (55v) and the payment of bailiffs' and lawyers' annual fees, and Sheppey included the cost of rent gathering.

Manorial courts: There are few signs in these accounts of customary dues such as labour services or reliefs from manorial tenants except suit of court. Unlike Morton, who used the traditional duties (*precaria*) of manorial tenants for cartage[37], the wardens hired carriers and often paid the tenants to carry goods. Manorial courts were held twice each year in both North Witham and Swayfield. Stewards were appointed from time to time to hold the courts. Henry Toky steward held all courts from the beginning until 1500, but thereafter, it was a matter of appointing someone for each occasion. Sometimes, one of the tenants was asked to hold the court (3v, 9). The warden attended on many occasions: once, the tenants did not come, and on another occasion, the warden arrived for the court but "*the steward cam' nott*" (9, 22). Sometimes the cost of hiring horses for these visits is included under this heading, but more often it is in casual costs. How the courts were held in 1500-1502, when Taylor recorded '*nil*' costs under this heading, is not clear. But from Sharpe's time, it seems the courts were left to the lawyers (see below) who received an annual fee rather than a separate fee for each court held.

Suits and amercements: The warden as landlord was cited into several neighbouring manorial courts in Stretton, North Luffenham (the prior of Brooke and the king's court), Easton on the Hill (the king), Wilsthorpe (lady Eyland) and Corby, Lincolnshire (lord Grey of Codnor); also in the abbot of Peterborough's Langdyke hundred court (with its duty of attendance, '*borosoken*', 56v) in virtue of property in Pilsgate and Wothorpe. In Stamford, he was summoned to St Cuthbert's court (St Leonard's priory), the abbot of Peterborough's two lesser courts, John Wykes' court and the king's court. After the acquisition of new property, he was also called before lady Busshey's manorial court at Thistelton (Rutland). From time to time he attended such courts in person. Payments were made in these courts for fines and '*essoyns*' (excuses for non-attendance and other infringements); presumably some of these are for repeated permissions for some of his tenants to continue to act in ways which contravened manorial customs.

---

[36] a thousand is not a thousand - see glossary

[37] *Morton* p xxxii

Sometimes the warden paid someone (usually a tenant) to attend on his behalf. The complicated network of land-holding involved a large number of official interactions, the costs of which remained relatively steady during this period.

Royal taxes

One burden which I think was felt to be particularly heavy was the payment of royal taxes on behalf of some of the tenants. The royal tenths and fifteenths granted to the king by parliament were collected from time to time, and an occasional royal aid was also to be expected. It is clear that many, perhaps most, of the tenants were responsible for paying their tax after assessment. When the warden wished to hold the Easter 1497 manor court in Swayfield, he was unable to do so

> *for the tenaunts wer afor the kyngs commissionars for the kyngs ayde and so ther was no cowrt kept as hyt aperyth in the cowrt Rollys* (9)

In that year, the warden agreed to pay this tax for some of the tenants[38] (9v): *I John taylyor payd thes prests for the seyd ayde* for some tenants in North Witham, Stretton, Easton, Swayfield (twice), Wilsthorp and Barham, to a total of £3 11s 1½d. He was due to pay the tax for properties which were in his hands for *reparacions* (18) and for some if not all of the Stamford town properties, but not for the rural tenants. When he came to pay again in the following year, 1497-8, he wrote that this was not to be a precedent (17):

> *Item I payd toward the kyngs xv in helpyng owr tenants off Swaffeld they nat to haf hytt off in dewete bott off benyvolence*

The king's aid is not heard of again until 1513-14 when the warden paid 20s "*to the eyd of the kyngs dwtey*" for the Stamford properties; in 1515-16, at "*martlemas*" [Martinmas, 10 November], he paid the same sum (117), and in 1516-17, the same again (122v).

REPAIRS TO PROPERTIES: BUILDING ACCOUNTS

But the activity which came to dominate a large part of the life of the warden was that of maintaining the properties on the estate. The building accounts of the *'Reparacions'*, as they were called, filled the pages of the account book.

It appears that most of the Browne's Hospital estate properties were held on tenancies which incurred the Hospital rather than the tenant in repairs - like the almoner at Peterborough, the warden "bore the responsbilty for repairs" for

---

[38] The royal tax of 1497 was the first such tax since 1490, and as such, the warden had no precedent to go on. See M Jurkowski, C L Smith and D Crook 1998 *Lay Taxes in England and Wales 1188-1688*, London: Public Record Office pp 124-134. The subsidy taken by Henry VII in 1504 does not appear in the account book since there is no account for that year; the fifteenth and tenth in 1512 was paid in 1513, and the fifteenth and tenth granted by parliament in 1515 in two parts was paid for the Stamford properties by the warden; the rural tenants presumably paid their own tax.

many rural and urban tenancies[39]. There were some properties which do not appear in the list of *reparacions* - these may have been held on terms whereby the tenant paid for all repairs. But for most of them, the warden was responsible for even minor repairs - in 1498-9, the sum of 8d was spent on repairing the barn doors and field gate of a property in Wilsthorpe (22v). But many repair bills were very substantial - indeed, at times an almost complete rebuilding was undertaken.

Date and wardens	**Number of properties (urban and rural) under repair**	**Amount spent**[40]
1495-6 Coton	U7; R8	13 10 5½
1496-7 (part) Coton	U4; R2	7 4 7½
1496-7 (part) Taylor	U5; R9	5 15 0
1497-8 Taylor	U6, R10	17 15 9
1498-9 Taylor	U5, R20	5 9 2
1499-1500 Taylor	U11, R6	8 0 10 ¾
1500-1 Taylor	U9, R13	12 7 0
1501-2 Taylor	U7, R0	11 10 10 ½
1502-3 Taylor	U12, R31[41]	30 17 7 ½
1503-4 (part) Taylor		
1506-7 Sharpe	U11, R11	10 13 6
1507-8 Sheppey	U6, R9	14 4 11
1508-9 Sheppey	U7, R7	10 15 8
1509-10 Sheppey	U10, R10	24 9 9
1510-11 Sheppey	U5, R10	7 5 11
1511-12 Sheppey	U not listed, R3	7 14 5
1512-13 Sheppey	U1, R3	2 11 6
1513-14 Sheppey	U not listed, R4	2 8 8
1514-15 Sheppey	U4+, R9	10 15 6
1515-16 Sheppey	U4+, R10	9 4 4
1516-17 Sheppey	U3+, R4	5 7 10

The size of the task can be seen in the table above: the properties have been divided (as the accounts divide them) into urban and rural, and repairs to the almshouse have been included (they cannot easily be separated out from the other repairs). The numbers of properties in the list above are somewhat misleading, since on occasion repairs to several properties in one village are lumped together under one heading. And the size of the repairs varied greatly.

---

[39] *Morton* p xxxiv

[40] Where totals exist in the account book, these have been accepted without checking; in other cases, the separate totals have been calculated. There will be errors but the figures give some impression of the scale of the enterprise

[41] It is possible that some repairs undertaken in the previous year are included in this account; some repairs were listed in a subsequent year to the year they were undertaken when accounts came in late.

Sometimes the tenant did the repair and was either refunded the costs or allowed rent off in lieu (6, 6v, 13, 27v, etc):

> *Item I allowyd wyllam skarboro off north luffnam for iij days sklattyng that he payd to yong Robard whythed of eston hym and hys servar A° Regni Regis henrici vij xv°* [1499-1500] (34v)

Sometimes the warden contributed towards the cost of an improvement, the swinecote at Easton, for example (53); the warden contributed 5s for a new chimney for Richard Campion, the warden's rent collector, in his house at Swayfield (27v).

A very wide range of buildings were involved, domestic, commercial and farm. Few halls are mentioned and as far as I can see no solar, but an occasional cellar (48v) was involved (*selar*, 49, is probably a cellar, not solar). There were many chambers including a corn chamber (which may however be 'corner chamber', 40v, 111). Outhouses such as bakehouses, brewhouses, kitchens, a malthouse, a milk house, and many penthouses were built or repaired. Lean-tos seem to cause frequent problems. A very large number of kilns, ovens and a few furnaces required constant attention (the kilns may be malt kilns in the barley lands of south Lincolnshire). Mill houses required a great deal of attention. Wells needed ropes and chains. There were dovecotes in almost every village and many in the town as well, as were swinecotes and hogstyes in both urban and rural areas. Above all, privies were cleaned out: one such *sege* was rebuilt in a garden and given a thatched roof, and at the Angel and the Crane and one other large house in Stamford, a *'withdrawght'* inside a chamber was dealt with. Garden and boundary walls were repaired with stone, mud or thorns, at least once with dry stone walling (32v, 40).

All parts of the buildings received attention. Many chimneys were added or repaired. Roofs, gables, louvres, gutters (of lead and stone) and shared (common) sewers, doors and gates with their thresholds, entries and porches are listed. Farm buildings occur frequently, especially barns, great barns and long barns: a barn of three bays was built for 30s for the tenant in North Luffenham, although another barn of three bays cost only 10s (95, 109). Stables with cribs and mangers also occur.

All kinds of building work were undertaken and supplied with materials. Thatching, slating, *hylling* (covering) occur most frequently. Roofing (making trusses) and many other kinds of timber work (joists, 'couples' and beams etc) occupied many hours of work. Pargetting, daubing (more frequently whitewashing, I suspect, than plastering; the bedesmen were engaged in daubing), pointing and plastering are paid for: the "*borning, bettyng, syftyng, redyng, and schotyng*" of lime plaster (44v; see 46) is recorded. Wattling was undertaken for walls. Buildings were *'undersett'*. There was much cleaning up after the work or after a disaster.

The warden then was running a major building business. He negotiated wage rates and hired (and no doubt fired) local tradesmen to undertake work for him.

He directly paid the workmen (12v) including their assistants at agreed daily rates and oversaw their work (17, 18, 30v, 32v). Taylor sometimes paid for the work and then accounted for it in the accounts of Robert Beomond (23):

> *her foleth certen Reparacions maade and overseyne by me jhon taylor' warden and they are putt in the accompt' off* Robard *beomond for hys discharge* (32v)

As time went on, more work was done on piece rates - by the rood (defined as 3 feet, 101) or by *'bargeyn'* or contract (*'a grete'*, i.e. by agreement):

> *Item payd to john hygen the carpentar for hys bargeyn agreyte to make iiij schopp wyndows leyng off somertre and trasyngs* [summers and joists] *abof ij peyntes* [penthouses] *and iiij dors xs* (39);

but to the end, day rates for tradesmen and lower day rates for their *'servars'* were the norm. The warden had become something of an entrepreneur with an eye, not to profit but to austerity, saving costs.

All this required building materials. The warden himself mobilised resources and arranged for their carriage to his two yards, one at the Hospital itself and one in Scotgate, the northern suburb of Stamford, which was close by, and to and from the building sites. No doubt the local tenant assisted with finding men and materials, but the accounts show clearly that in most cases, the warden was in direct control. He often bought items himself:

> *Item I john taylyor warden bowgt off yong cordale of eston for stor' off byldyng of the lyflode iij* Rode *bord and a quarter with the cariage metyng* [measuring or recording] *and cowchyng* [storing] *in owr barn* (34v)

The 1509 *'stoors'* account starts with no less than ten items which "*I boyghte*" (86), and the 1508 account shows the warden buying timber from several different sources ("*I boyht*", 79v).

And, as the *'stoor'* items show, he purchased materials in bulk (98v) - nails by the thousand in a wide variety of formats (penny, twopenny, threepenny, fourpenny, fivepenny, clout, splints, vart etc); different kinds of stone (bastard stone, broad stone, freestone, wall stone, quoins), sometimes in large quantities (167 loads of stone on one occasion, 19), from Clipsham and Barnack and other sources (e.g. Easton and Oundle); slates by the thousand and crests in smaller numbers from the Hospital stone pits in Wothorpe (paying the tenant for them) and from pits in Easton on the Hill and Collyweston, some perhaps second hand ("*battered and bored*", 110v). Mortar, sand (including yellow sand) and lime both by the seam and in the stone to be burned, flowed into and out of the yard; but bricks are rare - half a thousand for building a chimney top (52v). Timber, new and second hand, spars, *trasons* (joists), eaves boards, heart and sap laths and great balks, were purchased, and straw, stubble and reeds were acquired by the sheaves or bundles, and rope for thatching. A great deal of lead for gutters and drains was used, by the fother and web, and metal work, especially hinges, hasps, door bands and solder. In particular, locks and keys occur time and again. We see 5000 nails and

3000 laths bought at one time (56v), and on at least one occasion, a discount for the bulk purchase of nails was given (122v).

It has been questioned whether a person like the warden commissioning building works needed to know the precise meanings of the words they were hearing and using; but my impression is that when the wardens wrote words such as sidetrees, summertrees and rooftrees, wallplate and groundsill, '*couples*' (trusses), frank post, spikings, *stulps*, *trasons*, he did know what he was talking about. And some of the terms used are clearly local dialect: *cayle* and *bastard stone* are terms used in local quarrying[42]. True, he had great difficulty in spelling some of these words (see glossary), but I feel certain that when he bought specialist timbers, he could recognise them and know what they were used for.

A great deal of his resources went on cartage - the prices of carrying heavy loads from place to place varied greatly[43]. The cost of carrying wood fuel from Wolfhouse manor which is relatively close to Stamford was greater than the cost of the faggots themselves. Stone, timber, lime, thatch, lead all needed to be moved into and out of store. The Hospital had no cart of its own - so local traders and farmers over a very wide area were pressed into service, many of them tenants.

Building equipment and tools of all kinds from ladders (long and short) to scaffolding hurdles, sieves and scuttles, bowls and buckets, handsaws, a wimble (gimlet) and a '*wyndull to hold nails*' (44) were acquired, used and thrown away or occasionally sold when no longer required. All this was stored on the almshouse site and in the barn and yard in Scotgate to be used for the '*reparacions*' of the properties belonging to the Hospital under the direct supervision of the warden. From time to time, building equipment was moved from almshouse to barn (53v). Here could be found shovels, wheelbarrows and riddles (32v) and perhaps the stone sledge (18). New sand was set '*beside our own sand*' (38v). Larger timbers were stored in the barn, smaller and worked timbers at the Hospital (47). The Hospital grounds (including Browne's house next door which formed part of the site and continued to be occupied by the Elmes family who of course supported the family almshouse) was also a workyard; the accounts speak of materials brought in and sent out through 'the large gate' and the 'field gate' - the two entrances to the site which can still be seen on North Street. For example, some of the existing roof timbers from the Angel were taken down, carried through the streets to the almshouse site, rebuilt and repaired there, and the trusses carried back through the streets to erect on the Angel:

> *Item to the seyd Bacon for cariag off old tymbur from the seyd awngell to the almoshows and off the new rofe aftyr hytt was framyde to the seyd awngell* (46v)

---

[42] I am grateful to Stephen Hart, architect, who gave me a copy of a valuable set of notes of a talk 'Collyweston and its Trade', by Bob Osborn, quarryman of Collyweston, Northants, in 1976 in which several local terms are given with their meanings.

[43] See *Morton* pp xxxvi-vii

All this makes sense of the statement in Margaret Browne's will (1489) that

> *I will that alle my tymbre, borde, Iryn, stone, lede, Nayle, Lath and alle other stuf perteynyng to bilding or Reparacion being within my place or elswhere be preserved and kept to my said brother for the Reparacions of the tenementis that stonden in feoffees handes*[44]

Behind each of the reparation entries lay a set of documents, separate bills which contain details of the work done and costs; these were called *les parcelles*. In this, the wardens were carrying on from where William and Margaret Browne had left off, and no doubt this account book owed much in its format to the books kept by the Browne family. Indeed, we have by chance one indication of this management system. One of *les parcelles* happens to survive from the period befoe the wardens took over - a bill by Thomas Stokes dated August 1494 or 1495 for work done to the New Tavern in Stamford. Because it is a rarity, I have printed it in full here:

TNA, SP46/123/57
mense Augt A° x° R[egis] henr vij [10 Henry VII: either 1494 or 1495]

Costez necessarie made by me Thomas Stokes in the hous of Watkyn of the Newe Taverne viz

In primis for a loode of (pavyng *ins*) stoone	xvjd
Item for a loode of (gravell *del*) Sande	vjd
Item for pavyng wythin the hous and wythoute over and beside *xvjd* taken by distres by thalderman[1] at sondry seasons (for noon' pavyng *ins*)	ijs
Summa	iijs xd
Item for tymber for a pale in the gardeyn Nayles henges for a gate and for werkmanship of the same pale	ixs xd
Item payed for borde Nayles and werkmanship of a pentes over the welle	iiijs
Summa total of the parcells abovesaid with the *xvjd* for severall distressez	xixs

verso

Rem ([2]iij iiij xix li xiijs vjd *del*) lviij li xs iiijd
Surplus cxxxj li xd

Rem iij[c] xxvij li ixs vjd

----

[1] The Alderman here is the Alderman (i.e. mayor) of the town, and the distresses may be for failing to provide street paving (*for noon pavyng*).
[2] The figures here are uncertain - it could be iij iiij[xx] xix (i.e. either £79 or £99) but both are deleted

This would no doubt have been copied into or summarised in Stokes' annual account; similar *parcelles* lay behind every reparation account in this book.

[44] Rogers, Wills p 287

The regional economy: The Hospital then was a major player in the urban and rural economy, not just in Stamford but in the region. Tradesmen not only from Stamford but from the surrounding area were contracted to do work for the estate. It would appear that the villages immediately around Stamford possessed a range of skilled artisans which the town drew upon as if they were resident in the town – villages which appear to have become to some extent urbanised, almost suburbs to the town. Easton on the Hill, Collyweston, Ufford, Wittering, Barnack and Casterton provided masons; carpenters from Ryhall, slaters from Easton, a thatcher from Belmesthorp, a wright from Tinwell, were all employed by the warden. The Hospital's hinterland lay within about eight miles' distance of Stamford. It may be significant that, so far as I can see, no craftsmen or suppliers were sourced from Grantham, Spalding or Bourne, but Oakham and even Oundle provided workers or materials. The nearest the Hospital got to Grantham was 'Woolsthorpe by North Witham', as it was called. Stamford in the late medieval period (as later) looked to the south and west more than to the north. But the challenge to the wardens and their agents was to identify over that area the best and most cost-effective supplier of goods and services at a distance from the town: who would be the best carpenter or carter to undertake work at Warmington or North Witham; and can plasterers be brought from Oakham to work in Stamford itself? At times, the wardens paid someone to do the purveying of goods and services for them: Thomas Johnson in 1497-98 was paid 12d "*for overseyng off thys Reparacion and porveying off all thys stuff*" (18), but this was unusual in the early days; later the wardens clearly employed agents at times for this work.

Materials too were acquired from all over the place, not just at the midlent fair and the Simon and Jude fair[45] (122v), and the prices of various commodities can be seen to change during the 25 years of this account. The price of one pound of pepper for instance, used in the payment of rents, can be traced in most years; in Stamford markets, it rose sharply in 1498 from 16d a pound to 28d a pound and reached double its price (32d a pound) in 1501-2 before it fell back to near previous levels in the later years of this account. Cumin however remained more stable at 3d a pound, only occasionally rising to 5d a pound.

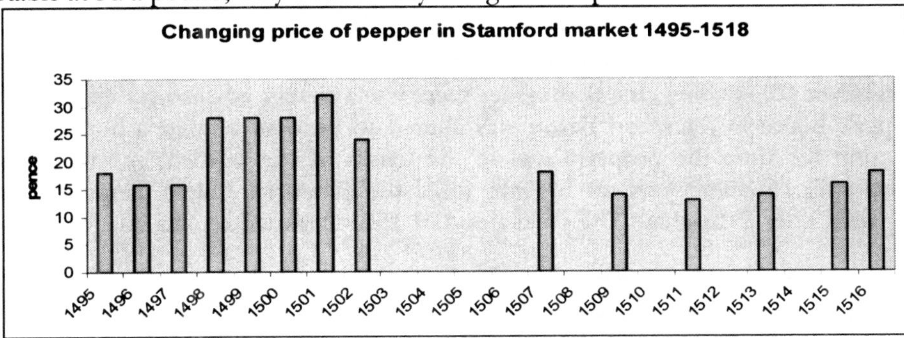

[45] There is one reference to a midsummer fair (122v) which did not exist; this may have been a mistake for mid-lent fair.

Wages however seem to have been more variable[46]. It is possible to measure the changes in wages in this account book in detail, and a quick glance is suggestive. In 1495-6, day rates appear to be relatively standardised: masons and carpenters were paid 5d or 6d per day, slaters 5d and thatchers 4½d; their 'servers' were usually paid 4d. By 1515-17, the picture is more complicated. More, probably most, of the work was by contract price or by the rood, not by daily wages; and in most cases when day rates are given, they included the server as well as the craftsman. And some rates are so high that they lead to the suspicion that the craftsman had to provide the materials within that price. Rates were variable. Masons and carpenters on the whole got 6d a day but occasionally 5d. The big change came with the slaters and thatchers. While thatchers were on the whole getting more than before, 5d or at times 6d, and at least once a contract amounting to 20d a day for a thatcher and his server (presumably however providing the materials), slaters clearly had to bargain for their wage rates: two slaters and their server(s) got only 14d and (on another occasion) 16d for two days work (i.e. 7d or 8d to pay for the slater and his assistant), but on another occasion 2s 4d was paid for two men and their *servars* for the same period. Labourers were on the whole receiving less – sometimes 3d a day. Some of the low wages may of course be for children or young people or for women or other low paid workers; there are no signs however of reduced wages being paid for short winter days of work.

Carpenters, masons, plumbers, plasterers, slaters and thatchers, wrights, glaziers, painters and tinkers, with their 'servers' and on occasion apprentices (45, 48), were all employed, sometimes several miles away from their homes. At times they were listed by their residence rather than by name - the mason of St Clement's parish, the smith of St Mary's parish, the plumber of St Andrew's parish, the slater that dwells in St Peter's parish, etc; were they perhaps the licensed craftsmen for that parish? On occasion, what appear to be partnerships can be seen, like Hygen of Belmesthorpe and Wright of Ryhall working together on several different sites over several years. Some workmen like John Hygen carpenter were almost full-time employees of the Hospital. Its commercial patronage must have been significant.

Building work: While much of the work was small-scale regular maintenance, some consisted of restoring properties when one tenant left and another tenant took over (28, 47, 66v etc). Sometimes there was a change of use - for example, a roper's house in Stamford Baron was altered to become a miller's house (47). During the time the property was in the hands of the warden, the rent was 'decayed', i.e. there was no income from the property. Other property was repaired after a disaster. The great flood of 1501-2 caused repairs and 'cleaning

[46] For the current debate about wages, see John Hatcher 2011 Unreal wages: long-run living standards and the 'Golden Age' of the fifteenth century, in B Dodds and C D Libby (eds) 2011 *Commercial Activity, Markets and Entrepreneurs in the Middle Ages: essays in honour of Richard Britnell* Boydell, pp 1-24, and the rejoinder by James A Galloway in *The Ricardian* vol 23 (2013) pp 110-111.

up' to some property for two years[47]. Surprisingly, there were few recorded fires - in North Witham and in Swayfield only; these properties remained damaged for several years (87, 92, 108). The greatest hazard as seen in this account book was of buildings 'falling down'. Time and again walls, lean-tos, penthouses, rooms and especially barns in both rural and urban settings fell down and were re-erected (e.g. 45-46v, 81v, 82, 109, 124). The brewhouse, penthouse and chimney at the Angel all fell down during the midlent fair 1503, damaging a *'maschfatt'* (46v), and took a long time to be restored; six years later, the penthouse fell down again (81v).

Some of the projects were on a massive scale. The Crane was probably the biggest undertaking. This inn stood in St Peter's parish; one of its walls abutted the castle. In 1497, John Golyn of Easton on the Hill took on a new tenancy and the occasion was used for a major enhancement of the property at a cost of £2 4s 8d; a further 4s 10½d was spent in 1500-1 when a wall fell. Yet in 1501-2, when Golyn's contract was cancelled ("*I expendyd at john golyns hows when I brak the indenture bytwene hym and the almoshows*", 43v) and Robert Cave replaced him, another major overhaul of the building was undertaken, costing £6 19 1½d, before the keys were handed over to the new tenant (39v). From this, we can see in this inn a hall ('new built'), 'shops' in the parlour, a high chamber, a long kitchen and great chimney, a well, a stable, a *thakk hows* (perhaps a privy), two privies (*seges*), a great gate towards the street and another great gate to the paved courtyard, steps, penthouse, a capon pen and hogsties in the little garden. The Angel (formerly in St Mary's Street) was also a very large inn. However, it would appear that in Stamford, with its numbers of large inns, the landlords of these two inns were not "among the rich and influential members of the town" as they were in other towns[48]; for both of these inns appear to have been hard to let, frequently changing their tenants.

One of the more interesting accounts points to the rebuilding in North Witham of a large barn (82v). It appears that while inserting (*drayng*) a first floor (*hows*) into an existing barn, the weight of this floor caused the building to collapse. The re-erection included no less than 27 'couples' (roof braces), suggesting the building would have been about 40 feet in length. The building may still survive in North Witham (where a number of buildings dating from the late medieval period remain although these have not yet been surveyed). In North Luffenham, Rutland, the farm bought by William Browne and held by the bedehouse does remain almost untouched[49].

---

[47] For floods at this time, see Anne Sutton 2013, 'Pondre the universalle wele of the cuntre': Richard III, bridges and floods, *The Ricardian* 23 pp 21-36. For the great flood of 1499-1500, see M K Jones 1986 Lady Margaret Beaufort, the Royal Council and an early fenland drainage scheme, *Lincolnshire History and Archaeology* vol 21 p 14.

[48] See J Hare 2013 Inns, innkeepers and the society of later medieval England, 1350-1600, *Journal of Medieval History* 39 (4) pp 477-497.

[49] It was recently surveyed by Nick Hill of English Heritage

Browne's Hospital: The repairs done to Browne's Hospital itself gives us an insight into the building. The chapel and its windows received attention from time to time (123), and church furniture and vestments for the chapel were supplied and repaired - a chalice made in London and sent there again for mending (17, 22), tapers for the altar, images of St Blasius and St Anne (65v), and books which required covering (38). There were bells in the chapel with a rope (86). The steeple to the Hospital was repaired (17v), as was a chamber over the cloister (86). The warden had a hall with a chimney (13), a parlour with a double door (66), a chamber (56v), an entry (13v), and a separate garden (22v); the confrater had a chimney to his chamber (22v). There were on site a kitchen (40v), a counting house (66) and a privy building (56v). The bedesmen had a garden of their own (46), and the bedeswomen had their own hall (40v). In the outbuildings were a woodyard (22v), a well with chains (44v), a stable (40), a storehouse (66) and a schoolhouse[50] (65v). There was a gate towards the highway (13, 13v) and a large gate and a field gate (13) to the rear.

The amount of money and time these repairs must have taken can only be imagined. It would have been enough to strain a fit man without other commitments. The warden had to develop strategies to manage the system and build up networks of workers and helpers to assist with these tasks over a wide area. None of these networks and assistants proved to be long-lasting in this period.

DISPUTES AND DISTRAINTS

As if such repairs were not enough, the warden had to cope with the stresses caused by the disputes he and his tenants got themselves into.

It was the estates which caused most of the numerous disputes in which the warden found himself embroiled. The section of the annual account headed 'casual costs' reveals something of the extent of these, but it is important to appreciate that the disputes listed in this account book are only a part of all the issues the warden had to deal with, those which involved him in direct payments.

Disputes: The tenants became involved in a large number of local disputes. Thus the warden went to Swayfield when Hugh Holm (perhaps related to Bartholomew Holmes the bailiff) was indicted at the sessions in Billesfield, Lincs, "*when [he] cast owt the hey owt off alen toppars barn*" (Toppar was a tenant of the Hospital in Swayfield) (30v). Master Cuff of Carlby sued the Hospital "*when he was hurte*" (70). The year 1509-10 is revealing: the warden was amerced "*for a*

[50] I have been wondering whether this is in fact a schoolhouse: it is the only mention of a school at all; and the phrase *Reparacion off ye stor howse or off ye scole howse* (65v) might lead one to wonder if it were a coal house - but again there is no mention of coal here except in London. On the whole, I stick with schoolhouse.

heghe [hedge] *at carlbe* [Carlby] *at master greysley cowrte at brasboro* [Braceborough] "; in the manor court of Swayfield

> *I had dywerse men of ye contre for to se weder yat colwell deyd* [did] *me wrong or not os in fellyng asche apon a dyk bank and for settyng of a kyln wall*
>
> ...
>
> *Item I toke a swyt of gorgius penbere* [George Penbury] *and of hew holme for sertyn mony yat the[y] howte* [owed] *to yis hows so I tok a wryte ... and ij alyas capyas* [writs of distraint] (85v).

There was a dispute with the abbot of Peterborough (80v), a boundary disagreement[51] in Stamford with Thomas Morrand, vicar of All Saints and the Hospital's patron, recorded in the king's great leet in the town (81), and a lengthy dispute with Sir John Hussey over land, a dispute which took the warden to London twice to "*make the end betwyx s' john huse and me*" (111):

> *Item for goyng to london ... to speyk with master hosse master breknall and with master pygot to mak aneynd off owr land' betweyn master hwsse and hws - they myghte not tend'* [attend to] *hyt yen* [then] *bot they promysyd me they wold make aneynd heyr at a sysse* [session] (117v)

In 1517-18 is recorded:

> *expens' made for apperance at lugborgh aforne my lorde of lincoln officers at ye swte* [suit] *off Bawchon* (125v)

There are several payments to lawyers to settle or withdraw disputes:

> *I peyd to master Archer for stopyng ye swyt betwyne jorge penbury and hwe holme yat I had taken ageyn yem* (91v)

Distraints seem to have been the normal way for such disputes to burst into the open. In 1502, Christopher Browne seized some cattle at Swayfield which caused the tenants much concern (37v; see below); and at the same time, a distraint was taken at Counthorpe:

> *I payd to the clerk of the cownseyll off my ladys for j lettur to master thomas Grymysby for the distrayne takyn in the closse of coynthorp iiij day of maij* (38)

A second letter had to be sent to Grymmesby. The warden paid the abbot of Peterborough 10s to have an indenture of agreement after a distraint at Pilsgate (73). Some cattle of a tenant were taken at Wilsthorpe (17) and a cow at Barham (27), and the warden had to give his personal surety before the distraint could be lifted. In 1506-7, Sheppey (acting for Sharpe the then warden who was busy with the gild dispute) *went to london to spek with Syr Jon hose for owr stres yat was takken at swafeld* (72v).

---

[51] This may not of course have been a *dis*agreement but an agreement registered in the king's court.

Most of these disputes centred on Swayfield and North Witham in Lincolnshire, but some of the Northamptonshire property could also cause trouble.

It is worth detailing one of these disputes to see more clearly the weight of responsibility which the wardens felt. In Sheppey's first year, 1507-8, the abbot of Peterborough had taken a distraint in Pilsgate (73).

> *when ye abbot of peterborow had takyn owr stres at pyllysgat, Master Ratlyff send thomas tawerner to ye abbott and so for hys sake he delywerd ye stres to a dey* [that is, he assigned a day for hearing the case], *and so I went to spek with Master pygott and he gaf me cownsell to go up to London to spek with Master breknal* [the abbot's counsel] *and hym togedyr ... hyt has cost me for goyng to peterborro vij tymes to agre[e] with ye abbot and I taryed yer sumtyme iij deys ... I went to spek with Master breknal on ye mundey in yowl weyk* [Yule week]
>
> *I weant to ber ye indentur yat was betweyn ye abot and me to Master pygot yat yt might be mad after cownsell at london*
>
> *Item for goyng to London at after crystonmes* [Christmas] *for to haf had an end with ye abbot, and hys atorney was not yer* [there] *and so I was dyssapwentyd* [disappointed]. *Item to speyk with master torn'* [Turner or attorney?] *and with master mollysworthe ... I went to Peturborow befor crystonmes to wyt wedder* [know whether] *owr wrytyng wer com home fro London or not; hyt was not ... I was yerfor* [therefore] *feyn to go spek with master pigot and he seyd hys man had lost ye cope* [copy]... *[I paid] for makkyg a new copy of ye sam indenture* (80v)

The warden thus became fully informed on legal documentation - indentures of agreement, writs of all kinds. He sent messengers to collect 'evidences', an acquittance from Misterton, copies of court rolls etc. Such documents had to be exactly worded, which could lead to much frustration: the agreement between the Hospital and the abbot had to be sent to London to ensure it was fully correct, but when it was lost by the lawyer's clerk, a copy had to be made and again sent to London. They would all be stored in the chest in the Hospital counting house.

Lawyers: And successive wardens became acquainted with lawyers and their ways, both locally and in London. Linked together through their London inns of court, nevertheless most had local connections in Lincolnshire or Northamptonshire. Thomas **Archer** of Hougham, Lincs, came from New Temple; he held offices in Lincolnshire, including coroner of the county (1502, 1511) and duchy of Lancaster receiver of the Long Bennington group of estates (1508-9). He worked however mainly in London. Sir John **Hussey** was from Gray's Inn, the son of Sir William Hussey of Sleaford, Lincolnshire, Chief Justice of the King's Bench. He too held many offices, including the stewardship of Stamford, but his main arena was the royal household and king's council; he eventually became lord Hussey but was executed in 1537. Clearly, he was not an easy man to deal with - he was given to violence at times.

But the main group were focussed round the Inner Temple where William **Elmes** had trained. Robert **Brudenell** of Stonton Wyville, Leics, and Deene, Northants, was from an Inner Temple lawyer family; serjeant at law, he was one of the most eminent (and most expensive) lawyers of his day, retained by many lords and institutions, including Peterborough abbey. Later he became knighted and served as Chief Justice of Common Pleas, but even in the days when he was consulted by Browne's Hospital, he was in the first flight of English lawyers. John **Molesworth** of Helpston, Northants, however, was a young lawyer at the time he was consulted, having just moved to Inner Temple from Clement Inn; he went on to become escheator of Northants and Rutland, and coroner for the abbot of Peterborough's liberty. Most importantly, the Hospital sought out Thomas **Pygot**, also of Inner Temple. Thomas was clearly sympathetic to the Hospital, for he had married Elizabeth, the widow of William Elmes. The Elmes family relocated from Stamford to Whaddon, Bucks, where Pygot lived and where he was JP and clerk of the crown. Pygot sponsored his stepson John Elmes into the Inner Temple. A serjeant at law, like Archer, he was a duchy of Lancaster official. The connections between members of this group can be seen as both William Elmes and Thomas Pygot appointed Robert Brudenell as executor of their wills[52].

The interaction between the wardens and lawyers was often intense. In London before the king's council, Archer became attorney for the warden and was retained on an annual fee (55v, 63), and the warden went to see him at his home (Hougham, Lincs), as also Brudenell at Stonton Wyville, Leics. Sharpe met the lawyers of the king's council and their clerks, not just in London but also in Cambridge where he had to stay for four nights (63v-64). Sir John Hussey was both a supporter and an adversary; the warden went to see him in Sleaford, in Cambridge and in London.(61v, 63v-64, 72v). In the immediate neighbourhood, we can see the lawyers on Lady Margaret Beaufort's council in action on several occasions. The lawyers of the abbot of Peterborough had to be met and persuaded; Masters Breknall (the abbot's counsel), Brudenell and Molesworth were consulted, some frequently. Archer and Pigot in particular became the lawyers of preference. Payments were made to their servants and gifts given to the lawyers as well as their fees. Wine (at least once Rhenish) was often flowing: in 1506-7, the warden paid

> *ffor wyne to s' John husey at after crystemese when he was at M Rathclyffys* (62)

In 1508-9,

> *I spent with archer when he was heyr at mysomer term … I gaf hym a grot to drynk for to be delygent betweyn my lord* [abbot] *and me* (80v)

Wine was presented to the sheriff "*yat I myghte be sped*" (93v). The warden spent 10s *ffor a newyerys gyffth* [New Year's gift] for Sir John Hussey (61v), *a crown gyltyd and ameld* [enamelled?]

---

[52] J H Baker 2012 *Men of Court 1440-1550* Selden Society Supplementary Series vol 18

THE GILD VERSUS THE HOSPITAL

The disputes which forced the wardens to engage lawyers were often disputes concerning the Hospital's tenants, over unpaid rents, fines for not attending courts, distrained cattle or goods, or encroachments of neighbours. Most of these disputes came to the wardens unsought. But the biggest dispute may in part have been self-inflicted - that between Christopher Browne on behalf of the gild of All Saints and the Hospital..

In order to understand what was at issue, it is necessary to remember the origins of the Hospital. When William Browne as Alderman of the gild of All Saints in the parish church of All Saints in the Market founded the Hospital in 1475, it was intended to be a combined gildhall and almshouse, named Clement Hospital. The first floor room (the Audit Room) was not the hall of the bedesmen; that hall lay in the buildings behind on the north side of the courtyard range. It was an elaborate gildhall with pantry, buttery and access to the kitchens. At a later stage, Browne decided to endow the Hospital from his own estate and re-name it as Browne's Hospital. While the gild did have some property, it was clearly not well endowed. I doubt that Browne ever considered that the relationship between gild and Hospital would not continue after his death[53].

As we have seen, Thomas Stokes took over as patron after Browne's death in 1489, working closely with William Elmes, the new Alderman of the gild. After the death of Stokes in 1495, Elmes became patron of the Hospital as well as Alderman of the gild. But Elmes died young in 1504, and for the first time, there was a break between the Hospital and the gild: Christopher Browne became gild Alderman, while Henry Wykes vicar of All Saints in the Market became patron under the statutes drawn up by Stokes.

There was already bad feeling between the Hospital and Christopher in a personal capacity. As we have seen, Christopher took a distraint on the Hospital tenants in Swayfield in 1502, which caused considerable upset to tenants and warden (John Taylor). But matters became worse when Christopher became gild Alderman in 1504, and it may be that the issue was forced on the warden by the behaviour of Christopher Browne; we know that he could be obstinate (see below).

The opening rounds: Exactly what sparked this off is not now known. The dispute had been going for some time before mid-1506 when Christopher Browne tabled his bill of complaint in chancery and the warden was summoned to London, for in his counter-plea, the warden wrote that

---

[53] It is possible that William Browne founded the gild; there is no sign of it before 1475; and Christopher Browne (as senior member of the Browne family) became its Alderman after the death of Browne's grandson and heir, William Elmes, in 1504. Christopher had already been at odds with William Browne; see Rogers, *Noble Merchant* pp 267-9.

> *the said Christofre hath put your said besechers to great coosts and chargs as for sut making for the same with the counsaill of your derest lady and moder the countesse of Richemount and Derby,*

but

> *the said Christofre was commaunded noo further to entromedle with the said houses* [i.e. the buildings].

The appeal to the council of Lady Margaret Beaufort at Collyweston nearby accords with the growth of the jurisdiction of that council in the region; the warden appealed to that council at other times during this account book period (see above)[54]. And, although Christopher was a member of her council[55], he did not receive a favourable answer in this court, and so he took his case to chancery (Christopher was in favour at Henry VII's court) and asked for a subpoena to the warden.

The chancery hearing 1506: The surviving bill of complaint of 22 May 1506 refers to only one issue, that of a sum of £20 which the Alderman said the Hospital owed the gild. The classic procedures were followed: Sharpe gave his 'answer to the bill of complaint', Browne gave a 'replication' and Sharpe gave his rejoinder[56]. Sharpe's attorney answered Christopher's charge by claiming that the matter should be heard in another court and not in chancery. He said that Sharpe had no knowledge of any such loan to his predecessor but that the matter did not concern the Hospital; if such a loan had been made, it must have been for Taylor's personal use and not for the use of the Hospital "*as shall playnly appere by bokes of accomptes therof*[57]". Taylor should be summoned. Christopher responded by reaffirming his initial complaint that the money had been borrowed and it was used for the Hospital, so the current warden must respond. Sharpe similarly reiterated his response.

The court of Requests: But (it would seem at the same time, although the documents are undated) Sharpe lodged a counter-suit against Christopher in the newly established Court of Requests[58]. In this, he mentioned three matters. First, the gild was claiming access to part of the Hospital premises which was against the statutes and deeds of the Hospital. Secondly, there was the sum of £20 which the warden now admitted had been given to the Hospital by William Elmes for the support of the Hospital but he averred that it was intended for

---

54 See also Jones, Lady Margaret Beaufort, the Royal Council and an early fenland drainage scheme, cited above note 47.

55 For full biography of Christopher Browne, see Alan Rogers, The parliamentary representation of Stamford 1467 to 1509 *Nottingham Medieval Studies* (forthcoming).

56 TNA C1/357/15-18; see Appendix IV

57 I think this refers to this book of accounts

58 I am grateful to Dr James Ross, then of TNA, for help with the details of the court procedures.

Elmes to be prayed for; this suit (he said) had already been dismissed by the council of Lady Margaret Beaufort, but Christopher was now maliciously pursuing it "*in your comen place*" [i.e. chancery]. Thirdly, Christopher was demanding a chief rent of 50s from Swayfield, "*Whiche your said Oratours aught not to paye unto hym, as it is evidently knowen both by the countreye ther as also by certain their deds; yit he herewith not satisfiede dailly sueth your said besechers to their expresse wronge and uttre undoing forever*" unless 'your grace' be moved with pity.

Christopher Browne's *'aunswer'* and the replication by Sharpe are now missing, but some of the contents of that replication can be seen from Christopher Browne's rejoinder to that replication[59]. Christopher confirmed what he said in his (now missing) 'answer'; and he claimed that the warden had now admitted that a loan of £20 towards the costs of the almshouse had been made by Elmes[60], so it should be repaid. He alleged that William Browne by his will had given the gild full control over their gildhall with buttery, pantry and kitchen. Thirdly, he reiterated what he had said in his 'answer' that the warden had given (*'seised'*) the chief rent of 50s from the manor of Swayfield to Christopher "*and they whos astate he hath in the said maner* [of Corby]". He went on to deny the allegation of the (missing) replication that Browne "*upon the foundacion of the said almeshous gave the said hall buttry pantry and kechyn with all other bildyngs the[n] called Clement now called Brounes Almeshous to the predecessours of the said now warden and to his successours*"; and he also denied "*that the said Aldermen and their bredren* [of the gild] *have occupied the said hall buttry pantry and kechyn onely by the sufferaunce of the said Warden and his predecessour, but* [he asserted that the gild] *hath occupied the same as in their owne title and right".*

The warden spent seven weeks in London during November and December 1506, ferrying between the city where he stayed, and Greenwich, Westminster, Wansbridge[61] where he met the dean of the king's chapel and Sir John Hussey, and even once to Richmond (again the dean). His activities are listed in detail (to the extent of recording that he burned coal there rather than the wood fuel at home). He met his attorney Master Archer several times, Sir John Hussey (steward of Stamford as well as member of the king's council) at least twice, Master Pygot, Master Breknall counsel for the abbot of Peterborough among other offices, Sir John Digby (with Pygot), the dean of the king's chapel (Dr Symeon), Mr Richard Sutton and Dr Hatfield (see Appendix V).

The decree: Nothing further is heard of the chancery suit but a decree was issued on Friday 18 December 1506:

Md yat uppon yat day ye kynkys [king's] *honorabull councell gaff centenc' and mad an*

---

59 TNA REQ 2/93/5; see Appendix IV

60 See Appendix VI

61 I have been unable to locate Wansbridge but it may be near Wandsworth or on the river Wandle to the south of the Thames. The warden rode there rather than go by boat.

> *End bytwyxth ye bedehowse and ye gyld off all alow'* [gild of All Hallows] *for all maters as hyt apperythe in the decree* (61)

We learn later that the decree was made

> *by your moost honorable counseill M doctour Symeon Dean of your most honorabill chappell, M doctour Hatton and M Richard Sutton,*

and so it is clear that the decree came from the Court of Requests which was virtually a sub-committee of the king's council under the dean of the king's chapel.

The decree dealt with the issue of the loan or gift of £20 which Sharpe was ordered to repay to the gild, but there is no indication concerning a decision about the chief rent. The warden also lost the charge relating to access, and thus early in the New Year, he recorded (62)

Item in expensys when ye alderman and ye honest men off ye town of stanfford whas at takyng off off ye loke off owr pantrey dore	*vjd*
Item in Wyne to M alderman [Thomas Lacey] *and M Rathclyff*	*iiijd*
Item to Wyllyam Smythe ffor drawyng off ye loke	*ijd*
Item to M Lacy[62] *sum ffor makyng off an enventory off ye goods belongyng to ye gyld off all halows wythin the bedehowse*	*iiijd*

The second pleadings (Court of Requests) midsummer 1507: However, it seems that while Sharpe released the gild's goods, he still refused to store them in the Hospital, and he did not pay the sum of £20; so Christopher Browne applied to the royal council again for the warden to appear to answer why he had not fully implemented the decree. In his (undated) bill of complaint[63], Browne stated that Sharpe had failed to implement the decree of "*your moost honorable counseill*", and asked for a writ of privy seal against Sharpe.

Thus Sharpe again went "*to london at medsomer terme when Mayster brown callyd hus uppe with a pryvy sigell.*" Again he ferried between Greenwich, Richmond and Westminster from a base in London. Among those he consulted was his attorney Mr Archer, whose clerk was paid "*ffor wrytyng off my answer to ye seyl*[64] *off complaynth*". Thus we have the 'answer' of Sharpe to the bill of complaint but not any further proceedings, the replication and rejoinder. In his answer, Sharpe said that he was willing to implement the decree as it stood but that the decree did not mean that he "*ne his successours shuld in eny Wise be charged ne chargeable with the kepyng of eny of the godes of the seid Gild*". He said he had given Christopher an indenture of surety to

---

[62] It is not clear if this is Thomas Lacy the Alderman of Stamford or Henry Lacy under-steward of the town and prominent local government official.

[63] TNA REQ 2/8/114a and b; see Appendix IV

[64] This word is not certain; I think it is an elision of two words, 'seyd bill', becoming 'seyl'

pay the £20 but that Christopher refused to return it "*to thentent that he by means therof hereafter myght eftsones troble and charge the same Warden and his successours*".

The only indication we have of the decision of the court to this second suit is the statement (68v):

> *Md yat the kyngs counsell hath decred yat the ... alderman off ye gyld off all hallose shall hav or receve off Robert beomonth* *xv li*

Thus Robert Beomond, the Hospital's former bailiff who still owed the Hospital large sums of money, was ordered to pay £15 of the sum of £20 to the gild: which must have been the only comforting decision the warden received from the whole of this affair, for it is doubtful whether the Hospital had the wherewithal in cash in hand to pay the debt. Christopher Browne and the gild would have to get the money out of Beomond.

The issues:

We can add further to the three issues at stake.

a) access: The removal of the padlock suggests that the gild did gain more or less free access to their own gildhall for future feasts, but there is no direct evidence. We know that the gild survived to the Reformation[65].

b) the debt of £20: John Taylor, in copying up the accounts of John Coton, inserts quite separately a note of the receipt of this sum (2):

> *In primis memorandum that my predecessor forsayd syr John Coton Receyvd off Mastyr Wyllam Elmes forsayd patron off thys almeshows ffor a stoor or a stok aforehand to hafe fo[r] to pay in tyme off neede as hytt aperyth in the booke off payments wrytyng in the begynnyng with the hand off the seyd S' John Coton for thys present yer* *xx li*

Later, he recorded in his own annual account for 1502

> *Item ther was borod off all halo gylde afortyme* *xx li* (41);

and occasionally it is mentioned as being in the stock or surviving balance of the Hospital (see Appendix VI). Taylor had surrendered and the gild clearly won on this issue.

c) **chief rent:** It would also seem that the warden lost his claim in respect of the chief rent. Margaret Browne's inquisition post mortem in 1489 reported that she held the manor of Swayfield of lord Grey's manor of Castle Bytham by fealty and a rent of 50s 4d[66]. Henry lord Grey of Codnor died in 1496, leaving

---

[65] The gild properties came to the Cecil family; Hartley and Rogers p 17. We might note here that the account book refers several times to a gildhall close to the church of All Saints and next door to the vicarage of All Saints (e.g. 45), which might be a temporary building used for this purpose during the dispute.

[66] *Calendars of Inquisitions Post Mortem* (*CIPM*) *Henry VII* vol i p 230 (551)

illegitimate children, so the entailed estate fell between three co-heirs, descendants of his grandfather Richard lord Grey of Codnor who had died in 1418. However, Henry's third wife Catherine lady Grey[67] (daughter of William lord Stourton and widow of Sir William Berkeley) continued to hold the estates for at least ten years (probably until her death); thus the chief rent would have been due to her or her estate officials. The formulaic nature of many of the entries in this account book is revealed by the fact that the rent is said to be paid to 'lord Grey', even though there was no longer a 'lord Grey'[68].

In claiming in 1502 that the chief rent should be paid to himself and "*they whos estate he hath*", and taking some cattle from the Swayfield tenants as a distraint, Christopher Browne was apparently claiming to be one of the feoffees of either lady Grey or one of the co-heirs. Taylor responded by writing that the rent was due '*to lord Grey's servants*' (41). Sharpe reverted to the standard phrase, stating that the chief rent was paid to 'lord Grey', and so it remained until the end of the account. However, it is clear that the recipient of the chief rent after the decree was Christopher Browne and his co-feoffees, for somewhat later Browne took another distraint which caused warden Sheppey a great deal of trouble and travel (described below), so that in the end, Sheppey bought out the chief rent from Christopher Browne and Sir John Hussey who was presumably another of the feoffees[69] (106).

The substantive issue

But behind these three issues (on which Browne won in each case) lay a much more serious issue which is never directly addressed but which can be seen in almost every piece of writing in this book – who owns the Hospital and its estates? All the documents relating to William Browne's administration of the Hospital, both as Clement Hospital and later as Browne's Hospital, emphasise that Browne managed it alone, that he paid for everything himself without anyone else being involved, and that he accounted to no-one. The same was true of Thomas Stokes, and the statutes that Stokes drew up contained no mention of the gild; careful provision was made for the patronage of the Hospital without calling on the gild. And it is this which explains the strong wording of the Narrative (see below) at the beginning of the account book, with its stress on

[67] Lady Grey borrowed from the gild of St Katherine, Stamford, the gild's hearse for her husband's funeral; *Act Book of St Katherine's Gild, Stamford 1480-1532* edited Alan Rogers, Stamford Survey Group and abramis academic publishers 2011 p 100

[68] John lord Zouche of Harringworth (who fought against Henry Tudor at Bosworth, was captured, attainted but restored in 1495) was one of the co-heirs; and in May 1505, John Busshe esquire claimed to be another descendant entitled to part of the inheritance. It seems Elizabeth Pole was the descendant of the third co-heiress. *Complete Peerage* vi pp 130-133; *CIPM Henry VII* ii 904 (pp 575-6), 966 (p609); either GEC is in error about the descendants or Busshe is a false claimant.

[69] It is significant that Sheppey went to London on Sharpe's behalf to talk with Hussey about the distress taken at Swayfield for a sum of 40s, see 72v; Hussey may have been involved in the first distraint for this chief rent.

William and Margaret Browne alone having founded the house and maintained it "with no-one over him" and that "he gave account which related to this house to no other person"; that after the deaths of William and Margaret, Thomas Stokes "ruled this almshouse" and "he rendered no account of this house to anyone during his lifetime". When John Coton took over, Taylor stated that he too was subject to "no other person … [nor did he] render account for his administration". And in the annual accounts from 1495 to 1504 copied up by Taylor, every page was carefully audited: *summa lateris* or *summa pagine* [70]…, followed by *probatum est per me* Henry Wykes (vicar of All Saints) who is described as

> *auditor and supervisor off thys and off every accompts off thys almos hows for hys tyme accordyng to the statutes off thys almos hows* (6v).

In October 1507, after the harrowing year spent in London arguing with the gild, Sharpe's account was audited by Henry Wykes vicar of All Saints,

> authorised supervisor and auditor for my time of each such account concerning the administration of all the goods and the office of warden of the same house as appears in the statutes of the said house … these being witnesses: sir Thomas Forster dean of Stamford, sir Robert Sheppey and sir William Hawkyns confrater of the said house and many others (68v).

The same formula is repeated in subsequent audits of accounts (78 etc).

It can hardly be doubted that Christopher Browne on behalf of the gild was claiming the power to audit the accounts of the Hospital (after all, his predecessor as Alderman of the gild William Elmes had audited the accounts). The issue of gild control had probably been raised as early as 1502, for in that year, the warden paid for three copies of the Hospital statutes to be made (38), perhaps to give one or more copies to Lady Margaret Beaufort's council. It is likely that it was this claim that led the warden to exclude the gild from its own gildhall. But equally it cannot be doubted that the decree of the Court of Requests of December 1506 had given the current Hospital administration reassurance of their independence of the gild, despite giving the gild once more access to its gildhall.

What is more doubtful, however, is the story that Taylor told of the origins of the Hospital. Taylor opened the account book with a three-page 'narrative' of the founding of the Hospital which deliberately sets out to exclude the gild which is never mentioned. But the fact that the money given to the first warden was admitted by the later wardens to have come from the gild and was to be repaid to the gild, and the fact that the gild seems to have won access to its gildhall, must suggest that the gild had a larger part to play in the building and maintenance of Clement Hospital in its early years than Taylor allowed for. It is surely this which caused Stokes and Taylor to reiterate the fiction that the

---

[70] 'total of this side' or 'page' 'approved by me Henry Wykes'

foundation of Browne's Hospital dated from 1494, that Stokes was the founder and that Coton was the first warden.

The role of Henry Wykes, vicar of All Saints in the Market, in all of this is intriguing. There is no sign of a gild chapel in the parish church, so the Hospital chapel presumably was the gild chapel. There is no sign of a gild chaplain or any other parish chaplain, so probably the vicar (Henry Wykes) served the gild as chaplain; the vicar (Thomas Stokes at that time) was certainly taking services in the Hospital chapel from 1476 when he was sued by the rector of Great St Michael, Stamford, on the grounds that the Hospital chapel lay in St Michael's parish. Yet Henry Wykes was named by Thomas Stokes in the statutes as the patron of the Hospital after the death of Elmes. Now Wykes was a close member of the Browne circle; as we have seen, he had been appointed vicar by Thomas Stokes and he was feoffee and executor for Browne, Stokes and Elmes; his brass is the only non-Browne-family brass in the Browne burial chapel in the parish church.

From the start, Wykes was closely involved in the Hospital administration. During the first year, he was instructed or authorised by Elmes to pay sums amounting to £20 to Coton, the warden, for cash in hand. Elmes seems to have been weak, absent or ill – he allowed Christopher Browne to harass the Hospital tenants in Swayfield over the disputed chief rent in 1502. But from 1504, when Elmes died, Wykes was patron and clearly supported Taylor against the gild. He meticulously signed every page of Taylor's copied up accounts. His loyalty to the parish gild in his own church of which he seems to have served as chaplain must have been sorely tried.

TRAVEL

The frequent law suits and other disputes, the holding of manor courts, the collection of rents and the overseeing of the property repairs meant that the warden was constantly travelling. From the start, he went long distances to "*ask rent*" (17). My impression is that every year, the warden spent more of his time away from the Hospital, presumably leaving the day-to-day administration to the confrater William Hawkyns. It is important to realise we only see those travels which incurred expense, but since for much of the time horse hire was essential, many journeys are recorded. Later, '*costs of keeping our horse*' appear as a separate item in the accounts. Keeping a horse (like a car) required accommodation (a stable was built in the Hospital in 1501-2, 40), fuel (*horsmete* and livery), maintenance (harness and shoeing, 10v, 65, 80) and repairs (*horse leche*, 65).

To give a flavour of the kind of burden undertaken on behalf of his tenants and the maintenance of the estate, we can take the account of some of the journeys made in 1510-11 (93-93v). Once again, Sheppey faced a distraint, once again

Christopher Browne was at the heart of the trouble, and once again Swayfield was the disturbed village.

The tenants reported that Christopher Browne had taken another distraint of their cattle, and the warden "*went to Swayfield to see what cattle were taken; it cost me 5d to content them for they were very wroth. On the morrow*", three of the tenants and the warden went to meet master Hussey (Browne's co-feoffee) at Deeping "*to desire him to see a remedy for us, but he came not there that day*", so the three tenants "*came with me home that night; and went again on the morrow and spoke with him; he promised he would do the best he could. He sent Thomas Stoke* [junior, nephew of Thomas Stokes I and a clerk in the royal exchequer[71]] *to Master Browne to have the distress delivered, but he* [Browne] *would in no wise deliver it.* [Therefore], *I was fain to go to Sleaford* [Hussey's residence] *and three of these men with me to see if any remedy would be there. It was three days before we could know what we should do*".

"*A week after Candlemas, I was fain to go to London, for the tenants had so great labour with bearing their* [confiscated] *cattle mete* [food] *and drink that [they] cried out to me, so that I was irked of them; I was surety for them for nine days. And I paid for a writ* [to the sheriff of Lincolnshire]. *When I was come home with this writ of replegear* [to release the cattle], *then I went to the sheriff to have a warrant to one of his bailiffs to have the cattle delivered; he dwells beyond Spilsby*[72], *so I lay at Swinstead*[73] *the first night at this side of Boston; [I went on the] morrow to Boston and the same night at Frysby*[74] *where the sheriff lies. The under-sheriff was not at home, he was at Lincoln, so I was fain to hire me a guide. I paid at Horncastle and at Lincoln the same night at supper. ..., I paid for wine for the sheriff that I might be sped ..., and paid the sheriff for serving a writ* [against Browne] .... *[I had] breakfast there on the morrow and spent washing my gown and grooming my horse ... At Ancaster homeward and at Swayfield that night before I came home .... [I went to] Corby when the distress was borrowed and I spent on the king's bailiff and on other men that had a down on us ...*" (93-93v)

It is no wonder that the Hospital bought out the chief rent from Browne, Hussey and the other feoffees (106).

It is impossible here to provide a complete itinerary of all the journeys shown in these accounts, but we can indicate the kind of journeys successive wardens made. Travel to Swayfield and North Witham for the twice-annual manor courts occur in most years, sometimes a wasted journey if the steward or the tenants did not turn up (43v). He attended other courts as summoned (30v). He travelled for land transactions - to Greetham to purchase some land, to North Witham several

---

71 See Rogers, Eton's First 'Poor Scholar'

72 Sir Robert Dymoke of Scrivelsby, Lincs, who should have been sympathetic, since he was named on the bederoll of the Hospital

73 A manor belonging to Elizabeth Elmes, William Browne's daughter

74 Firsby by Spilsby, Lincs

times for the sale of Swynhaw woods and to finalise the grant of property from Sir Thomas Delalaund (see Appendix III). He was constantly at North Witham and Swayfield, sometimes staying two or three days (17, 73) - to lease a close, to see where a gate should be placed, to measure lands (17, 20), to see his bailiff (17), to take possession of the property of his under-bailiff Arnold Morton who was arrested (53), to see for himself what his neighbour Colwell had done before he issued a writ against him (85v). He constantly met his tenants, going round to introduce Beomond as the new bailiff (17), rushing out to them when they suffered distraints (93). In 1496, Coton went on one day "*to Carlby, Wylsthorp and Barham xxvj day of October*". Taylor went to Barham to admit a new tenant (27) and other places to collect rents, distraining some tenants (17, 27, 80v). The warden went to oversee repairs many times (17, 30v etc), to buy supplies for the '*stoor*' and to sell wood (17). He was constantly seeking the help of lawyers and other officers - to Lyddington for the bishop of Lincoln's officials, to Collyweston for Lady Margaret Beaufort's court, to Sleaford for Hussey, to Lincoln for the sheriff, suffering disappointment when they did not turn up, like Hussey at Deeping (93). He made repeated journeys, complaining about "*goyng to peterborro vij tymes to agre with ye abbot and I taryed yer* [there] *sumtyme iij d*eys" (73).

London was clearly within their horizon. Taylor sent his bailiff Holmes and another man to London about the sale of Swynhaw woods (4); Sharpe went to London twice in 1506-7, once from late October to late December and again at midsummer 1507 for four weeks; during the same year, Sheppey went to London on his behalf (72v, 80v); in 1508, Sheppey dashed up to London to consult the lawyers Pigot and Breknall (73), and in 1514 again Sheppey went

> *to London to speyk with master hosse master breknall and with master pygot to mak a neynd* [an end] *off owr land' betweyn master hwsse and hws* [us] (111, 117v)

SOCIAL REFLECTIONS

The life of the warden of Browne's Hospital in the early sixteenth century must have been very stressful. Much of this travel was in winter-time along roads that were often impassable (save in London, there are no signs of river-borne travel, even to Boston and Lincoln). No wonder Coton died soon after taking over the reins of the estate, Taylor left after seven years, Sharpe left after three years (and an especially horrendous year in 1506-7), Sheppey seems to have been ill for his last three years and died after ten years in office.

The book, despite its formal nature, is more than simply an account book. The writers on many occasions provided details of their activities and even their feelings which are out of place in a more formal account book.. One warden tells us he was disappointed (80v) and 'irked' with the tenants with their constant complaining, for no doubt they laid their troubles at his door in much the same way that the escaped Jews did with Moses. The tones of frustration when he had

had a wasted journey because the steward or other official could not be found shine through the pages. William Elmes could not make some payments himself, because he had gone down with the "swetyng syknes" (10). And we know that Sharpe was ill in London:

Md yat I payd for leche crafts at london iijs iiijd (63v)

And we can see him fasting: on several successive Wednesdays in London, he recorded (58v)

In primis ffor my manys brekfast	*jd*
Item ffor hys dener	*ijd*
Item ffor hys supper	*ijd*
Item ffor my bred that day	*ob* (½d)

He paid full board for his man on these days while he himself ate only a morsel or had drink only.

The warden and women

And we can see something of his social interactions. If we are to believe this account book, the warden lived in a man's world. His main interactions with women were - so far as we know - limited mainly to the women attendants in the Hospital and women tenants. We know nothing about the families behind the warden, the confrater or inmates. But we need to remember two things. First, the document we are discussing was written by unmarried men and was used in a largely male-oriented socio-cultural context. So women occurred only occasionally and in certain well-defined roles. On the other hand, the Hospital was founded in part and certainly managed in part during its early days by Margaret wife of William Browne. Her interest in it remained until her death; after the death of her husband in April 1489, Margaret continued to run the Hospital, supervise the *reparacions* of the Hospital estates although they were in the hands of feoffees, probably appointed the women attendants, one of whom was her house-servant, and prepared another petition to the king for licence to endow the Hospital. She gave some woodland to the Hospital in her widowhood and remained active to within a week or so of her own death in October 1489.

It is unlikely that Elizabeth Elmes her daughter occupied the same position *vis a vis* the Hospital as her mother. Although on Margaret's death, Elizabeth entered into her Browne inheritance, including many properties in Stamford and the Browne house next to the Hospital, she is unlikely to have been in the town often, although she could still speak in her will in 1510 of "*my chambre in Stamford*". Her son William Elmes lawyer, Recorder and MP for Stamford, Alderman of the gild of All Saints and patron of the Hospital after the death of Thomas Stokes, seems to have lived in the Browne house. The only references to Elizabeth Elmes in the account book are to properties in her possession, not to her personally; and her manor of Wolfhouse in Rutland provided the Hospital every year with its fuel - at cost, of course. As we have seen, she left some legacies to the Hospital in her will; they show her continued interest in the almshouse.

There was however one way in which women influenced the actions of the warden considerably. William Elmes died as a young man in 1504, and his widow Elizabeth [Iwardeby] married another Inner Temple lawyer Thomas Pygot; and Pygot became a favoured lawyer used by the warden in several of his legal disputes[75]. It is not too much to assume that Elizabeth [Iwardeby/Elmes] Pygot retained an affection for the Hospital from the days of her first marriage; her arms are frequently to be found quartered with the Elmes arms in the glass in the gildhall (now the Audit Room).

The women attendants: The two women attendants were included in the total number of bedesfolk. Mathilda and Elizabeth Huntley (perhaps sisters or sisters-in-law) were in the Hospital from at least 1495. Almost certainly they were appointed by William and Margaret Browne. The only thing we know about them is that 'Mawde Huntley' was a servant in the household of Margaret Browne before she transferred to the Hospital and received a legacy of clothing in Margaret's will[76]. They were to be paid the same stipend as the men, i. e. 7d per week, with accommodation including their own kitchen and hall. Their tasks prescribed by the statutes were to wash clothes, obtain and prepare the food and to wait on the bedesmen:

> "the women of the aforesaid Almshouse for the time being be and carry themselves as the Dames [mother figures] of the said house and so bear themselves in washing and other things befitting honest women and (so far as is decent) be altogether attentive and useful to the aforesaid poor men in their necessities".

Their burden of prayers was reduced accordingly:

> "and both of the said poor women, on account of their close occupation in serving the rest of their fellows, shall be bound to say two [instead of three] Psalms of the Blessed Mary every day at least"[77].

They were regarded as fully part of the community; in 1498, when Sir Thomas Delalaund made his grant to the Hospital, Mathilda and Elizabeth Huntley 'poor women' appear in the list of witnesses to the title deed alongside the ten 'poor men', promising to pray for Delalaund.

---

[75] Thomas Pygot sergeant of the coif was overseer of the will of Elizabeth Elmes in 1510, TNA PROB 11/17/2; see Rogers Wills pp 293-4. See E W Ives 1983 *The Common Lawyers of Pre-Reformation England: Thomas Kebell, a case study* Cambridge University Press p 473; Baker, *Men of Court* cited above.

[76] Rogers Wills p 287: *Item I geve to Mawde Huntley a blak goune lyned with blak bokeram, a kirtill furred with foxe and conye, a blak cloke lyned with blak in the sholders, a smok, a kerchief.*

[77] Wright pp 47, 41

Elizabeth Huntley died 8 January 1503. She was not replaced immediately - John Taylor left the almshouse in February 1504 without having made a new appointment. The two and a half year gap in the accounts from 1504 to 1506 makes it impossible for us to suggest when she was replaced by one Margaret. Mathilda also must have died or left the Hospital in this two year period, and in this case was clearly not replaced. For when on or about 12 March 1512, "*Margaret departtyd from yis hows to heyr son*" (fol 97), the Hospital was left without any woman attendant at all. Katherine Goldsmith was not appointed until 16 April 1512; in the meantime, the warden "*peyd for waschyng of clothys and for dyhttyng* [preparing] *of met and serwyyng yem v wykks*" (97), a total of 18d, half of the 35d which he would have paid one woman for five weeks in the Hospital. No other woman was admitted during the remaining time of this account (to 1517). It must have been a major task for one woman to look after two clergymen and the bedesmen, even though their numbers fell at times to six or seven, once to no more than five.

The warden and elite women: Women hardly occurred among the landlords to whose officials the warden paid chief rents. Lady Eyland for the farm at Wilsthorpe and lady Busshey of Thistelton are the only ones named. The king's officials were managing Stamford, although nominally for part of this period it remained among the estates of queen Elizabeth (she died in February 1503 and Stamford reverted to the crown). The most important 'political' woman the warden would have had to deal with was Lady Margaret Beaufort, mother of Henry VII, whose presence from time to time at Collyweston nearby was greatly felt in the town[78]. She was very sympathetic to different forms of religious observance, supporting the anchoress in St Paul's who had been the beneficiary of William Browne's generosity and encouraging another anchoress at St Michael's nunnery in Stamford. Apart from the Christopher Browne affair, there were other occasions when the warden applied to her ladyship's good offices. In 1501-2, Taylor went to Collyweston twice to get letters from the clerk of her council to Thomas Grimsby over the distraint Grimsby had taken in Counthorpe (38, 42v); and in 1506-7, Sharpe obtained "*ye letter* [to the abbot of Peterborough] *commyssyd ffrom ... my ladys grace ye kyngys moder*" (64) concerning the new land in Carlby. Lady Margaret's council was clearly a power in the land which could be useful on occasions and could never be ignored.

The warden and women tenants: Several of the Hospital properties were held by women. Jenett Holmes widow (who may be related to Bartholomew Holmes, the Hospital's first bailiff in south Lincolnshire) and Margaret Jamys widow both held properties in Swayfield (51, 108). As time went on, the number of female tenants seems to have increased. When Whytwick died sometime before 1511-2, his widow took over (112v). The wife of John Thomas held a shop in All Saints parish, but whether she were a widow or held that shop during the lifetime of

[78] M K Jones and M Underwood 1992 *The King's Mother: Lady Margaret Beaufort, countess of Richmond and Derby* Cambridge University Press; see Rogers, '*Noble Merchant*' p 105

her husband is not clear (92). When "Branden's wife" applied to take over a tenancy of the house next to All Saints vicarage in Stamford in 1499-1500[79], Christopher Browne acted as her surety (26v).

We can see very few women traders. Agnes Sharpe recently widowed sold a bucket, wheelbarrow and shovel to Taylor (44), perhaps her dead husband's equipment. Sometime between 1499 and 1503, John Hikson tenant in Scargills in Swayfield died, and John Taylor went to Greetham, Rutland, seeking to purchase her Carlby property; the transaction was eventually effective. Whytwell's wife in Easton sold some *'sparrs'* to the Hospital during the work being done on their property (123v). There is only one mention of women crafts: in 1516-7, Sheppey paid "*for a Coveryng to the Canopye with a sylk frynge with skowryng and dyghtyng of the same to Agnes Claypole*", perhaps related to John Claypole who had held a shop in All Saints parish of the Hospital (123).

Miscellaneous

The book throws light on many aspects of life at the time. For example, candles were bought to provide "*candle light to work withal*" (49v). We know that the Angel and the Crane both had signs outside (46v, 33v). Cherries were bought to entertain M Brudenell the lawyer "*at master Elmys place*" (either next door to the Hospital or at Wolfhouse) (9v); beef, mutton and fish as well as ale were provided for workmen on several occasions (64v, 80 etc). The strength of the parishes in late medieval Stamford is clear to see[80]: not only are tradesmen defined by the parish they lived in but the properties owned by the Hospital were as frequently named by the parish as by the tenant: 'the house in St Andrew's parish', 'the furthest house in St Peter's parish' etc. Tithes and 'halylofe' payments from many properties were dispensed at due times of the year. Clothes were washed and horses were groomed: the word *'dighting'* is used to cover both meanings as well as to prepare food (93v, 97). Payments are made to the bells at Stretton (37, 42v). The warden paid for "*crying two foals*" in Bourne and Grantham (86v), while the Hospital made a charge (*'prest'*) to the "morris fools" to perform before the crowds in the market place below the Hospital (84). But few festivals can be seen here - Christmas and Yule are merely dates by which events can be located.

It is strange that, in relation to the borough council of Stamford, the Hospital seems to have been in something of a bubble. There are very few references to the borough elites. The Alderman (i.e. mayor) [Thomas Lacy[81]] was called on to

[79] This is the house which may have been a gildhall for some time, which may account for the involvement of Christopher Browne.

[80] The borough Hall Book shows quite clearly that the parishes had replaced the six wards of the Domesday Stamford, Stamford borough records, Stamford Town Hall, HB vol. i. For example, taxes were collected by parishes; searchers of the markets were appointed for the parishes, etc

[81] Stamford Town Hall records, HB i fol 84r

supervise the removal of the padlock from the gild pantry in the Hospital in 1507 (62); and he or Henry Lacey, a prominent councillor, deputy-steward for the town, who also served as steward on occasion for the Hospital, drew up the inventory of gild goods in the pantry, but both may have been engaged on behalf of the gild, not the Hospital. William Radclyffe, former Alderman and MP and founder of the town's grammar school, appears from time to time, entertaining Sir John Hussey and intervening with Lady Margaret Beaufort for the Hospital (38, 62, 73). Thomas Williams of St Martin's parish in Stamford Baron helped the Hospital accounts when Sheppey was ill. But that is all[82].

The crisis of 1517-18

The year 1517-18 was a crisis year for Browne's Hospital. As in Hamlet, all the leading characters are killed off and someone unknown comes in to sort out the mess, so Browne's Hospital experienced a wholesale change of personnel. The warden Robert Sheppey died; so too did John Taylor, *eminence gris* behind the Hospital for more than twenty years. So too did William Hawkyns, the elusive confrater, perhaps a stabilising force in this period of the Hospital's history; he seems to have died in 1516 (117v). Richard Dykelun and William Tylle took over as warden and confrater respectively; both were apparently Cambridge university men[83].

There may not have been a longer period of stability for the wardens, for ten years later (by 1526), Master Thomas Foster[84] [sic] the former rector of St Michael's church, dean of Stamford and auditor was named as warden, with *two* supporting clergy, Dom William Tealle and Dom William Higden as stipendiary priests. It is not clear how this occurred; perhaps Higden was the gild chaplain in the parish church of All Saints in the Market[85]; for the Hospital made its return to the clerical subsidy in this year under the parish church of All Saints, which

---

[82] One "goodman of the borough" is paid for some pointing done, 87v; I take 'goodman' here to be a surname. Robert Hans, fishmonger, town councillor and former Alderman of the borough, sold some thatch reed to the warden to be used at North Luffenham (5v), but Hans lived next door to the Hospital to the east, Alan Rogers (ed) 2003 *William Browne's Town: Stamford Hall Book 1465-92* p 53; for biography of Radclyffe, see Rogers, Parliamentary representation.

[83] For Dykelun, see note 20 above. One William Till, Tyll, was at Eton 1468-70 and King's College, Cambridge, 1470-72, Venn's *Alumni Cantabrigiensis* p 588; the Eton connection is important, for Thomas Stokes founder of the Hospital after William Browne had been at Eton and King's College; see Rogers, Eton's First 'Poor Scholar'. However, it is unlikely (but not impossible) for this Tylle to be the confrater, for he would have been aged about 64 when he became confrater and 81 when he died in 1535.

[84] Throughout the account book, he is Thomas Forster; he may be the Cambridge student 1505-9, Venn's *Alumni* sub nom, but Venn says this man died in 1518, while Thomas Forster was warden of Browne's Hospital in 1526.

[85] Salter *Clerical subsidy 1526* p 61; in the gild certificate of 1548, there was no separate chaplain for the gild; *Calendar of Patent Rolls* 1548-9 p 358. The Hospital income devoted to the clerical element in 1526 was £17 p.a., so the second chaplain received £5 p.a.

may have been the stratagem which enabled it to survive the closure of other Hospital-chantries in the attack on chantries. But three years later, 1529, John Muston appears as warden and remained warden until at least 1535. William Tille (Teyle) was confrater from 1518 until at least 1535. Thomas Colson and John Gilpyn were the Hospital's bailiffs in 1535[86]. Oh, for the second account book for the Hospital to tell the story of how it weathered the storms of the Tudor revolution. If it ever turns up in some remote archive, do let me know.

THE BOOK

We can now see the genesis of this account book. It was created by John Taylor in Stamford during and for the law suit against the gild, probably in November 1506 while Sharpe was in London (see Appendix VI). It was intended to be tabled in court but it was not retained among the court records; Sharpe took it back to Stamford. Thereafter, the book continued to be used by the wardens. On his return, Sharpe did not copy up his first two and half accounts, but his final account drawn up in October 1507 covering the year 1506-7 (including the two visits to London) is presented here. Subsequent wardens continued to use the book for the annual audit of their accounts.

The book is of 125 folios, 21½ cms wide and 31½ cms high. Two or more pages have fallen out between folios 104 and 105[87], so that the end of one account (1513-4) and the beginning of the next account (1514-5) are missing. Sheppey (and his accountants, for at times he was too ill to write up his own accounts) almost filled the book; his successor started on the final pages with notes towards an annual account. Two final pages have been lost but the last surviving page shows signs of having been exposed for a long time. The binding dates from the early eighteenth century when Richard Rawlinson owned the manuscript; it consists of the blank side of an early parchment.

The original folios were unnumbered; in the eighteenth century numbers in ink were added to every fifth folio. More recently pencil numbers have been added

---

86 LAO, BHS 7/12/29; *Valor Ecclesiaticus* vol iv p 142.

87 Dr. Bruce Barker-Benfield of the Bodleian Library has kindly supplied the following note concerning the manuscript's structure. He observes that the tight binding makes collation difficult, but suggests the following tentative analysis, disregarding the 18th-century flyleaves: "Quires I-III^{12} (fols. iv + 1-11, 12-23, 24-35), IV^{12+1} (fols. 36-7, 38b, 38a, 39-47, with a slip now foliated 38b added before 38a), V-VI^{4} (fols. 48-51, 52-5), VII-VIII^{14} (fols. 56-69, 70-83), IX^{8} (fols. 84-91), X^{6-1+1} (fols. 92a, 92b, 93-6, where the second leaf is cut out leaving an unfoliated stub, to which a smaller slip foliated 92b is now pasted), XI$^{8-1}$ (fols. 97-103, the 6th leaf mostly cut away leaving a large unfoliated stub after fol. 101), XII$^{24-2}$ (fols. 104-25, the 23rd and 24th leaves lost at end after fol. 125). Uncertainty is strongest at the proposed short quires at V-VI (evidently an area of anomaly) and the large final quire at XII. However, some support is provided by the watermark evidence, whereby leaves carrying the watermark (a hand surmounted by a star throughout) are conjoint with unwatermarked leaves, in folio format."

from 1 to 125. There are two inserted items; these have been given the numbers 38b and 92b (note that 38b does not come *after* 38 but after 37v and before 38; however 92b comes after 92, i.e. between 92v and 93). The first of these is a very small (but very important) note inserted by Taylor relating to Christopher Browne's distraint at Swayfield. The second was originally a loose sheet of paper which was tucked into the book for safe keeping and ended up between folios 92 and 93, where it is now fastened to a stub. This is a new rental of the Hospital property and can be dated to 1517; it is quoted on folio 125. I have therefore put a note in the transcript at folio 92 but included the text after folio 125; to have put the text in at folio 92-93 would antedate it by some seven years.

Language: The language is English with Latin for the headings and some of the more formal elements such as the audit. There is no French here; French seems rare in late medieval Stamford documents[88]. The Brownes and their circle were highly literate: Browne used a letter 'B' on his seal and merchant's mark, and he and his wife had mottoes in English. There are many inscriptions in the glass in the Hospital; there are long Latin epigraphs on the brasses of the Browne family and on the brass plaque in the Hospital. The Hospital circle assumed people could read. But the English of these accounts is highly variable in spelling, displaying signs of what has been called 'written orality', trying to cope with technical terms in the local dialect. Some words clearly defeated the wardens (see Glossary). Sheppey on occasion played with words; in the account for 1509-10 and again in 1511-12, he alternated the word 'the' and 'ye' in the entries recording weekly payments to the bedesmen and women - *'Item the xij dey'* is followed by *'Item ye xix dey'* and so on for the whole year (84-85, 96v-97v).

EDITORIAL CONVENTIONS

The Latin has been given as written with minimum extensions and put into italics; most items have been translated or summarised in an attached footnote, but common form Latin phrases which occur frequently are left untranslated to preserve the original format, with a footnote translation on the first occurrence. Some of the more common Latin phrases are included in the glossary. However, the Latin Narrative on folios 1-2 is here only in an English translation; a note directs the reader to the Latin text which has been printed in *Antiquaries Journal.*[89]

The English is given as written in the book. I have retained the 'y' (representing the thorn 'th') where it occurs. Some writers used the yogh **ȝ** frequently for 'y', 'g', z, even for 'w' or other consonant - frequently in 'gate' ('Pillsȝate'). I have

[88] But note an unusual French memorial slab to Henry Elyngton rector of St Paul's 1400, R Greenhill 1976 *Incised Slabs* ii pp 455-482.

[89] P A Newton 1966 William Brown's Hospital at Stamford: a note on its early history and the date of the buildings, *Antiquaries Journal* 46 pp 283-286.

transcribed this uniformly as 'y'. Sheppey uses the letter 'w' to mean 'w', 'u', or 'v' - thus 'Pwlwr' is 'Pulver'. The letters 'f' and (long) 's' are frequently mixed up, and the vowels 'a', 'e' and 'o' are sometimes used interchangeably. Where an obvious letter or part of a word has been omitted, this has been supplied, but normally where a word has been contracted, I have retained the symbol (e.g. *lokk*) since it not certain if the contraction is for a final 'e' or a final 's'. The abbreviated form of 'tenant' with a contraction could be either 'tennant' or 'tenaunt'; since there is one occasion when the form 'tennant' is written in full, I have adopted 'tennant' throughout. Capitals are particularly uncertain, especially 's' and 'w'; they are used without any rhyme or reason; an initial 'r' is usually in capital form. The gaps between words again is uncertain - e.g. 'a mercements', 'a batements', 'be fore' etc. Editorial interventions are in square brackets. Some explanatory notes have been added to ease the reader's access to the meaning of a particular word or phrase, but for most words that require explanation, please see the glossary. Where the meaning of a word, name or placename is uncertain or unknown, I have included it in the glossary and index but without a definition.

Formatting the text has proved difficult - the layout is often informal. Different groups of payments have been bracketed together in the original and sub-totals provided in many different places, above, below, in both margins, sometimes repeating the page total. Marginal notes or sub-totals have been included in the printed text at an appropriate point with a footnote to indicate the original location in either the right-hand or left-hand margin. Where marginal sub-totals occur through a continuous section, one footnote at the beginning indicates this. Sub-headings are as in the text but have been uniformly indented. An occasional line-space has been inserted to break up a long piece of text to ease the reader's task. In one case (the two London visits), I have added formatting - the first words of each new day have been emphasised so that each day can more easily be identified; in the original text, identification of each day is easier than in the printed version.

Deletions and insertions in the original text have been placed in round brackets with the abbreviation *ins* for 'insertion' or *del* for 'deletion' - e.g. "for iij (pownds *ins*) wax"; "vjs (vijs *del*)". Not every mark that looks like a deletion, erasure or correction has been included, since some appear to be blots made by wet ink. Again later marginal notes such as 'nota' have been omitted.

The annual accounts in the original do not start on a new page each time but run on. However, to make the changes clearer, I have started each annual account on a fresh page; and a date has been added to the top of each page to indicate which year the account relates to.

THE TEXT OF BODLEIAN LIBRARY, MS. RAWLINSON B.352

ACCOUNT BOOK FOR BROWNE'S HOSPITAL, STAMFORD, 1495 TO 1518

THE TEXT OF BODLEIAN LIBRARY, MS RAWLINSON B352

[In late 1506 (see Appendix VI), John Taylor, vicar of St Martin's church, Stamford, and former warden of Browne's Hospital, wrote this 'narrative' of the founding of the Hospital by William and Margaret Browne. It was intended for the law suit which the then warden, William Sharpe, was attending in London. The aim was to show that the gild of All Saints, Stamford, who had their gildhall in the Hospital, played no part in the foundation or subsequently and had no part in the administration of the Hospital estates.
It was written in Latin but since the text has been printed[40], I have only included a translation here]

fol 1

In eo qui est Alpha fit primum nostro intencionis
Et in eo qui est Omega fit finis nostro conclucionis
[41] *Amen*

Here follow certain things worth remembering (*memorata digna)* collected and recorded in the form following by Master John Taylor secular chaplain and Master of Arts who was at one time the second warden of this almshouse.

To the praise of the most holy and undivided Trinity Father and Son and Holy Spirit, of the glorious Virgin Mary and all the saints; And for the assurance (*certitudinem*) of those present and the perpetual memory of those to come, it is firmly committed to memory, That a certain right honourable (*prehonorabilis*) man named William Brown merchant of the staple of the town of Calais and of this town of Stamford, in his time the most pre-eminent (*prestantissimus*) comburgess, and his wife named Margaret Browne most closely joined (*coniunctissima*) with him in the same (*prefatam*) praise to God, erected from the foundations (*a fundamento*) [and] built this said almshouse (in a place called Cleymont, which place was before a most vile dung-pit) and other excellent works (*alia egregia*) which now are seen and will continue to be seen with the help of God, they both completed and perfected this building during their mortal lives in the year of Our Lord 1475, alternatively the fifteenth year of the reign of king Edward the fourth. In which year the same donor (*prelibatus*), that most humane of men (*vir humanissimus*) William Brown, from what had been given to him, appointed in this same almshouse out of devotion to God two priests, secular chaplains, to celebrate divine service and twelve paupers to be sheltered (*confortandos*) out of love for God, and during his whole life he sustained and maintained these priests and paupers at his own expense and costs. And since (as if it were unworthy) no-one was over him (*nullus sibi preerat*) in this almshouse during his life, he

[40] P A Newton, William Brown's Hospital at Stamford: a note on its early history and the date of the buildings, *Antiquaries Journal* vol 46 (1966) pp 283-86

[41] "In Him who is the Alpha is our first intention; And in Him who is the Omega may our final end be. Amen"

therefore gave the account which related to this house to no other person, and he set over this house no person other than himself to rule it in that time. But because the eternal spirit of life (*spiritus vite ineternum*) shall not remain in man, as he is flesh, the said William Brown was fulfilled (*expletis*) in the service of God for not a few years but yet as if broken by old age (*senio confractus*), went the way of all flesh; and that he rendered his spirit devotedly to God, those who then were present bore witness with pious lamentations, in the year of Our Lord 1489, on the 12th day of the month of April, dominical letter D. Not long after (and sorrow comes to him who resists the will of God) his said most devoted wife in the same year breathed her last breath of life on the 29th day of the month of October; on whose souls may God have mercy, Amen.

Moreover, in the second place, it is to be noted that after the death of the aforesaid William and Margaret by their will and common consent, a certain right honourable man of illustrious memory by name Thomas Stok (Master of Arts, secular chaplain, canon of the cathedral church of York, and rector of the church of Eston by Stawnford, of worthy memory and uterine brother of the said Margaret Brown) ruled this almshouse during his life worthily, and he sustained the priests in the charges of William Brown and Margaret his consort in this almshouse and the poor men there. Further, he placed this almshouse with all its appurtenances in mortmain, having petitioned and obtained a licence from the lord king Henry the seventh as appears by letters patent of the lord king in the tenth year of this king,

fol 1v

alternatively in fact anno Domini 1494. Into which same almshouse he instituted, admitted and inducted into real possession dom John Coton secular chaplain into the office of first warden in this house[42]. And also dom William Hawkyn secular chaplain into the office of first confrater in this house. Further the said Thomas Stok composed, established and duly promulgated certain statutes concerning the constitution, ordering and governance of this said house, the said warden and confrater and their successors; and he also set the number and arrangements of the twelve paupers of either sex in this house as appears more fully in his book of statutes.

However, since the said Thomas Stok during his lifetime (notwithstanding the admission of the said warden and confrater) reserved to himself full authority to compose (*condendi*), interpret, declare, correct the statutes and to see everything done which belongs to this almshouse, this by virtue as if principal and governor, he rendered no account of this house to anyone during his lifetime. But as the prophet said, 'Who is the man who lives and shall not see death?' Therefore like his other fathers, so this venerable man the said Thomas Stok duly paid (*persolvit*) the debt of the human condition, And from this miserable world departed to the Lord full of good works in the year of Our Lord 1495 and on the 23rd day of the month of October.

---

[42] Marginal note: 'John coton first warden'

After whose death the said John Coton actively executed his said office, namely warden in this almshouse, to pay, receive, administer, preside over, correct what needed to be corrected and did such other things that belong to his office in this almshouse from the feast of the Nativity of Our Lord in the said year and occupied this his office in this house for one whole year and a little more, because death snatches men unexpectedly: 'For that hour is not conceived when the son of man shall come'.

Therefore the said John Coton died, overtaken by Death in the year of Our Lord 1496[1497], on the tenth day of the month of January. And no other person during his lifetime was burdened to render account for his administration correctly.

After the said dom John Coton, John Taylor secular chaplain was elected, admitted and inducted into real possession of the office of warden in this almshouse in the year of Our Lord 1496[1497], on the 22nd day of January by the venerable and trustworthy man William Elmes patron and most worthy supervisor of this almshouse (as the statutes then required)[43].

Because truly as it is written in the book of the statutes of this house, each year in the month after the feast of St Michael the archangel, the warden of this house for the time being will render his faithful account of his administration; Therefore in exoneration of my conscience and also that the state of this house should be better and more fully known to the assurance of the living and as an example and perpetual memory to those to come; I the said John Taylor second warden of this almshouse, although unworthy, proceed to my account in this wise.

* * *

[Account for the year Michaelmas 1495-1496: Taylor copied up Coton's first account but it is clear that it was still incomplete, for Taylor himself made some of the payments and allowances]

Thys is the first accompt' off thys almos hows aftyr the deth off mastyr thomas stok fownder of the seyd hows ffor j holl yer, that is to sey from the fest

fol 2

[44]*de anno* R' R' *henr' vij xj*

off seynt myhell tharchangell in anno dni m° cccc° lxxxxv unto the seyd fest in the yer off owr lord god m° cccc° lxxxxvj°. Or ellys aftyr an other dat' ffrom the fest off seynt myhell tharchangell in the yer off the Reygne off kyng harry the vij the xj yer unto the fest off seynt myhell in the Reygn' of the sayd kyng the xij yer.

---

43 Marginal note: 'John Taylor the second warden'

44 'In the eleventh year of the reign of king Henry VII'

1495-1496

Recept'

In primis memorandum that my predecessor forsayd syr John Coton Receyvd off Mastyr Wyllam Elmes forsayd patron off thys almoshows ffor a stoor or a stok afor'hand' to hafe fo to pay in tyme off neede as hytt aperyth in the booke off payments wrytyng in the begynnyng with the hand off the seyd S' John Coton for thys present yer xx li

Summa Recept thys yer bysyde the Rent xx li

Item the Rentale off Robard beomond baylyff off j part off owr lyflode this yer as hytt aperyth by the booke off hys accompts thys yer extent to the summa off xxxvij li vs ijd ob
Item the Rentale off Bartylmew holm off Swafeld baylyff off the other part off owr lyflode for thys yer as hytt aperyth by the boke off hys accompts thys yer extent to the summa off xxiiij li viijs vd
Summ' total off the extent off owr lyflode thys yer lxj li xiijs vijd ob
Summ' total off my holl charg that is to say the stok and extent off owr lyflode thys yer lxxxj li xiijs vijd ob

Off thys summa I Jhon taylyor[45] ask off myn awdytors allowanc by thes parcells foloyng
In primis the seyd S' John Coton my predecessor hath payd ffor diverse chargs and payments to hymself, hys confrater S' Wyllam Hawkyn, to the beydmen and beydwomen off thys almoshows and other chargs as hytt aperyth by the boke off hys payment wrytyn with hys own hand thes parcells foloyng undyr thys form

Mensis Januarii

In primis payd to the beydmen the vij day	viijs[46]
Item payd to the seyd por'men the xiiij day	viijs
Item payd to the for seyd men the xxj day	viijs
Item payd to the por'men the xxviij day	viijs
ffebruarii	
Item payd to the por'men the iiij day	viijs
Item payd to the seyd por men the xj day	viijs
Item payd to the por men the xviij day	viijs
Item payd to the por men the xxviij day	viijs

[47]*Summa soluciones istius lateris* iij li iiijs
probatum est per me henricum Wykys

---

[45] Taylor is accounting for Coton's payments

[46] Each of the ten men and two women were receiving 8d per week instead of the 7d of the statutes; see Appendix III. Payments were usually made on Friday of each week.

[47] 'Total of payments on this page; proved by me Henry Wykes'. The audit note on each page is in the hand of Henry Wykes.

Folio 2 in John Taylor's distinctive hand: the end of the Narrative (first four lines); a statement about the sum of £20 received by the warden from Henry Wykes; and a copy by Taylor of the beginning of Coton's first account 1495-6, the receipts and the first payments to the bedesmen and women. The probate signature of Henry Wykes concludes the page (Bodleian Libraries, University of Oxford).

fol 2v

Adhuc de compoto Anni R' R' *henr' vij xj*

Mensis Marcii

Item payd the iiij day to the beydmen	viijs
Item payd to the por men the xj day	viijs
Item payd to the pormen the xviij day	viijs
Item payd to the pormen the xxv day	viijs
Item payd the moren after the anunciacion off owr lady to my ffelawe and me ffor owr quarter wag' afor servyd	iij li

Mensis Aprilis

Prima die Aprilis payd to the beydmen	viijs
Item payd to the beydmen the viij day	viijs
Item payd the xv day to the pormen	viijs
Item payd to the seyd beydmen the xxij day	viijs
Item payd to the pormen the xxix day	viijs

Mensis Maij

Item payd to the beydmen vj day	viijs
Item payd to the pormen the xiij day	viijs
Item payd to the beydmen the xx day	viijs
Item payd to the beydmen the xxvij day	viijs

Mensis Junij

Item payd the beydmen the iij day	viijs
Item payd the beydmen the x day	viijs
Item payd the beydmen the xvij day	viijs

[48]*Mortuus est Robartus Johnson huius domus compauper*

Item payd the beydmen the xxiiij day	vijs iiijd
Item payd the morn aftyr seynt John Baptyst day to my felaw and me ffor owr quarter afor servyd	iij li

Mensis Julij

Item payd to the beydmen the fyrst day	vijs iiijd

[49]*Intravit et admissus est Willielmus Hesull in numerum pauperum*

Item payd to the beydmen the viij day	viijs
Item payd to the beydmen the xv day	viijs
Item payd to the beydmen the xxij day	viijs
Item payd to the beydmen xxix day	viijs

Summa solucionis istius lateris xiiij li xiiijs viiijd
probatum est per me henricum Wykys

[48] death of Robert Johnson bedesman

[49] admission of William Hesull as bedesman

fol 3

Adhuc de compoto anni Regni Regis henrici vij xj

Mensis Augusti

Item payd to the beydmen the v day	viijs
Item payd to the beydmen the xij day	viijs
Item payd to the beydmen the xix day	viijs
Item payd the beydmen the xxvj day	viijs

Mensis Septembris

Item payd the ij day to the beydmen	viijs
Item payd the beydmen the ix day	viijs
Item payd the beydmen the xvj day	viijs
Item payd the beydmen the xxiij day	viijs
Item payd the beydmen the xxx day	viijs
Item payd the morn aftyr myhelmas day to my ffelaw and me ffo the quarter afor servyd	iij li
Summa	vj li xijs

Summa soluciones custodi et suo confratri			ix li
Summa soluciones pauperibus per manus custodis hoc anno	xv li	xs	viijd
Summa utriusque solucionis	xxiiij li	xs	viijd[50]

Her foloeth certen expens payd thys (yer *ins*) by the handys of the seyd S' John coton as hytt aperyth by hys book of hys wrytyng off thys yer

In primis payd for j vestment haloyng thatt cam ffrom eston[51]	iiijd
Item payd the xxix day off april to the person off seynt myhels in stawnford ffor j pencion annuall of thys almos hows accordying to the composicion of the same	vjs viijd
Item payd for a spruse cofer in the cowntynghows for to kepe in money	xxd

her foloeth dyverse allowance and payments maade by the ij baylyffs Robard beomond and bartylmew holm as hytt aperyth by the books off accompts off them boothe for thys yer

decayse allowyd to Robard beomond

[52]In primis ij tenements at Walkote j yer	xixs
Item at Wyrthorp j howse j yer	vjs viijd
Item j sklatpytt in Wyrthorp felds at Bulgate	vjs viijd
Item at eston owr ladys Rent assyse	ijs
Item at Staunford the hows next the vycar of all halos	xxs

---

[50] 'total of both payments'. This line has been squeezed into the text

[51] Easton on the Hill was the benefice of Thomas Stokes, the former patron of the Hospital.

[52] Decays and abatements are reductions in rents allowed temporarily for various reasons. Throughout the whole book, a marginal note *Walkot* has been added in a later hand against almost all entries mentioning Walcot; these have been omitted from this edition.

Item the hows next by hytt half j yer xs
decayse alloyd Bartylmew holm
Item j medo plott in Swafeld callyd hawkeyng xxd
Summa off dekays thys yer iij li vjs

Summa lateris x li vjs viijd
probatum est per me henricum Wykys

fol 3v

Ad huc de compoto Anni Regni Regis henr' vij xj
Chef Rents allowyd Robard Beomond in hys accompt
In primis the tenements in stawnford sum tym to the duke off york now to the kyng xxixs
Item the closs in Bredcroft to the kyng j li pepur pric' thys yer xviijd
Item the awngell in stawnford to the gyld off corpus Xti [Corpus Christi] of Stawnford xijd
Item the hows in seynt myhel parysch to seynt leyonards of stanford (for ij yer *ins*) vjs vjd
Item the hows at the malere brygg in all halo parysh to John Wyks ixd
Item the hows in seynt marten parysch by the water syde to gye thorney of carlby iijs
Item j hows in the seyd parysch next the chyrch to the abbey off peterboro iijd)
Item j hows in the seyd parysch on the same seyd [side] next byyend thatt)
to the abbey aforeseyd iiijd)
Item j garden in the seyd parysch toward the Nonnys [nuns] of stawnford)
chef [rent] to the seyd abbey ijd)
[53]Summa ixd

Item the ferm place at pyllysgat to the abbey off peterboro ixs iijd ob qa
Item j part off j closse in pyllysgate feld hyerd of gye thorney afor'seyd vd
Item the tenement off Warmyngton to boro abbey aforseyd iiijs
Item the same place payth to the scheryfsgeld off northamtonschyr vjd
Item the tenement in Bernak payd now to Master Vincent ixd

Item the ferm at northluffnam payth to thomas Basset iijs viijd)
Item the seyd place payth to lord sowch jd ob)
Item the seyd place payth to the prior off Brooke iijd ob)
Summa iiijs jd

Item the hows in Eston wher Bryan stokley dwellyth payd to the kyng xxd)
Item the same place payth to the charter hows in coventre ijs viijd)
Item the hows in Eston wher John Wrygt dwellyth payth to the kyng)
j li comyn and jd Summa iiijd)

[53] This and the following 'summa' are written in the right-hand margin against the items bracketed.

Item for the closse bylongyng to the seyd hows by indentur payth to the college of tatursale xvjd

Summa vjs[54]

chef Rents allowyd Bartylmew holm in hys accompt

In primis the maner off Swafeld payth to lord grey thys yer ls iiijd

Item the hows next the parsonage in northwith[am] payth to S' thomas delaland vs and ij capons Summa vs vjd

Item the tenement in barham payth to the kyng jd

Item the land of the same payth to the erle off Westmorland ob

Item the hows and land at Wylsthorp to lady eyland that I payd myself iijd

Summa off chef Rents thys yer v li xviijs iijd qa

Costys in kepyng off owr cowrts Swafeld and northwithom

In primis allowyd Bartylmew in hys accompt for (ij *ins*) cowrts at Swafeld ijs vijd ob

Item I John taylyor Warden allowyd Wyllam scherschaw off northwithom in hys Rent ffor ij cowrts kept at northwithom as hyt aperyth by the cowrt Rollys - fyrst for the cowrt kept aftyr myhelmes vjd

Item for the cowrt kept aftyr pasce xxiijd

Item payd to herry toky steward off owr cowrts for hys fee off thys yer xiijs iiijd

Summa in costs off cowrt xviijs iiijd ob

Summa lateris vj li xvjs vijd ob qa

probatum est per me H' Wykys

fol 4

Ad huc de compoto Anni Regni Regis henrici vij xj

Sewts mercyments[55] and fynys to dyverse lords

In primis allowyd Robard beomond in hys accompts for arrerages of mercyments att stretton ijs viijd

Item for the cowrt off the prior off brook at northluffnam mercyment at j cowrt iiijd

Item for j essoyn att j other cowrt of the same prior jd

Item for j fyne att the kyngs cowrt ther xijd

Item ffor j fyne at the kyngs cowrt at Eston vjd

Item ffor langdyk cowrt for ij yer mercyments ijs

Item allowyd bartylmew owr baylyff in hys accompts for lord greys cowrt at corby viijd

Item allowyd by the same accompts for the kyngs cowrt at stretton thys yer viijd

Summa off mercyments and arrerages vijs xjd

[54] markings indicate this total refers to the last four entries except John Wright's house

[55] amercements are fines imposed for breaches of manor customs; essoins are payments for permission to be excused

Item alloyd Robard beomond in hys accompts for j m[l] kydds from wolfhows to thys almoshows for the makyng off the seyd kydds vs xd
Item ffor cariag' of the same m[l] kydds to the almoshows xs

Payments by Robard beomond to the beydmen of thys hows
In primis the seyd Robard was allowyd in hys accownts ffor money payd to S' John Coton warden off thys hows j weke wages of the beydmen the fryday afor seynt andrew day vijs[56]
Item for the same cawse the fryday afor seynt nycolas day vijs
Item for the same cawse the fryday aftyr owr ladys day the concepcion vijs
Item for the same cawse the fryday next aftyr vijs
Item for the same cawse the fryday on cristmas evyn vijs
Summa off the payments xxxvs

Casuall costs for thys almoshows
In primis I John taylyor warden allowyd Wyllam scherschaw off northwithom in hys Rent thys yer as aperyth by a byll for costs at metyng with Master delaland at cristmas when S' Wyllam Hawkyn was ther with M elmes iijs vjd
Item Robard beomond is allowyd in hys accownts thes parcells foloyng ffor expens' att northwithom and stretton ffor Master elmes vd
Item expendyd at Beltons hows by the comawdment of S' John Coton warden ijd
Item payd to bartylmew holm for expens' rydyng to London for Swynhaw wode vjs viijd
Item payd to Wyllam ffreman for expens' Rydyng to London vjs viijd
Item for horse hyer v days xxd
Item for ij haly lovys for the ij howsys next the vycar off all halos vjd
Item for the halylofe for the barn in Skofgate ijd
Summa off casuall costs xixs ixd

Summa lateris iij li xviijs vjd
probatum est per me henricum Wykys

fol 4v

Adhuc de compoto Anni Regni Regis henrici vij xj
off thyngs bowgt for the stoor off thys almoshows
Item accowntyd by Robard beomond ffor iiij m[l] nayle bowgt at mydlent fayr ixs iiijd
Item payd to turton sawer for sawyng off leghys the xviij day off junii xjd
Summa off thyngs of stor off hows xs iijd

Reparacion in the almoshows it self payd by Robard beomond
In primis payd on whytsonday evyn ffor iij sem lyme spent at the almoshows ijs
Item the ij day off September payd for mendyng off glass wyndows xd

---

[56] This was at the statutory rate of 7d per week, not 8d; see Introduction.

Item the iij day of September payd to a plommar for sowderyng the leds of the chapell and other places ijs iiijd

Summa vs ijd

Reparacion in stawnford at the awngell by Robard beomonds accompts

Item payd to thomas wyng for caryag' off sklatt and sand to dyverse places vjs
Item to Robard hamulden ffor cariag' off j lode ston and j lode erth to the awngell vijd
Item payd to thomas gudale for vj days mason wark ther ijs vjd
Item to Robard yate for servyng the seyd mason v days and half xxijd

Summa xs xjd

Reparacion at the hows in seynt andrew parysch by Robard beomond the tennant beyng Robard grene

Item payd to thomas gudale ffor iiij days wark xxd
Item to hys server iiij days xvjd

Summa iijs

Reparacion at the hows in the pultre merkett next Bullok schop accowntyd by the seyd Robard beomond

Item payd on seynt andrew day to thomas gudale ij days mason werk xd
Item to hys servar Robard yates for ij days viijd
Item to the seyd mason for iij days wark xvd
Item to hys servar Robard yates for iij days xijd
Item j lode ston and j lode erth vijd
Item allowyd cramp that was the tennant for j lok iiijd
Item for clensyng off the drawgt sege xijd

Summa vs viijd

Reparacion at the hows in all halo parysch next the vycarag' except j hows that is to sey wher John sabyn dwelt By Robard Beomond

Item payd xxvij day off august to the seyd mason for iiij days xxd
Item to hys servar Robard yates for iiij days xvjd
Item to the seyd mason for x days wark iiijs ijd
Item to hys servar x days iijs iiijd
Item for ij lode ston and ij lode erth xiiijd
Item to Robard andrew off Ryall for ij lode stobull iijs
Item payd to ij women for havyng in the seyd stobull ijd ob

Summa xiiijs xd ob

Summa lateris xlixs xd ob
probatum est per me h Wykys

fol 5

Ad huc de compoto Anni Regni Regis henrici vij xj

Reparacion at the hows next the vycar off all halos and at the hows next malere bryg In Robard beomond' accowmpts

In primis ijC led nayles	iiijd ob
Item ij corbys ffor ij ledes	iijs viijd
Item jC led naylys	ijd ob
Item j plommer to mend the led ther and the led at malere brygg	viijd
Item payd to thomas gudale the mason ffor vij days werk ther and at the barn in skofgate and at the seyd hows at malere brygg	ijs xjd
Item hys servar Robard yates vij days	ijs iiijd
Item payd to John wrygt ffor ij days wark	xijd
Item payd to thomas fazyakurley for iiij lode erth	xijd
Item j payr bonds for j wyndow	jd ob
Item for caryag off j lode strawe	ijd
Item payd to kesten the thakkar for ij days and half thakkyng the hows next the swyncote	xjd ob
Item hys servar ij days and half	ixd
Item to Robard yates for syftyng off sande	iiijd
Item for iij lode erth and iij lode ston at the barn in Skofgate	xxjd
Item j lode ston and j lode erth to the hows at the malere brygg	vijd
Summa	xvjs xd

Reparacion at wyllam Bakers hows in seynt peter parisch. In Robard beomonds accownts

Item payd to thomas gudale the mason for viij days werk and half	iijs vjd ob
Item to Robard elys the mason iiij days werk and half	xxijd ob
Item Robard yates to serve them v days and half	xxijd
Item Robard Bryce mason v days wark at the oven	ijs jd
Item thomas gudale mason x days wark at the oven	iiijs ijd
Item Richard Uffyngton mason v days wark at the oven	ijs jd
Item Robard elys mason ix days wark at the oven	iijs ixd
Item Robard yates to serve them x days and half	iijs vjd
Item payd to Robard hamulden for cariag' off ij lode ston from eston to the seyd oven and ij lode erth and iiij lode cayle	xviijd
Item payd to syngar off Sowthorp for iij lode ston to the same oven	xijd
Item for ston that was bowgt for the seyd oven	xijd
Item for iij lode ston from eston	vjd
Item payd to syngar off Sowthorp for other iij lode ston	xjd
Item for plaster spent at the seyd hows	iiijd
Item j sem lyme spent ther at the seyd hows	viijd
Item to john wylson for sklattyng wark at the seyd hows	vd
Item to j wrygte ther and att the awngell	vd
Summa	xxixs vijd

Summa lateris xlvjs vd
probatum est per me henricum Wykys

fol 5v

Ad huc de compoto Anni Regni Regis Henrici vij xjo

Reparacion at stawnford and stretton by Robard beomonds accompts

Item x sem lyme spent at stretton by Robard whythed sklatter pric' vjs viijd
Item xij sem lyme spent at stawnford by the seyd Robard viijs
Item payd to the seyd Robard on cristmas evyn opon Rekonyng xxs
Item to john wrygte the yongar for v days wark at stretton ijs jd
Item for j bord that the seyd John Wrygt bowgt ther iijd
Summa xxxvijs

Reparacion at northluffnam by the seyd Robard beomonds accompts

Item the iiij day off februarii payd to Robard hans of staunfford for Reede spent ther xxd
Item skarboro the tennant was allowyd for Reparacions by a byll vijs iiijd ob
Summa ixs ob

Reparacion at eston and Wyrthorp by Robard beomonds accompts

Item payd to Robard kesten off Wyrthorp for thakkyng at geylys garrad hows and at fox hows the weyvar viij days and half iijs vjd ob
Item to hys servar howgh dawntre viij days and half ijs vjd
Item to Robard kesten for teryng off j florth in Bryans hows xd
Item to howgh dawntre hys servar vijd
Item payd to Rychard corby ffor iiij lode stobull spent at eston iiijs ijd
Item to John undyrwode ffor j lode stobull xvd
Item viij sem lyme that was spent at eston wyrthorp and stawnford vs iiijd
Item for the cariag' off the lyme that was spent at eston and wyrthorp xiiijd
Item to thomas cristofer for cariag' off j lode ston and j lode mortar to wyrthorp iiijd
Item to Rawlyn sklatter for j lode ston jd
Item payd to Bryan stokley for lath to the seyd teryng at eston ixd
Summa xxs vjd ob

Reparacion at Pylsgate by the seyd Robard beomonds accompts

In primis to thomas godale the mason for vij days wark and half ijs iijd ob
Item Robard Bryce the mason for x days wark ther iiijs ijd
[57] Item Ric' Uffyngton the mason x days iiijs ijd
Item Robard yates the servar x days iijs iiijd
Item for j boll and j skotyll to the same wark vd ob
Item to Robard kesten thakker for v days wark xxijd ob
Item hew dawntre hys servar iiij days xijd
Item the seyd thakkar ix days wark and half iijs vjd ob
Item John Baker ix days and half to serve hym ijs iiijd ob
Summa istius partis xxiijs ijd ob

Summa lateris iiij li ixs ixd ob
probatum est per me h Wykys

[57] This line inserted

fol 6

*Ad de eodem compoto Anni Regni Regis Henrici vij xj^o^*

At pylsgate *ut supra*

Item thomas gudale the mason iiij days wark and half	xxijd ob
Item pers laborer hys servar iiij days and half	xviijd
Item payd to Jhon Whypp for vj lode ston spent ther	xviijd
Item Robard Kesten x days wark	iijs ixd
Item wyllam Cristofer hys servar x days	ijs vjd
Item the seyd thakker v days wark	xxijd ob
Item wyllam hamulden hys servar v days	xvd
Item payd to the seyd wyllam for vj lode ston from Walcote pytts	iijs
Item for iiij lode ston from Eston pytts	xvjd
Item for viij lode erth	ijs
Item payd to herry okley for xx lode stobull	xxvjs viijd
Item for viij lode ston to the gavell of the same hows	xvjd
Item vij lode mortar to the same hows	xiiijd
Item half sem lyme to the same place	iiijd
Item for ij fre stonys for the same wark	ijd
Item j pece tymbur for the wark	iijd
Item for hedghyng off the closse perteygnyng to the former stuff and warkmansschypp	iijs iiijd
Summa istius part'	liijs xd
Summa total off Reparacion at pylsgate thys yer	iij li xvijs ob

Reparacion att stretton allowyd in the accompts off Bartylmew holm baylyff

In primis ffor cariag' off x sem lyme bord' and ledghys	ijs
Item for cariag' off iij lode sand	vjd
Item for wands to the kyln and making of the hyrdyls	ijs viijd
Item for iij pec' off tymbur to the barn dorrs	iiijd
Item for thakkyng off the hey barn	viijd
Item for stapulls and bands off yrn [iron]	ijd
Item for making off j wall in Skelyngtons entre	ijs viijd
Summa	ixs

Reparacion at carlby by the same accompts

Item John stanley the tennant is allowyd for Reparacion as hyt aperyth by hys byll	vijs
Item for other Reparacion that was Rekynd	ijs
Summa	ixs

Summa lateris iij li xjs xd
probatum est per me henricum Wykys

fol 6v

Ad huc de compoto Anni Regni Regis henrici vij xj *Et hic finis*

Item I John taylyor allowyd wyllam sclorry off Wylshorp in hys Rent thys yer for mendyng off off [sic] the grynde off yrn off hys barn dor jd ob
Item for j lode off ffen thak spent ther xvjd
Item I had ij horsys and j kow dystreynd for the rent and cowd nat sell hem to the valew therfor I ask for abatement of the pric' off j horse viijd
Item of the pric' off j other horse ijs viijd
Item of the pric' off j kowe xxd
Item of the pric' of the dong in the yarde xijd
Summa vijs vd ob

Item the seyd Robard beomond baylyff is allowyd ffor hys fee thys yer xxvjs viijd
Item the seyd bartylmew holm baylyff is allowyd for hys fee thys yer xvs xd
Summa off baylyfs fees thys yer xlijs vjd

Summa total off expensys thys yer that is to sey off payments to the warden and hys confrater/ for the beydmens wages/ other expenses/ decayse/ chef rents/ costs off cowrt mercyments and fynys/ payments/ casuall costs/ off thyngs bowgt ffor stor of hows/ Reparacions/ Allowance/ and baylyfs fees liiij li viijs iiijd qa

Summa superplusagii off the Rents thys yer is vij li vs iijd qa off the whych superplusag' s' herry wyk' vycar off all halos in stawnford owt to hafe for beyng auditor and supervisor off thys and off every accompts off thys almos hows for hys tyme accordyng to the statutes off thys almos hows iij li vjs viijd the whych summa off iij li vjs viijd the seyd s' John Coton fyrst warden my predecessor hath payd to the seyd s' harry Wyk' vycar as hyt aperyth by the booke off the payment of the seyd s' John coton afor' thys accowmpt was maade contrary to the statuts off thys hows for (it *ins*) schuld haf ben payd aftyr the accompt' maade all thyngs els allowyd[58]. And so ther Remaynyth off the superplusag' off Rents off thys yer ffor to encrese the forseyd stok off xx li ageynst the next accowmpt' iij li xviijs vijd qa And the summa off the stok Remaynyth styll xx li

Summa off the stok and superplusag' togedyr is xxiij li xviijs vijd qa
probatum est per me hen' Wykys

[58] For this statute provision, see Appendix III

fol 7
[1496-97. This account includes the last few months of Coton's wardenship and the accounts of John Taylor for remainder of the year]

de Anno Regni Regis henrici vij xij° Compotus secundus
Her foloeth the second accompt' off thys almos hows accowntyd and rekynd by the the [*sic*] seyde John taylyor second warden off thys hows ffor j holl yer that is to sey from the fest off seynt myhell tharchangell in the yer off owr lord god m^{l} cccc° lxxxxvj° unto the seyd fest [of] seynt myhell in the yer off owr lord god m^{l} cccc° lxxxxvij°. Or els aftyr another date ffrom the fest off seynt myhell tharchangell in the yer off the Regne off owr sofereygne lord kyng herry the vij the xij yer unto the seyd fest off seynt myhell in the yer off the Reynge off the seyd sofereynge lord the xiij yer.

In primis the seyd John taylyor chargeth hymself with the summa off the stok and superplusag' of the last accompt' as hytt aperyth in the fote off the seyd accompt xxiij li xviijs vijd qa
[59]Item he chargeth hymself with money Receyvyd off Bartylmew holm by byll indentyd ffor the sale off owr wood off Swynhaw vj li xixs viijd)
Item the seyd warden Receyvyd [o]ff wyllam scherschaw for wod of the same sale iijs)
Item off thomas grene baylyf to master delaland ffor wod of the same sale ijs vjd)
[60]vj li vs ijd
(Item Receyvyd for the Reversion off j strayd calf at Swafeld xijs *del*)
Summa total off the stok superplusag' and new Receyts xxxj li iijs ixd qa

Item the Rentale off Robard beomond baylyff off j part off owr lyflode thys yer as hytt aperyth by the book off hys accowmpt' thys yer extent to the summa off xxxvij li xvijs ixd ob
Item the Rentale off Bartylmew holm off Swafeld baylyff off the other part off owr lyflode for thys yer as hytt aperyth by the book off hys accompt' of thys yer extent to the summa off xxiiij li viijs vd
Item he is charged with hey thatt he sold at Wylsthorp thys yer vjs viijd
[61]Item for the reversion off a strayd calf at Swafeld xijd
Summa off the extent off owr lyflode thys yer lxij li xiijs xd ob
Summa total off both thes summa lxxxxiij li (xxjd ob qa *del*) xvijs vijd ob qa

Off thys grete summa I john taylyor ask allowance off my awdytors by thes parcels foloyng
In primis the seyd s' John coton my predecessor hath payd to hym self hys confrater and to the beydmen as hytt aperyth by the book off hys payment

[59] note in left-hand margin 'wode solde'

[60] sub-total in right-hand margin; the sub-total should read 'vij li vs ijd'

[61] line inserted

wrytyn with hys own' hand thes parcells foloyng undyr thys form

Mensis Octobris

In primis payd the beydmen the vij day viijs
Item payd the xiiij day viijs
Item payd to the beyd men the xxj day viijs
Item payd the same day for j li wax and making the tapurs on the awter[62] viijd
Item payd to the beyd men the xxviij day viijs

[63]*Summa soluciones istius lateris* xxxijs viijd
probatum est per me enricum Wykys

fol 7v

de compoto anni Regni Regis Henrici vij xij°

Mensis Novembris

Item payd the iiij day to the beydmen viijs
Item payd to the beydmen the xj day viijs
Item payd to the beydmen the xviij day viijs
Item payd to the beydmen the xxv day viijs

Mensis Decembris

Item payd to the beydmen the second day viijs
Item payd to the beydmen the ix day viijs
Item payd to the beydmen the xvj day viijs
Item payd to my felaw and me for owr quarter wag'
aforservyd (vjs viijd *del*) iij li
[64]Item payd to the beydmen the xxx day viijs

Mensis Januarii

Item payd to the beydmen by the hands off s' John coton the vj day viijs

Item memorand' that the x day off Januarii in the yer off owr lord god m[l] cccc° lxxxxvj° the forsayd fyrst warden off thys almos hows s' John coton departyd by naturall deth in thys almos hows owt of thys wrechyd world to the grete mercy off god. And therfor the xiij day off Januarii was payd to the beyd men for her wag' by the hands off s' harry wyk' then beeyng vycar off all halo chyrch viijs

Item payd to the beydmen by the seyd s' harry wyk' the xx day off Januarii viijs
Item memorandum that the xxij day off Januarii the yer off owr lord god abofe wryten Anno Dni m° cccc° lxxxxvj° the aforerehersyd Master John taylyor secular preest was lawfully admyttyd (off the Ryght wyrschypfull patron off thys almos hows, Mastyr Wyllam Elmes)[65] to be warden off thys almos howse And so

[62] despite the statutes, the warden is charging the Hospital for wax and tapers for the chapel; see Appendix III

[63] Total of payments of this page

[64] the payment due or made on 23 December is missing

[65] the parentheses are clear in the original text

the seyd John taylyor succedyd the seyd s' John Coton, unto the whych John taylyor was delyyverd [erasure] by the vycar aforseyd of that money that Remaynyd in s' John Cotons hands xiiijs viijd owt off the whych summe off money the seyd John taylyor warden payd to the por beydmen for her wag' fyrst aftyr hys admission the xxvij day of Januarii viijs

Mensis ffebruarii

Item payd to the beydmen the iij day viijs
Item payd to the beydmen the x day viijs
Item payd to the beydmen the xvij day viijs
Item payd to the beydmen the xxiiij day viijs

Summa solucionis istius lateris ix li viijs
Probatum est per me henricum Wykys

fol 8

De compoto Anni Regni regis Henrici vij xij°

Mensis Marcii

Item payd to the beydmen the iij day viijs
Item payd to the beydmen the x day viijs
Item payd to the beydmen the xvij day viijs
[66]*Mortuus est Richardus Sutton huius dom' paup'*
Item payd to the beydmen off thys almos hows the xxiiij day vijs iiijd
Item payd to the beydmen the last day off March vijs iiijd
Item payd to my confrater s' wyllam Hawkyn and myself owr quart' wag' iij li

Mensis Aprilis

[67]*Mortuus est henricus walch huius dom' pauper*
Item payd to the beyd men for her wag' the vij day of april vjs viijd
Item payd to the beydmen the xiiij day vjs viijd
[68]*Admissus est et intravit thomas Reynold huius dom' pauper*
Item payd to the beydmen the xxj day vijs iiijd
Item payd to the beydmen the xxviij day vijs iiijd

Mensis Maii

Item payd to the beydmen the v day vijs iiijd
Item payd to the beydmen the xij day vijs iiijd
Item payd to the beydmen the xix day vijs iiijd
Item payd to the beydmen the xxvj day vijs iiijd

Mensis Junii

Item payd to the beydmen the ij day vijs iiijd
Item payd to the beydmen the ix day vijs iiijd
Item payd to the beydmen the xvj day vijs iiijd

---

[66] death of Richard Sutton, bedesman

[67] death of Henry Walch

[68] admission of Thomas Reynolds as bedesman

Item payd to the beydmen the xxiij day vijs iiijd
Item payd to the beydmen the last day off Junii vijs iiijd
Item payd to my confrater s' wyllam hawkyn and to me owr quart' wag' iij li

Mensis Julii
Item payd to the beydmen the vij day vijs iiijd
Item payd to the beydmen the xiiij day vijs iiijd
Item payd to the beydmen the xxj day vijs iiijd
Item payd to the beydmen the xxviij day vijs iiijd

Mensis Augusti
Memorandum that for dekay off owr lyflode and other cawsys and charges the wag' off the beydmen and beydwomen was chawngyd and abatyd from *viijd* j weke to *vijd* a weke so to contynew

[69]*Et tunc admissus est Rychardus Bulkley in numerum pauperum huius dom'*

Item payd to the beydmen the iiij day off August vijs
Item payd to the beydmen the xj day off August vijs

Summa solucionis istius lateris xiiij li xvjs
Probatum est per me h' Wykys

fol 8v

Ad huc de compoto Anni Regni Regis Henrici vij xij

Item payd to the beydmen the xviij day off August vijs
Item payd to the beydmen the xxv day off August vijs

Mensis Septembris
Item payd to the beydmen the fyrst day vijs

[70]*Mortuus est Willielmus Blakborn huius dom' pauper*

Item payd to the beydmen the viij day vjs vd
Item payd to the beydmen the xv day vjs vd
Item payd to the beydmen the xxij day vjs vd
Item payd to the beydmen the xxix day vjs vd
Item payd to my confrater s' wyllam hawkyn and to myself owr quart' wag' iij li
Summa vli vjs viijd

[71]*Summa solucionis custodi et suo confratro* xij li
Summa solucionis pauperibus hoc anno xix li iijs iiijd

Her foloeth dyverse allowance and payments maad by the ij baylyfs Robard beomond and Bartylmew holm as hyt aperyth by the book off accompts off them both for thys yer

chef Rents allowyd to Robard beomond in hys accompt
In primis ffor owr tenements in stawnford to the kyng xxixs

---

[69] admission of Richard Bulkeley; this line inserted

[70] death of William Blakborn

[71] Total of payments to warden and confrater; total of payments to paupers this year

Item for the clossys in Bredcroft j li pepur pric' thys yer xvjd
Item for the awngell to corpus christi gylde xijd
Item the hows in seynt myhell parysch and in seynt Andrews to seynt leynards xijd
Item the hows at the malere brygg to John Wyks ixd
Item the hows by the watersyd in seynt marten parysch to gye thorney iijs
Item ij howsys with j garden in the same parysch to the abbeye off peturboro ixd
Item the ferm at pylsgate to peturboro ixs iijd ob qa
Item certen lond within a closse hyerd off gye thorney vd
Item the hows and land in Barnak to master vincent ixd
Item the hows in Warmyngton to the abbey off peturboro iiijs
Item the same hows to the scherefsgeld off northamton vjd
Item the ferm at northluffnam to thomas Bassett iijs viijd)
Item the same ferm to lord sowch jd ob) Summa iiijs jd
Item the same ferm to the prior off Brooke iijd ob)
Item owr tenements in eston to dyverse lords as hyt aperyth in last accowmpts vjs

chef Rents allowyd bartylmew holm

In primis percroft in Swafeld payth to s' thomas delaland xijd
Item tenement in barham to the kyng and the erl of westmorlond jd ob
Item the maner off swafeld to lord grey ls iiijd
Item the hows in northwithom next the parsonage to s' thomas delalaund vs vjd
Item I John taylyor payd for the seyd maner of Swafeld *vs* and for the hows in northwithom *vs* notwithstandyng Bartylmew was allowyd hyt by hys auditors for he payd hyt nott Summa xs
Item payd for chef Rent at Wylsthorp thys yer to my lady eylond iijd
Summa off chef Rents thys yer vj li (viijs xd *del*) (ixs jd *ins*) qa

Summa lateris xj li xvs ixd qa
Probatum est per me henricum Wykys

fol 9

Adhuc de compoto Anni Regni Regis henr' vij xij°

decayse Allowyd Robard Beomond

In primis the howse at mallere bryg in alhalo parysch j quarter vs
Item j howse at Wyrthorp j yer vjs viijd
Item j sklatt pytt in Wyrthorp felds at Bulgate vjs viijd
Item at eston owr ladys Rent assyse ijs
Item ij tenements at walcott with land j yer xixs
Item the barn and the yard in Skofgat j yer vjs
Item ij closys in bredcroft batyd the Rent thys yer iijs vjd

decays allowyd Bartylmew

Item j medo plott in Swafeld callyd Brodyng iiijs

Item j medo plott callyd Hollyng xxd
Item certen leys or Ryggs in the feld iijs
Item j cotag at northwithom that the taylior dwelt in j quarter xd
Item the tenement at Wylstorp to my charg' in the kay [decay] xxs vjd
Summa off decayse (lviijs iiijd *del*) iij li xviijs xd

Mercyments for sewts off cowrts allowyd Robard beomond
In primis at northluffnam at the prior of Brooke cowrt vijd
Item for j fyn at the kyngs cowrt ther xijd
Item for the cowrt at langdyk hundreth xijd

Mercyments allowyd Bartylmew
Item ffor lord greys cowrt at corby viijd
Item for the kyngs cowrt at stretton viijd
Item I payd for j essoyn at the kyngs lete at stawnford jd
Item ffor j essoyn at stretton jd
[72]Summa off mercyments iiijs jd

costs off owr cowrts northwithom and Swafeld
(In primis for horshyer to northwithom cowrt aftyr myhelmes iiijd *del*)
Item allowyd scherschawe for costs off cowrt at the same tyme ijs
Item for the cowrt at pasche *h[abe]o nil* ffor the tennants wer afor the kyngs commissionars for the kyngs ayde and so ther was no cowrt kept as hyt aperyth in the cowrt Rollys
Item for horshyer to the cowrt schuld haf ben the same tyme iiijd
Item expendyd ther opon the steward and myself and som tennants vjd
Item for horshyer to Swafeld cowrt at pasce iiijd
Item for costs of the cowrt ther as hyt aperyth by the cowrt Rollys xxiijd
Item payd to herry toky owr steward off owr cowrts for hys fee of thys yer xiijd iiijd
Item payd for parchment to wrygt in owr cowrt Rollys iiijd
Summa off costs off owr cowrt thys yer xviijs ixd

Summa lateris (iiij li xiiijd *del*) v li xxd
probatum est per me henricum Wykys

fol 9v

Ad huc de compoto Anni Regni Regis henr' vij xij

Payments to the kyngs ayde ffor owr lyflode
In primis allowyd Robard beomond in hys accowmpts for the lyflode in stawnford xxviijs xd ob
Item for pylsgate and Barnak ijs
Item for eston and wyrthorp xd ob
Item for northluffnam ijs

allowyd Bartylmew in hys accowmpts

[72] this total is in right hand margin

In primis for Swafeld vjs viijd
Item for northwithom ijs vijd
Item for Wolsthorp ijs ijd
I John taylyor payd thes prests[73] for the seyd ayde In primis
for northwithom vjs vjd
Item for stretton xiijd
Item for eston xvjd
Item for Swafeld at on tyme vjs vjd
Item for the same whan I was ther at the cowrt iijs iiijd
Item I allowyd fabyon of Swafeld for the same ayd iijs iiijd
Item wyllam sclorry the tennant of Wylsthorp was allowyd for
the same ayd ijs xd ob
Item I payd for hows and land in Barham xijd
Summa off the payment to the kyngs ayd iij li xjs jd ob

Casuall costs for thalmos hows allowyd Robard beomond
In primis expendyd at northwithom for the prior off launde horsmete iiijd
Item for salt fysch ther the same tyme iiijd
Item for horshyer to Stonton to M Brudnell[74] and expens' for
M delalands mater vd
Item for 1 stryk peys for M brudnells hors at stawnford for the
same mater iijd ob
Item for 1 galon off wyn and 1 quart' the same tyme to hym and
M delalaund xvd
Item for 1 pynt wyn to M brudnell the same tyme at master Elmys place jd ob
[75]Item for cherys the same tyme jd
Item for expens' to okham to know the stynt off the kyngs ayd for Rutland iiijd
Item for horsmete for 1 colt off wyllam sclors off Wylsthorp that
was dystreyned viijd
Item for the halylofe for the barn in Skofgate ijd
Summa (viijs *del*) iiijs

Item ffor makyng off j m[l] kydds at Wolfhows for the almos howse vs xd
Item payd for cariag' off the same to Robard grene of seynt Andrew parysch viijs
Summa xiijs xd

Summa lateris iiij li viijs xjd ob
Probatum est per me henricum Wykys

[73] MS torn

[74] Brudenell lived at Stonton Wyville, Leics, Ives *Common Lawyers* p 454

[75] the first seven items are bracketed together with the word 'Summa' but no total is given.

fol 10

Adhuc de compoto Anni Regni Regis henrici vij xij

Casuall costs payd by John taylyor warden

In primis payd to s' thomas forster parson off seynt myhels in stawnford for the pencion vjs viijd

Item I allowyd scherschaw in hys Rent of thys yer for expens' and costs at northwithom at the meetyng with master delaland for owr mater at pasce ijs

Item for horsmet and mans mete when I cam fyrst with master Elemes to master delaland for the mater off Swynawh [sic] woode ijs viijd

Item I payd to master Robard brudnels man for hys labors to me in the same mater the last day off Junii viijd

Item payd to thomas seyvell for hys costs Rydyng to master Elmes in owr erands and cawsys for the same mater for vj days *viijd* j day summa iiijs

Item for horshyer to northwithom the xviiij and xix day off Julii ffor owr cawsys with master delalawnd viijd

Item for horsmete the same tyme iiijd

Item I payd to Ardern master brudnells clark by the comawndment off master Elmes beying seke in the swetyng syknes for hys labors in wryttyng owr seyd maters off master delalaund xxij day off Julii vjs viijd

Item payd for j box and Red wax for master brudnell to cary owr byll indentyd off owr seyd matter bytwene master delalaund and us jd ob

Item payd for horshyer to northwithom to mete with master brudnell at northwithom for the same mater opon seynt bartylmew day and the moro after vjd

Item for costs off horsmet the same tyme viijd

Item I payd to george pendulbere servant to master delaland in hys mastyrs name for to fynysch owr maters bytwene hym and us awardyd by the prior of lawnd and master off Burton lazarus in Recompense of hys cost and chargs x li

Summa xj li iiijs xjd ob

Item in other cawsys by thes parcells In primis spent at Ryall at sygt off certen tymbur and bord bowgt off herry gervys ijd

Item I payd to skarboro son off northluffnam for tellyng me when the commissionarys schuld sytt at okham for sessyng off lyflode for the kyngs ayde in rutland ijd

Item I Rewardyd Bartylmew holm owr baylyff at hys fyrst payment that he payd to me by byl indentyd for the yer abofe wryten ijd

Item I payd for j sadylcloth to Ryde withall vjd

Item I expendyd at Swafeld in overseyng dyvers thyngs ther xij day off Maii viijd

Summa istius part' xxd

Summa lateris xj li vjs vijd ob

probatum est per me henricum Wykys

fol 10v

Ad huc de compoto Anni Regni Regis henrici vij xij

Item payd for the halylof ffor owr barn in Skofgate ijd
Item payd for papyr iijd ob
Item expendyd at Swafeld the xix day off Julii ijd
Item I gaf the masons that wrowgt at fabyons howse the same day jd
Item I payd for j lok and j key for the cofer with ij keys in the chapell vd
Item I expendyd att eston overseyng dyverse tenements xiiij day of august ijd
Item I expendyd goyng to barham and Wylsthorp the last day of august ijd
Item for horshyer to meyte Swynhaw woode the j day of september iiijd
Item I expendyd at northwithom opon me and the man that met [measured] the wod and opon thomas godale mason that Rode with me vjd
Item I gaf j Reward to the man that met the wod hys name was thomas aman by mesur it was xiij akers j Rode and half and xij poles large mett xijd
Item, I payd to the marbuler for the plate off laton that stands at the grese fote in the cloyster of thalmos hows with the gravyng bygynnyng thus *H nova structura* iijs iiijd
Item for expens' to carlby Wylsthorp and barham xxvj day of october iijd

Summa of thys part vjs xd ob

Summa total off casuall costs xj li xiijs vjd

Thyngs bowgt off Robard beomond for stor off the almoshows and allowyd hym in hys accompts

In primis ij lokks with j key for S' Wyllam Hawkyn chawmbyr dore xvjd
Item for x m[l] lath nayle at mydlent fayr ixs ijd
Item iiij m[l] smale spykyngs viijs
Item j dosen payr dor bands iijs
Item ij dosen payr and half wyndow bands ijs xd
Item j sadyll and j brydyll for stoor of thalmoshows iijs viijd
Item iij Rood' boord off herry Jarvys off Ryall xixs
Item of the seyd herry Jarvys certen tymbur pric' xxvjs iiijd
Item for cariag' off ij lode tymbur from thomas fazyakurleys hows iiijd
Item for cariag' off iiij lode fre ston to thalmos hows from the hows in cornstall viijd
Item for iij mortar bollys and hopyng off them iiijd
Item for ij syffys to syft sand ijd
Item for iiij m[l] clowt nayle vs iiijd

Summa iiij li ijd

Summa lateris iiij li vijs ob
Probatum est per me h Wykys

fol 11

Adhuc de compoto Anni Regni Regis henr' vij xij°

Reparacion at the Awngell allowyd Robard beomond in hys accompt

In primis payd to hew Douch for j lode sand	iiijd
Item to j tennant mendyng dyverse guttars	viijd
Item j sem lyme and half spent ther	xijd
Item undyrsettyng the hows whan the ostyy wall ffell down	vd
Item to thomas goodale the mason for x days wark	iijs ijd
Item wyllam scherwyn the mason iiij days wark	xxd
Item denys the mason v dais wark	ijs jd
Item to Robard yate for clensyng the grownd and servyng them xij days	iiijs
Item payd to Rychard cleyr for servyng thes masons vij days	ijs iiijd
Item j wrygt to mend the sygne off the awngell and j withdrawgt	iiijd
Item j skottyll	ijd
Item wyllam scherwyn the mason ij days and half	xijd ob
Item denys the mason ij days and half	xijd ob
Item to hew douch for x lode ston ffrom eston pytts	iijs iiijd
Item ij lode fyllyng ston	iiijd
Item xvj lode mortar erth	iiijs
Item payd to hew douch for caryag' away off xviij lode Ramell	ijs xd
Item j sem lyme spent ther	viijd
Item thomas godale the mason iiij days werk ther and (j half *ins*) in other places	xxijd ob
Item Robard yates hys server iiij days and half	xviijd
Item to John wrygt for mendyng the tavern dor	vd
Item for mendyng off j payr off jeamaws for the sam dor	jd
Item to hewgh douch ffor j lode ston	iiijd
Summa	xxxixs xjd ob

Reparacion at the hows in cornstall belongyng to the awngell allowyd Robard beomond in hys accowmpt of thys yer

In primis payd to Robard grene ffor xij lode mortar to the new wallys	iijs
Item payd to hym for caryag' off old tymbur from the seyd hows to the barn	iijd
Item payd to wyllam Edmund ffor ij lode sand for the sklatters ther	viijd
Item for hyer off j bockett for to draw watyr	iijd
Item payd to John cob mercer for ix sem lyme (and half *ins*) for the sklattyng	vjs iiijd
Summa	xs vijd

Summa lateris ls vjd ob
probatum est per me henricum wykys

fol 11v

Ad huc de compoto Anni Regni Regis henrici vij xij°

Reparacion of the hows in cornstall in seynt georges parysch bylongyng to the awngell maade by me John taylyor warden *Anno supradicto*

In primis payd to John wrygt for takyng down off the old Rofe	ijs ijd
Item ij laborers takyng down the old wallys iij days	ijs
Item to godale the mason v days werk	ijs vjd
Item ij laborrers v days werk	iijs iiijd
Item for j syff to syft sand and mortar	ijd
Item for j soo to ber in water	viiijd
Item to the mason iij days	xviiijd
Item ij laborers iij days	ijs
Item the mason vj days	iijs
Item ij laborrers vj days	iiijs
Item the mason iij days and half	xxjd
Item ij laborers iij days and half	ijs iiijd
Item the mason iiij days	ijs
Item ij laborers iiij days	ijs viijd
Item the mason ij days and half	xvd
Item ij laborrers ij days	xvjd
Item j laborer half j day	ijd
Item payd to John Smyth for vj lode mortar	xviijd
Item payd for tymbur to the seyd hows	iiijs viijd
Item payd to lylly the carpentar for settyng up the new Rofe	viijs
Itrem for cariag' of the seyd new Rofe	vjd
Item to the mason ij days furryng the govells	xijd
Item ij laborers ij days	xvjd
Item payd to John Smyth ffor [carriage?] off old tymbur and skaffold tymbur	ijd
Item payd to Robard Whytehed off eston the yonger for j lode of evys sklatt	vs
Item for the caryag' off the same from eston	iiijd
Item payd to the seyd Robard Whythed for hyllyng the sayd hows	xiiijs iiijd
Item payd off j lode sklatt from Bryans hows of eston	iiijd
Item for cariag' off iij lode sklatt from thalmos hows	vijd
Item j lode sand for the seyd wark	vd
Item j sklatter to mend Barnard Rychmans hows ageyn	xjd
Item half sem lyme to the same mendyng	iiijd
Item for cariag' away off the Rammell that was left	ijs vjd

Summa lateris iij li xiiijs ixd
probatum est per me henricum Wykys

fol 12

Ad huc de compoto Anni Regni Regis Henrici vij xij°

Reparacion at alys hosyers the hows next the vycarag' of all halos By Robard Beomond

In primis j lode sand iiijd
Item for caryag' awey off Ramell from her dor vjd
Item ij sem lyme and half spent ther xxd
Item j lode thornys for the hedgh in the garden viijd
Item for caryag off the seyd thornys vjd
Item for hedghyng off the seyd thornys iijd
Summa iijs xjd

Reparacion in dyverse places in stawnford By Robard beomonds accompts

Item for hokys stapulls lokks and keys at the hows next cleypoll schopp viiijd
Item for splentyng off j govell ther iijd
[76]Item for j lode erth ther iijd
Item for mendyng off j glasse wyndow at the hows in seynt myhell parysch xijd
Item payd to thomas godale the mason iij days and half pavyng at wyllam Baker xxjd
Item hys servar Robard Baro iij days and half xiiijd
Item payd to yardley for vj lode gravell for the same pavyng ijs
Summa vijs jd

Reparacion at eston and wyrthorp By Robard beomonds accowmpts

Item j lode sand to Bryans hows iiijd
Item hew dawntre for syftyng the seyd sand iijd
Item j lode stobull spent at Wyrthorp xviiijd
Item kesten the thakker with hys servar ij days and half xxd
Item j sem lyme and half spent at Bryans hows xijd
Item ffor cariag' of the seyd lyme to eston iijd
Item payd to john wrygte the elder for x days wark at eston and Wyrthorp iiijs ijd
Summa ixs ijd

Reparacion at thomas hondslows in seynt marten parysch by the seyd Robard beomonds accompts

Item payd to hew douch ffor j lode erth iijd)
Item to Robard kesten off Wyrthorp for j day and half teryng ther vijd ob)
[77][Summa] xd ob

Att netyltons hows in the same parysch By Robard beomond

Item to Robard yardley for cariag' off ij lode plaster and j lode tymbur from the almos hows to the seyd hows off netyltons vjd
Item to John wrygt the yongar for tymbur wark off j florth ijs vjd

---

[76] this line inserted

[77] right-hand margin

Item for j syff and j skotyll iiijd
Item to thomas godale for makyng off the plaster florthe iijs
Item to Robard yate hys servar ijs
Summa viiijs iiijd

Summa lateris xxixs iiijd ob
probatum est per me h wykys

fol 12v

Ad huc de compoto Anni Regni Regis henrici vij xij

Reparacion at Pylsgate by Robard beomond
Item for hoks and henghelis vijd) Summa
Item for ston to an oven vd) xijd

Reparacion at northluffnam by Robard beomond
Item for ston to an oven iiijs
Item for cariag' off the same ijs ijd
Item half sem lyme iiijd
Item j mason x days wark iiijs ijd
Summa xijs

Reparacion at Warmyngton in Robard beomonds accompt
Item for hedghyng and dychyng off j closse ther vs iiijd

Reparacion att Swafeld allowyd in Bartylmewys accompt at ffabyans kyln hows
In primis ij masons xij days wark *vd* j day summa xs)
Item j servar to them xij days *iijd* j day summa iijs)
Item for dyggyng off ston iij days *iij[d]* j day summa ixd)
Item j mason v Rode wark and half *xijd* j Rode summa vs vjd)
Item for fellyng off sparrs in northaw wod vjd)
Item for cariag' off iiij lode tymbur to the seyd hows iiijd)
Item for cariag' off the seyd sparrs iij lode vjd)
Item for wryght wark vs vijd) Summa
Item jC Reede iijs) xxxixs ixd
Item for cariag' of the seyd Reede xd)
Item for Redyng the seyd hows xvjd)
Item ij dos[en] thak Rope xvjd)
Item ij lode strey xxd)
Item for cariag' of the seyd strey iiijd)
Item j thakker v (vj *del*) days *vd* j day summa ijs jd)
Item servar vj days *iiijd* j day summa ijs)
Item j woman to draw thak vj days *ijd* j day summa xijd)

payments by myself
Item I John taylyor warden payd to the seyd wark In primis)
to the wryght vjs vjd)
Item for strey to the seyd hows allowyd fabyon xjs) xxs vd
Item for cariag' off mortar to the wallys (iij days *ins*) ijs vjd)
Item for cariag' off mortar erth to Rygg withall vs)
Summa iij li ijd

Summa lateris iij li xviijs vjd
probatum est per me h wykys

fol 13

Adhuc de compoto Anni Regni Regis Henrici vij xij

Reparacions at other plac' in Swafeld in Bartyllmews accompt'
Item j mason iij Rode and half at John holmes hows iijs vjd
Item for wrygt wark at the same hows vjd
Item ij wrrygts j day to mend Robard torpar' chawmbyr xd
Summa iiijs xd

Her foloeth certen Reparacions maade and payd by me John taylyor warden for thys yer abofwryten at John lynleys hows at northwithom
In primis iiij lode stray to thakk iiijs
Item for drayng off the seyd strey *ijd* j lode summa viijd
Item for cariag' of the seyd strey vjd
Item j thakkar iiij days and half *iiijd* [78] j day summa xxijd ob
Item hys servar iiij days and half *iiij[d]* j day xviijd
Summa ixs ob
Memorandum that off thys summa off *ixs ob* the seyd john lynley abates *ijs* at hys cost as he promysyd bysyd hys Rent thys yer and so the summa Remanyth cost to thys almos hows vijs ob

Reparacion of the chymney in the prests hall of the almos hows
In primis ffor wollyng Ropys for skaffoldyng ijd
Item half sem lyme iiijd
Item for makyng off the skaffold viijd
Item thomas godale the mason v days wark ijs vjd
Item j laborer ij days viijd
Summa iiijs iiijd
Item j lode erth to mend the wardens entre ijd
Item for temperyng off the seyd erth iiijd
Item for leyng off freston and cowchyng the seyd erth vjd
Summa xiijd

[78] error for '*vd*' per day

Reparacion of the entre dor ther

Item payd to John wrygt for hys labor	xvd
Item to the playsterer	xijd
Item for hespys stapuls and lathys	iijd
Summa	ijs vjd

Item payd to a plommar for sowderyng the leds off the chapell (xxv day *ins*) off January xijd

Reparacion of the cloyster wall toward the hyewey

Item di' [half] sem lyme	iiijd
Item thomas godale the mason ij days	xijd
Item ij laborers j day	viijd
Summa	ijs

Summa lateris xxijs ixd ob
probatum est per me henricum wykys

fol 13v

Adhuc de compoto Anni Regni Regis henrici vij xij°

Reparacion off the town wall at owr feld yate

In primis for ij laborers to avoyd the ston and erth vj days and half	vs
Item thomas godale the mason ffor bateryng off ston ij days and half	xvd
Item ij laborers ij days and half	xxd
Item the mason ij days and half	xvd
Item laborers iiij days and half	(ijs iijd *del*) iijs
Item the mason iiij days and half	ijs iijd
Item ij laborers v days werk	iijs iiijd[79]
Item the mason v days	ijs vjd
Item ij laborers j day	viijd
Item the mason j day	vjd
Item ij laborers rakyng and clensyng mortar that was left	viijd
Item the masons for mendyng the gresyngs of the town wall	iiijd
Summa	xxijs vd

Reparacion off the chymney at Robard grenes hows in seynt andrew parysch

Item j mason ij days werk	xijd
Item hys server ij days	viijd
Summa	xxd

Reparacion at the wallys at Bredcroft clossys

Item j mason iiij days werk	ijs
Item ij laborers iiij days	ijs viijd
Item j heng lok for the dor off the dofcot	ijd
Summa	iiijs xd

[79] deletion illegible between 'iijs' and 'iiijd'

Reparacion at Barham

Item for caryag' off iij lode ston from stawnford xviijd
Item for ij lode mortar erth iiijd
Item thomas godale the mason v days wark off j grondsell ijs vjd
Item hys servar v days xxd
Summa vjs

Reparacion att stretton

In primis x lode ston with the cariag' ffrom clypsam iijs iiijd
Item v lode mortar erth xd
Item mason makyng ther certen wark a grete vjs viijd
Item j carpenter for mendyng off j wyndow ijd
Item for thakkyng the barn viijd
Summa xjs

Item I payd to the mason aforeseyd thomas godale for hewyng off Clxxxiij koyns off ffreston for to haf in stor for beyldyng iijs ixd
Summa iijs ixd

Summa lateris xlixs viijd
probatum est per me h wykys

fol 14

Adhuc de compoto Anni Regni Regis henrici xij Et hic est finis istius compoti

Item Robard beomond baylyff is allowyd hys fee for thys yer for hys labor xxvjs viijd
Item the seyd bartylmew holm baylyff is allowyd hys fee thys yer xvs xd
Item the seyd bartylmew is allowd for hedghyng the wod off Swynhaw the tyme off the sale xviijs
Item the seyd bartylmew holm is pardond and for gevyn off hys arrerage off thys yer as hyt aperyth in the foote off hys accowmpt consideryng hys extrem poverte and so consequently lost to thys almos hows the summa off iij li xvijs xjd ob Besyde other grete lossys that thys hows had by the sale off the sayd wod off Swynhaw as hyt evidently aperyth in the fote off hys accompt - [80]*vide ibi si vis et nota pro ballivo*

Summa istius part' vj li xviijs vd ob

Summa total off expens' thys yer that is to say payments to the warden and hys confrater, to the beydmen and beydwomen, chef Rents, decayse, mercyments, costs off owr cowrts, payments to the kyngs ayde, casuall costs, of thyngs bowgt for stor off buyldyng, Reparacions, baylyffs fees, and other lossys amowntyth to lxxxv li ixd ob qa

Summa in superplusage off the Rents thys yer [81]*habeo nil et ideo nil vicaro omnium sanctorum*

---

[80] 'Look there if you wish and note for the bailiff' [probably Beomond who replaced Holm].

[81] 'of surplus, I have nothing and therefore nothing to the vicar of All Saints'

Hyt aperyth thatt the stok and superplusage off the last accompt and off new Recepts thys yer that schuld haf incresyd the stok is decayed xxij li vjs xjd qa

Summa that Remaynyth fynally at thys accompt is viij li xvjs xd
probatum est per me henricum Wykys

fol 14v
[Account of John Taylor for the year 1497-98]

de Anno Regni Regis henrici xvij xiij° *compotus tertius istius domus*

her foloeth the iij accompt' off the seyd john taylyor warden of thys almes hows ffor j holl yer that is to sey from the fest off seynt myhell the archawngell in the yer off owr lord god m[l]cccc[o] lxxxxvij[o] unto the seyd fest of seynt myhell in the yer off owr lord god m[l]cccc[o] lxxxxviij[o] Or els aftyr an other date ffrom the fest of seynt myhell in the xiij yer off kyng harry the vij unto the seyd fest off seynt myhell in the xiiij yer off the seyd kyng.

In primis the seyd John taylyor chargeth hym self with the summa off the stok Remaynyng fynally of the last accompt' as hyt aperyth in the fote off hys seyd last accompt' viij li xvjs xd

Item he accomptyth ffor schreddyng off aschys and welos at Bredcroft the wyche he had to hys own use thys yer vjs viijd

Summa off the old stok and new increse ix li iijs vjd

Item the Rentale off the charge off Robard beomond holl baylyff off owr lyflode thys yer as hyt aperyth by the boke off hys accompt' extent to the summa off lxij li ijs vd

Summa off the extent of owr Rents thys yer lxij li ijs vd

Summa total off the stok and owr Rents also to gedyr is lxxj li vs xjd

Off thys holl summa I the forsayd John taylyor discharge myself byfor myn awdytors deputyd by the statuts as now beyng m wyllam elmys patron off thys howse and s' harry wyk' vycar off the church off all halos in stawnford by thes parcels foloyng

In primis the seyd John taylyor haf payd to himself hys confrater to the beydmen and beydwomen off thys almos hows aftyr thys form foloyng

Mensis octobris

In primis payd to the beydmen and women for ther weks wag' the v day vjs vd

Item to the seyd beydmen the xiij day vjs vd

[82]*M[emorandum] quod xiiij die intravit et admissus est thomas Bentley in numerum pauperum istius domus elemosinarie*

Item payd to the beydmen the xx day vijs

Item payd to the beydmen the xxvij day vijs

Summa solucionis istius lateris xxvjs xd

Probatum est per me henricus wykys

[82] Thomas Bentley admitted on 14 October

fol 15

de compoto pro Anno Regni Regis henrici vij xiij

Mensis Novembris

Item payd to the beydmen the iij day	vijs
Item payd to the beydmen the x day	vijs
Item payd to the beydmen the xvij day	vijs
Item payd to the beydmen the xxiiij day	vijs

Mensis decembris

Item payd to the beydmen the fyrst day	vijs
Item payd to the beydmen the viij day	vijs
Item payd to the beydmen the xv day	vijs
Item payd to the beydmen the xxij day	vijs
Item payd to the beydmen the xxix day	vijs
Item payd to my confrater s' wyllam hawkyn and to myself owr quart' wag'	iij li

Mensis januarij

Item payd to the beydmen the vth day	vijs
Item payd to the beydmen the xij day	vijs
Item payd to the beydmen the xix day	vijs
Item payd to the beydmen the xxvj day	vijs

Mensis ffebruarij

Item payd to the beydmen the ij day	vijs
Item payd to the beydmen the ix day	vijs
Item payd to the beydmen the xvj day	vijs
Item payd to the beydmen the xxiij day	vijs

Mensis marcij

Item payd to the beydmen the ij day	vijs
Item payd to the beydmen the ix day	vijs
Item payd to the beydmen the xvj day	vijs
Item payd to the beydmen the xxiij day	vijs
Item payd to the beydmen the xxx day	vijs
Item payd to my confrater s' wyllam hawkyn and to myself owr quart' wag'	iij li

Mensis aprilis

Item payd to the beydmen the vj day	vijs
Item payd to the beydmen the xiij day	vijs
Item payd to the beydmen the xx day	vijs
Item payd to the beydmen the xxvij day	vijs

Summa lateris xv li vjs
Probatum per me henricum wykys

fol 15v

Adhuc de compoto pro Anno Regni Regis henrici vij xiij°

Mensis maij

Item payd to the beydmen the iiij day vijs
Item payd to the beyd men the xj day vijs
Item payd to the beydmen the xviij day vijs
Item payd to the beydmen the xxv day vijs

Mensis Junij

Item payd to the beydmen the fyrst day vijs
Item payd to the beydmen the viij day vijs
Item payd to the beydmen the xv day vijs
Item payd to the beydmen the xxij day vijs
Item payd to the beydmen the xxix day vijs
Item payd to my confrater and to myself owr quart' wag' iij li

Mensis Julij

Item payd to the beydmen the vj day vijs
Item payd to the beydmen the xiij day vijs
Item payd to the beydmen the xx day vijs

[83]*Expulsus est Ricardus Bulkley huius domus pauper per Johannem taylyor tunc custodem huius dom' pro certis suis defectibus incorrigibilibus factis per eiusdem Ricardum contra statuta et consuetudines laudabiles istius dom'*

Item payd to the beydmen the xxvij day vjs vd

Mensis Augusti

Item payd to the beydmen the iij day vjs vd
Item payd to the beydmen the x day vjs vd
Item payd to the beydmen the xvij day vjs vd
Item payd to the beydmen the xxiiij day vjs vd
Item payd to the beydmen the xxxj day vjs vd

Mensis Septembris

Item payd to the beydmen the vij day vjs vd
Item payd to the beydmen the xiiij day vjs vd
Item payd to the beydmen the xxj day vjs vd
Item payd to the beydmen the xxviij day vjs vd
Item payd to my confrater and to my self owr quart' wag' iij li

[84]*Summa soluc' custodi et suo confratri hoc Anno* xij li
Summa soluc' pauperibus hoc anno xvij li xvijs
Summa utriusque solucionis xxix li xvijs

Summa lateris xiij li viijs ijd
Probatum est per me henricum Wyk'

---

83 Richard Bulkeley expelled by John Taylor warden for incorrigible offences against the statutes

84 Payments to warden and confrater £12; payments to paupers this year £17 17s; total of both payments £29 17s

fol 16

Ad huc compoto pro Anno Regni Regis henrici vij xiij°

Anuall charges

In primis payd to the parson off seynt myhells in stawnford for hys pencion thys yer vjs viijd
Item for makyng off j m[l] kydds at wolfhows wod for the beydmen vs xd
Item for cariag' of the seyd kydds to the almos hows xs

Chef Rents off the holl lyflode to dyverse lords allowyd Robard beomond in his accompts

In primis for dyverse tenements in staunford to the kyng by yer xxixs
Item for the clossys in Bredcroft j li peper pric' thys yer xvjd
Item the hows at mallere Bryg to John Wyks ixd
Item hows off the awngell to corpus Xti gylde xijd
Item the hows in seynt myhell parysch to the place of seynt leonards vjd
Item j hows in seynt andew parysch to the same place vjd
Item the hows in seynt marten parysch by the watyrsyde iijs
Item ij howsys and j garden in the same parysch to the abbey off peturboro ixd
Item Bryans howse in eston to the kyng xxd)
Item the same place to the charterhows in coventre ijs viijd)
Item j closse off john wrygts hows hyerd of the college off tatursale xvjd)
Item the seyd john wrygts howse to the kyng jd and j li comyn summa iiijd)
summa vjs
Item the ferm off pylsgate to the abbey off Boro ixs ijd ob qa
Item land within a closse off the same ferm hyerd off gye thorney of carlby vd
Item the hows in barnek to master vincent ixd
Item the place in Warmyngton to the abbey off Boro iiijs
Item the same place to the scheryfsgeld off northamtonschyr vjd
Item the ferm off northluffnam to tomas Bassett iijs viijd)
Item the same place to (s' *del*) lord sowch jd ob) summa
Item the same place to the prior off Brooke iijd ob) iiijs jd
Item the maner off Swafeld to lord grey ls
Item the closse callyd percroft in Swafeld to s' thomas delaland xijd
Item the hows in northwithom next the parsonage to the seyd s' thomas vs
Item the hows in twyford to the seyd s' thomas xijd
Item the hows in Barham to the kyng jd
Item the seid hows to the erle of westmorlond ob
Item the place at wylsthorpe to my lady eyland j li comyn ijd
Summa off chef Rent' v li xixs jd qa

Summa lateris vij li xixd qa
Probatum est per me henricum Wykys

fol 16v

Ad huc de compoto pro Anno Regni Regis henrici vij xiiij°

Decayse thys yer by the accompt of Robard beomond

In primis j howse att mallere bryg' j yer	xxs
Item the hows next the vycarag' half j yer	xs
Item j hows at Wyrthorp j yer	vjs viijd
Item j sklatt pytt in the same feld j yer	vjs viijd
Item ij howsys at Walcott j yer	xixs
Item the barn in Skofgate	vs ijd
Item the hows at Wylsthorp	xvijs ijd
Item owr ladys Rent at eston	ijs
Item the hows in seynt marten parysch wherin Rychard bykerton dwellyd	xs
Item ij closys in bredcroft batyd the Rent thys yer	iijs vjd
Item toll hows in Swafeld	iijs
Item hallyng closse in Swafeld batyd the Rent	iiijd
Item the land in carlby abatyd ffor gye thorney	viijd
Summa of dekays	v li iiijs ijd

mercyments for sewts off dyverse cowrts

Item for the cowrt off Peturboro at Langdyk	xijd
Item for dyverse cowrts at northluffnam	xixd
Item for lord greys cowrt at corby	viijd
Item for the kyngs cowrt at stretton	vd
Item for Robard eylands cowrt at Wylstorp	iiijd
Summa	iiijs

costs off owr cowrts att Swafeld and northwithom

In primis for horshyr to myhelmes cowrt	iiijd
Item for costs of the cowrt the same tyme	xxjd
Item for horshyr to the cowrt aftyr pasce	iiijd
Item for costs of the cowrt the same tyme	ijs
Item for horshyr to northwithom cowrt aftyr myholmes	iiijd
Item for costs off cowrt the same tyme	xxd
Item for horshyr to the cowrt of northwithom after pasc'	iiijd
Item for costs off cowrt the same tyme	xjd
Item payd to herry tokey owr steward for kepyng thes cowrts	xiijs iiijd
Summa off costs off cowrt	xxjs

Summa lateris vj li ixs ijd
Probatum est per me henricum Wyk'

fol 17

Adhuc de compoto pro A° Regni Regis henrici vij xiij°

Casuall cost' and charg'

In primis for horshyr to Swafeld to spek with Bartylmew holm	iiijd
Item j Reward to Richard Whytwyll to Ryde with me	vjd
Item I expendyd ther on hym and me	ijd

Item for horshyr to Wylsthorp to ask rent iiijd
Item for horshyr to Wylsthorp the xvij day of Januarij ijd
Item for fodyr for wyllam sclors catell thatt was dystreynyd iiijd
Item I expended at Wylsthorp opon me and thomas Reynold iiijd
Item payd to John Smyth for lodyng sclors cart a stress from Wylsthorp to stawnford vjd
Item for settyng off lxxx setts off welos at Bredcroft viijd
Item for tyeth off the seyd welos and schredyng of aschys viijd
Item for horshyer to Swafeld the xvj day off April iiijd
Item expendyd ther opon Robard beomond and me jd
Item I payd toward the kyngs xv in helpyng owr tennants off Swaffeld they nat to haf hytt off in dewete bott off benyvolence[85] vjs viijd
[86]Item I expendyd at carlby to know whan the cowrt schold be ther ijd
Item I payd to master brudenells man for j Reward toward hys costs when he browgt the indentyr of owr mater[87] with m dalalaund in parchment ix day of maij iiijd
Item for horshyer to Ryde with Robard Beomond to gyff hym autorite in hys offyce off baylywyk[88] the xij day off maij iiijd
Item expendyd the same day in dyverse places iijd
Item ffor horshyer to Wylsthorp to overse the Reparacion ijd
Item for horshyre to pay werkmen at Wylsthorp xxiij day off Junij ijd
Item expendyd ther opon the werkmen my hors and my self ijd
Item for horshyre to northluffnam ijd
Item for haloyng off owr chales vjd
Item for makyng off the same at london [*blank*]
Item for horshyr to latt m dalalaund see the indenture in parchment xxij day of august iiijd
Item I expendyd opon the masons wyrkyng at Swafeld the same day jd
Item for clensyng the comen sewar at wyllam Bakers vjd
Item for horshyre to seale the indenture off m delalaunds mater the xix day of september iiijd
Item for Red wax for the same sealyng ob

Summa off casuall costs xiiijs vijd ob

Summa lateris xiiijs vijd ob
Probatum est per me henricus Wykys

[85] the tax granted to the king by parliament at the rate of one fifteenth; Taylor paid the tax as a 'benevolence' and it was not to be a precedent

[86] marginal note 'fifteen dayes'

[87] Delalaund gave to the Hospital property in south Lincolnshire in return for his family being added to the bederoll of the Hospital; see Appendix III

[88] Beomond took over from Bartholomew Holm as bailiff in south Lincolnshire as well as in Stamford and south of the river Welland; Taylor shows him to the tenants.

fol 17v

Ad huc de compoto pro anno Regni Regis henrici vij xiiij°

ffor the stor off the almoshows bowyt by john taylyor warden
In primis for henglok' hespys and stapulls xd
Item ij yern [iron] Rakys vjd
Item for makyng off j bar jd
Item for cariag' off iij lode sklatt from the dofcote in Bredcroft xd
Item for sawyng off legyhys and evys bord xxd
Item for Reede for akyrlonds hows in stretton vijd
Item j dos[en] skaffold hyrdyls iijs iiijd
Summa vijs xd

ffor the stor off the almoshows by Robard beomonds accowmpt'
Item iij lode playster pric' the lode *ijs iiijd* Summa vijs
Item at mydlent fayr for j dos' lokks iijs
Summa xs

Reparacion at the new closse in exchawng with master delalaund
In primis payd to mylys toppar in ernest off hys bargeyn off dychyng jd
Item to the seyd mylys ffor hedghyng and dykyng the seyd closse conteynyng in lenghte Cij Rode by scherschaws seyng payd by scherschaw xxxjs
Item I payd the seyd mylys ffor hedghyng and dykyng off the same vjs viijd
Item for fellyng xxij lods thornys to the same hedghe xxijd
Item for cariag' of the seyd thornys *ijd* j lode iijs viijd
Item for fellyng staks and edyryng vj lode *ijd* j lode ijs
Item fellyng viij lods thornys to save the spryng from cattel viijd
Item for caryyng the seyd thornys xvjd
Item for leyng the seyd thornys in the dych viijd
Item scherschaw was allowyd for destroyng off hys closse when the sale wod off swynhaw was caryd thoro hytt ijs
Item for horshyr to northwithom to mete the seyd dych and aftyr my mesur hytt conteynyd in lenghth lxxxxxij [sic] Rode ut supra xx day off Junij iiijd
Item expendyd opon Robard beomond that Rode with me and opon my self than ijd
Summa ls vd

Reparacion at almoshows and wyllam Bakers hows by Robard beomond
In primis j plommar for schotyng iij webbys of led and leyng j gutter at s' wyllam hawkyn chymney iiijs vd
Item to the plommar for sowderyng leds of the chapel and leyng a gutter at wyllam Bakers chymney iiijs viijd
Item for j lok with ij keys to the wardens garden dor and hys confraters vjd
Item to John Wrygt for mendyng the stepull of thalmoshows ijd ob
Summa ixs ixd ob

Summa lateris iij li xviijs ob
Probatum est per me henricum Wykys

fol 18

Ad huc de compoto pro Anno Regni Regis henrici vij xiij°

Reparacion at Wylsthorp maade and payd by me John taylyor warden
Imprimis for j lode sklatt to the dofcote ijs vjd
Item for cariag'of the same from eston to stawnford iiijd
Item for cariag' off lyme and sand and part of the seyd sklatt to Wylsthorp viijd
Item payd to j sklatter mendyng the seyd dofcote ixd
Item for j lok to the dofcote dor ijd
Item to the kyngs xv ffor the hows and land the tyme off dekey xijd
Item j lode off fen thakk xvjd
Item v lode strey vs
Item j thakkar v days and half *iiijd ob* j day Summa ijs ob qa
Item j servar v days and half *iijd ob* j day Summa xixd qa
Item for drawyng off iiijC thak and half *ijd* jC Summa ixd
Item half dosen thak Rope vd
Item j spar to ley undyr the evys off the stabull jd
Item for the halylofe for the same hows in the tyme off the dekay jd
Item ij lode whete strey ijs
Item vij bonds thak Rope vjd
Item vj schevys Reede ijd
Item j thakkar ix days *vjd* j day Summa iiijs vjd
Item hys servar ix days *iiijd* j day Summa iijs
Item j laborer ix days *iiijd* j day Summa iijs
Item for caryag' off water ix days *iiijd* j day Summa iijs
Item for hyer off j scledd and j tub and horsehyer to drawe hyt xxd
Item for drawyng off xiijC thakk *ijd* jC summa ijs iijd
Item x lode erth to Rygg with all *jd* j lode summa xd
Item for cariag' off tymbur and bord ffor the barn dor ijd
Item for j grynd off yrn to the barn dor ijd
Item ij lode fen thakk ijs viijd
Item j Reward to thomas Johnson for overseyng off thys Reparacion and porveying off all thys stuff xijd
Summa xljs xd

Summa lateris xljs xd
Probatum est per me henricum Wykys

fol 18v

Ad huc de compoto pro A° Regni Regis henrici vij xiij°

Reparacion at dyverse tenement' in stawnford and pylesyate by Robard beomond
Item for wryyt wark at wyllam Bakers Robard Baros at pylsyate john thomas howse and the almoshows xijs vd
Item for wrygt wark abowt wyllam Bakers well ij days xd
Item j lode sclatt ijs vjd
Item ffor cariag' of the same to pylsyate vjd

Item ffor the halylofe for the barn in skofgatte ijd

Summa xvjs vd

Reparacion at stretton by Robard beomonds accowmpts

Item vj lode strey ffor thakkyng vijs viijd
Item j thakker iiij days ijs
Item iij servars and laborers iiij days iiijs iiijd
Item for watyll wand ijs
Item j wattyller ij days xd
Item j schredder ij days xd
Item v lode mortar to Rygg withall vijd
Item for thak Rope jd
Item for wythwand jd

Summa xviijs vd

Reparacion of the hows next the parsonage in northwithom by Robard beomond

Item v lode thakk vs
Item j thakker vj days and half iijs
Item j servar to hym vij days and half *iiijd* j day Summa ijs vjd
Item iiij lode erth to Rygg withall vjd

Summa xjs

Reparacion at Swafeld in dyverse places per R Beomond

Item for ledyng off ston and mortar to the lytyll howse in John holms howse and to the kyln hows iij days wark and half xd j day summa ijs xjd
Item payd for half j dosen thak Rop for holdernes hows iiijd ob
Item iij lode thakk to holdernes hows and John elyns iiijs ixd ob
Item to Christofer wrygt for ij days werk and half at the seyd howsys ijs viijd
Item to wympeny the mason for j wall makyng att fabyons and att stroxtons hows vjs iiijd

Summa xvijs jd

Summa lateris iij li ijs xjd
Probatum est per me henricum Wyks

fol 19

Ad huc de compoto pro Anno Regni Regis henr' vij xiij°

Reparacion at swafeld at Robard toppars hows by Robard beomond

In primis lx sparr' for the seyd hows viijs
Item ijC rede and xl schevys and labor abowt hys iiijs viijd
Item for cariag' off iiij lode sparrs from the wod xvjd
Item for caryag' off iij lode sparrs to the water and hom ageyn ijs
Item for cariag' off ij lode Rede from the fen xxd
Item j m[l] ffen thakk and j mans labor to bye hytt vjs xd
Item j lode fen thak xiiijd ob
Item for cariag' off ix lode fen thak ffrom the fen vijs vjd
Item j lode fen thak bowrt off thomas stroxton ijs

Item ij lode barly straw ijs
Item ij lode stobull iijs iiijd
Item ij dosen Bastyn Rope xviijd
Item for takyng down the hows and clensyng the grownd to the masons x days vs
Item for dyggyng and cariag' off Clxvij lode ston and mortar xxxjs ijd
Item for watelyng the seyd hows xxd
Item j warkman makyng an erth govell xijd
Item for fellyng splynts and cariag' off the same vjd
Item clensyng the grownd bytwyx the dors iijd
Item to wympeny the mason for xxvij Rode and half mason wark xxxjs viijd
Item to Christofer wrygt for makyng the seyd hows j gret' xxijs iiijd
Item to the thakkar v days and half ijs iijd ob
Item the same thakkar iij days and half xvijd ob
Item ij laborers beme fyllyng choppyng thak and servyng the thakkar vjs ixd
Summa vij li vjs jd ob

Reparacion at the crane in stawnford maad by the tennant John Golyn[89] and allowyd by me john taylyor warden in the accowmpts of the seyd Robard beomond

In primis for clensyng the hall aftyr hyt was beyldyd xijd
Item for fowyng and hafyng awey the ramell in the cowrt aftyr the sklatters had don ijs
Item for caryag' awey off the Ramell of ij hogstyes in the lytyll garden xxd
Item for clensyng off a sege in the seyd garden viijd
Item for makyng of j thakkyd hows over the sege ther xs
[90]*Summa istius part'* xvs iiijd

Summa lateris viij li xvijd ob
Probatum est per me h Wykys

fol 19v

Ad huc de compoto pro Anno Regni Regis henrici vij xiij° *Et hic est finis Reparacion ut supra de eodam*

Item for clensyng the seage in the hye chawmbyr viijd
Item forr caryyng awey the Ramell that was left in the garden aftyr the sklattyng off the chawmbyr xijd
Item for clensyng off the well viijd
Item for tymbur wark abowyt the seyd well xijd
Item for pytchyng off the water guttar from the well into the land xxd
Item for pavyng off the cowrt ijs
Item for sand and gravell with the caryag' to the same pavyng xxd
Item for makyng off j herth in the long kechyn ijs

[89] John Goylyn was also keeper of the Bulle inn in 1488, HB I 45

[90] this part of this major repair to the Crane inn was totalled; the repair continues on the next page.

Item for makyng and mendyng ij Rakks in the stabull viijd
Item for mendyng off ij mangers in the seyd stabull vjd
Item for makyng off j capon pen in the cowrt viijd
Item for makyng a peyntes over the seyd pen iijs iiijd
Item for mendyng the herth in the grete chymney aftyr brenyng [burning] off the playster ffor the beydhows viijd
Item for makyng off j schopp within the parlowr xs
Item for naylys to the same makyng xxd
Item for leyng in off j grownsyll at the grete gate toward the strete vjd
Item for lokks and haspys viijd

Summa istius part' xxixs iiijd

Summa total of thys Reparacion is xliiijs viijd off thys summa the seyd john golyn is allowyd be the advyse off john taylyor warden and s' herry wyks vycar off all halos in the presence off Robard beomond baylyff and to hys dysyarg [discharge] xls
Item the seyd Robard beomond is allowyd for hys fee thys yer xls
Item he is allowyd for j gown (thys *del*) ffor thes iij yers past vs

Summa lateris iij li ixs viijd

Summa total off payments to the warden hys confrater, the beydmen and women, chef rents, annuall chargs, decayse, mercyments, costs off cowrts, casuall costs, off thyngs bowgt for stor off howse, Reparacions and baylyffs fee lxiiij li (xvjs *ins*) (vjs *del*) iijd ob qa

Summa in superplusage off owr Rents thys yer *habeo nil et ideo nil vicario omnium sanctorum* etc
Summa finalis Remaynyng off the stok vj li ixs vijd qa
Probatum est per me h Wyks

fol 20

[Account of John Taylor for the year 1498-99]

de Anno Regni Regis henrici vij xiiij°   compotus quartus

her foloeth the iiijth accowmpt' off thys state off thys Almoshows accowntyd and Rekynd by the seyd John taylyor second custode othyr wyse callyd warden off thys seyd hows ffor j holl yer that is to sey from the fest off seynt myhell tharchawngell in the yer off owr lord god m^l^ cccc° lxxxxviij° unto the seyd fest off seynt myhell in the yer of owr lord god m^l^ cccc° lxxxxix° Or els aftyr an other dat' ffrom the fest off seynt myhell in the yer off the Reygne off kyng herry the vijth the xiiijth yer unto the fest off seynt myhell in the yer off the Reygne off the seyd kyng the xvth yer

In primis the seyd john taylyor warden chargeth hymself with the summa off the stok Remaynyng in the foote off hys last accownt as hyte aperyth vj li ixs vijd qa
Item he chargeth hym self for certen wod that hym self had to bren owt off the wode off swynhaw iijs iiijd
Summa off the stok now is vj li xijs xjd qa

Item he chargeth hym self with the charge off the Rentale off Robard beomond holl baylyff off the lyflode off thys hows as hyt aperyth by the boke off hys accompts of thys yer the extent is lxij li ijs vd
Summa off both charges to gedyr is lxviij li xvs iiijd qa

Off thys summa the seyd John taylyor asketh allowance for certen payments as hyt aperyth by thes parcells foloyng

Mensis Octobris

[91] *Admissus fuit et intravit willelmus Bacon in numerum pauperum istius dom'*

In primis payd to the beydmen for j weks wag' the vth day vijs
Item payd to the beydmen the xij day vijs
Item payd to the beydmen the xix day vijs
Item payd to the beydmen the xxvj day vijs

Mensis Novembris

Item payd to the beydmen the ij day vijs
Item payd to the beydmen the ix day vijs
Item payd to the beydmen the xvj day vijs
Item payd to the beydmen the xxiij day vijs
Item payd to the beydmen the xxx day vijs

Summa lateris iij li iijs
Probatum est per me henricum Wykys

[91] admission of William Bacon

fol 20v

de compoto pro Anno Regis Regni henrici vij xiiij compotus 4o

Mensis decembris

Item payd to the beydmen the vij day vijs
Item payd to the beydmen the xiiij day vijs
Item payd the beydmen the xxj day vijs
Item payd the beydmen the xxviiij day vijs
Item payd to my confrater s' wyllam and to myself owr quart' wags' iij li

Mensis Januarii

Item payd to the beydmen the iiijth day vijs
Item payd to the beydmen the xj day vijs

[92]*Mortuus est thomas Brygg huius dom' pauper*

Item payd to the beydmen the xviij day vjs vd

Item payd to the beydmen the xxv day vjs vd

Mensis ffebruarii

Item payd to the beydmen the fyrst day vjs vd
Item payd to the beydmen the viij day vjs vd
Item payd to the beydmen the xv day vjs vd
Item payd to the beydmen the xxij day vjs vd

Mensis marcius

Item payd to the beydmen the fyrst day vjs vd
Item payd to the beydmen the viij day vjs vd
Item payd to the beydmen the xv day vjs vd
Item payd to the beydmen the xxij day vjs vd
Item payd to the beydmen the xxix day vjs vd
Item payd to my confrater and to myself owr quart' wag iij li

Mensis Aprilis

Item payd to the beydmen the vth day vjs vd
Item payd to the beydmen the xij day vjs vd
Item payd to the beydmen the xix day vjs vd
Item payd to the beydmen the xxvj day vjs vd

Mensis Maii

Item payd to the beydmen the iij day vjs vd
Item payd to the beydmen the x day vjs vd
Item payd to the beydmen the xvij day vjs vd
Item payd to the beydmen the xxiiij day vjs vd
Item payd to the beydmen the xxxj day vjs vd

Summa lateris xiiij li xs iiijd
Probatum est per me henricum Wykys

---

[92] death of Thomas Brygg

fol 21

De compoto pro anno Regni Regis henr' vij xiiij° *Compotus quartus*

mensis Junius

Item payd to the beydmen the vij day vjs vd
Item payd to the beydmen the xiiij day vjs vd
Item payd to the beydmen the xxj day vjs vd
Item payd to the beydmen the xxviiij day vjs vd
Item payd to myself and my confrater owr quart' wag' iij li

mensis Julii

Item payd to the beydmen the v day vjs vd
Item payd to the beydmen the xij day vjs vd
Item payd to the beydmen the xix day vjs vd
Item payd to the beydmen the xxvj day vjs vd

mensis Augusti

Item payd to the beydmen the ij day vjs vd
Item payd to the beydmen the ix day vjs vd
Item payd to the beydmen the xvj day vjs vd
Item payd to the beydmen the xxiij day vjs vd

Memorandum that thomas Bentley beydman had lycens off the warden ffor j cawse lawfull to be absent iff he wold iiij weks

Item payd to the beydmen the xxx day vs xd

mensis Septembris

Item payd to the beydmen the vj day vs xd
Bentley cam ageyn
Item payd to the beydmen the xiij day vjs vd
Item payd to the beydmen the xx day vjs vd
Item payd to the beydmen the xxvij day vjs vd
Item payd to myself and to my confrater owr quart' wag' iij li

Summa istius part' xj li vijs xjd

Summa solut' custod' et suo confratr' hoc anno xij li
Summa solut' pauperibus hoc anno xvij li xvd
Summa utriusque solucionis xxix li xvd

Annuall charges

Item payd to the parson off Seynt myholl for the pencion off thys hows thys yer vjs viijd
Item for makying off m[l] kydds at wolfhows vs xd
Item for cariag' of the seyd kydds to the almoshows xs

Summa xxijs vjd

Summa lateris xij li xs vd
Probatum est nper me henricum Wykys

fol 21v

Adhuc de compoto pro anno Regni Regis henrici vij xiiij° compotus quartus

Chef Rents thys yer by Robard beomonds accompt

In primis for owr tenement' in stawnford to the kyng xxixs
Item for the clossys in Bredcroft to the [93] j li pepur ijs iiijd
Item the hows in all halo parysch at mallere brygg (to john wyks *ins*) ixd
Item the awngell to the gyld off corpus xti in Stanford xijd
Item the hows in seynt myhell parysch to seynt leonards of stanford vjd
Item the hows in seynt marten parysch by the watur syde to John thorney of carlby iijs

Item the hows in the same parysch with the porch wher bykerton dwelt to Boro abbey iiijd)
Item the hows next hyt on thys syde to the same Abbey iijd)
Item the garden in the same parysch toward the nonnys off stanford ijd)
[94]summa ixd

Item the ferm place at pylsyate to Boro abbey ixs ijd ob qa
Item the land in a closse off the same ferm to john thorney vd
Item the place at Barnek to master Vincent ixd
Item the place at Warmyngton to Boro abbey iiijs
Item the same place to the scherefs torn off northamton schyr vjd

Item the hows off Brian in eston to the kyng xxd)
Item the same place to the chartur hows in coventre ijs viijd)
Item the hows wher john wryght dwellyth to the kyng jd and j li comyn)
summa iiijd)
Item the closs that longyth to the same hows hyerd of the colleg off tatursale xvjd)
Summa vjs

Item the ferm at northluffnam to thomas Bassett iijs viijd)
Item the seyd ferm to lord sowch jd ob)
Item the seyd ferm to the prior off brooke iijd ob)
Summa iiijs jd

Item the maner off swaffeld to lord grey ls
Item a closse in the same town to s' thomas delaland of northwithom xijd
Item the hows in twyford to s' thomas delalaund xijd
Item the hows in northwithom next the parsonage to s' thomas delalaund vs
Item the hows at Barham to the kyng jd
Item the seyd hows to the erle off westmorland ob
Item the hows at wylsthorp to Robard eyland j li comyn vd
Summa off chef Rents thys yer v li xixs xd qa

---

[93] 'kyng' omitted

[94] this and the following two summa are in right-hand margin

Mercyments for sewt off cowrts

Item for langdyk hundreth xijd

Item att northluffham to dyverse cowrts xixd

Item for swafeld to lord greys cowrt att corby viijd

Item for stretton to the kyngs cowrt vd

Item for Wylsthorp to Robard eylands cowrt iiijd

Summa iiijs

Summa lateris vj li iijs xd qa

Probatum est per me h Wykys

fol 22

Ad huc de compoto pro Anno Regni Regis henrici vij xiiij^o^ compotus quartus

Costs off owr cowrt' at Swafeld and northwithom

In primis for horshyer to myhelemes cowrt at Swafeld viij day of october iiijd

Item for costs of cowrt ther the same tyme xvijd ob

Item I Rewardyd the quert[95] iiijd

Item for horshyer after pasce to Swafeld when the steward cam' nott iiijd

Item for expens' ther the same xviijd

Item for costs off cowrt an other tyme after that xvd

Item for horshyer to northwithom cowrt aftyr myhelmes xx day of November iiijd

Item for costs off cowrt the same tyme xd

Item pasc' cowrt at nortwithom *h[abe]o null*

Item for parchment to wrygt in the cowrt Rollys and streyts iiijd

Item payd to herre tokey owr steward' for kepyng thes cowrts hys fee xiijs iiijd

Summa xxs ob

Casuall costs

In primis expendyd to northwithom for the beydmens cawse to spek with M delaland for hys devocion of gevyng off iij tenements xd

Item payd to john cleypole for hys Awdytt of Bartylmew holm' baylyf iijs iiijd

Item expendyd to northwithom in the forseyd cawse an other tyme vjd

Item I payd to m delalands clerk ffor wrytyng off deds off the leyse viijd

Item I payd for makyng of the tapurs on the auter in the chapell viijd

Item for horshyer to peturboro to spek with thabbott for lycens off mortmayne iiijd

Item payd to the goldsmyth in seynt marten parysch for mendyng owr chales xijd

Item for haloyng a geyn the same chales vjd

Summa vijs xd

Decayse By Robard beomonds accownt

In primis the hows at malere brygg xs

Item the hows next the vycar off al halos iij quart' xvs

---

[95] probably 'quest', i.e. jury; see fol 81

Item j sclatt pytt at wyrthorp feld' vjs viijd
Item the hows next cleypols schope iij quart' vijs vjd
Item ij howsys at Walcote xixs
Item the barn in Skofgate iiijs vjd
Item the iij acr' medo abatyd Rent thys yer xijd
Item v akers erabyll land falo and ley ijs vjd
Item owr Rent at eston ijs
Item tenement in seynt marten parysch j quart' iijs iiijd
Item land at carlby for john thorney abatyd xviijd
Summa iij li xijs vjd

Summa lateris v li iiijd ob
Probatum est per me henricum Wykys

fol 22v

Ad huc de compoto pro anno Regni Regis henrici vij xiiij° compotus quartus

Casuall costs by Robard beomond
In primis for the halylof for the hows next cleypoll schop iijd
Item payd to thomas Reynold for goyng to Sowtluffnam to spek with the steward jd

Reparacion at the Almoshows allowyd Rob beomond
Item for hewyng off the wardens sparrs xijd
Item j sklatter to mend the gutter of the chymney of s' Wyllam hawkyn xijd
Item ij days j sklatter at the hows in the wodyard when the chymney was maad xijd
Item for makyng wrygt wark off j dor in to the wardens garden xijd
Item j mason j day at the same dor vjd
Item hys servar j day iijd
Item ij stryk lyme ijd
Item di[m] sem lyme for the sklatting at s' Wyllams chymney iiijd
Summa off bothes vs vijd

Reparacion at stawnford in dyverse placs By Ro Be

In seynt marten parysch
In primis for thornys to hedgh ij gardens ijs ijd
Item for fellyng the seyd thornys xd
Item ij men ij days hedghyng the seyd thornys xxd
Item for cariag' of the seyd thornys v lode ijs jd
Item j sklatter j day at thomas hondyslows vjd

at the awngell
Item j lode sand iiijd
Item j lode sklatt with cariag' ijs xd
Item j sklatter iiij days mendyng ijs
Item a laborer ther ij days viijd
Item j lode erth spent ther iijd

at thomas wrygts hows
Item for clensyng the yard when the leynto fell down ijd

at john thomas hows
Item ij lode walcott ston for the oven viijd
Item ij lode wyrthorp ston for the same iijd
Item j skatter j day at jhon thomas hows vjd
Item j sklatter j day att wyllam Bakers vjd
Item j sklatter j day at the crane vjd
Summa xvs xjd

at Wylsthorp
Item j wrygt to mend the barn dors and the feld yate viijd

Summa lateris xxijs ijd
probatum est per me h Wyk'

fol 23

Ad huc de compoto pro Anno Regni Regis henrici vij xiiij° compotus quartus

Reparacion at pylsyate Ro bemond
Item j lode sklatt ijs vjd
Item for cariag" off the same iiijd
Item j lode sand iiijd
Item ij days and j sklatter xvd
Summa iiijs vd

Reparacion at Barham made by the warden and Rekynd with Ro beomond
In primis j key for the lok on the hall dor ijd
Item makyng off iiij wyndows and the cariag' off them iijd
Item sawyng off ledghys for the same wyndows iijd
Item ij lode strey to thak the hows bowgt off the parson of gretford iijs jd
Item for cariag' of the same strey viijd
Item ij lode ffen thakk with cariag' iijs iiijd
Summa vijs ixd

Reparacion at wyrthorp and eston By Ro beomonds accompts
Item ij lode stobull xxd
Item for cariag' off the same xd
Item the thakkyng of the same straw (iij days *ins*) xviijd
Item servar to the thakker iij days xijd
Item ij lode stobull for the howsys att wyrthorp and eston ijs viijd
Item for the thakkyng of the same ijs viijd
Item j dos' thak Rope vijd
Summa xs xjd

Reparacion at eston - Ro beomond
Item for cariag' off lyme to Bryans howse vd
Item j lode sklatt ijs vjd

Item for cariag' off the same iiid ob
Item j lode sande iijd ob
Item for tymbur to Bryans swyncote xvd
Item for wrygtwark at the seyd swyncote ij days xijd
Item for sklattyng the seyd swyncote half j Rode ijs vjd
Item j sklatter iij days mendyng fawts ther xviijd
Item j sklatter ij days at john wrygts hows xijd
Item for wrygtwark off j peyr of yats at the same hows xxd
Item for ij lokks at the cotag in eston vjd
Item for mendyng the well at the cotag' wher the carver is iiijd
Summa xiijs iijd

Summa lateris (xxxvijs *del*) xxxvjs iiijd
probatum est per me h Wyk'

fol 23v

Ad huc de compoto pro A° Regni Regis henrici vij xiiij° *compotus 4*

Reparacion at wolsthorp by syde northwithom Ro beomond
In primis j wryyt to mend the barn vd
Item for cariag" off sparrs from northaw iiijd
Item for wattyll to the seyd sparrs iiijd
Item for wattyllyng the same wattyll iijd
Item j thakker j day and half vijd ob
Summa xxiijd ob

Reparacion at Swafeld by Ro beomond
at Robard toppars hows
Item ij lode playster for j chawmbyr florth iiijs vjd
Item to the [*deletion*] playsterar schotyng the seyd florth xxd
Item ffor the playsterars boord xijd
Item j laborer to serve the playsterar xijd
Item j thakkar ij days at the same hows vjd

at stroxtons hows
Item j wrygte and help to draw the barn iijs
Item for Rollys Borod at corby vjd
Item iij lode mortar spent ther vjd

at john elyns hows
Item j wrygt j days wark vd
Item for wattelyng ther viijd
Item for drawyng and servyng the thakker vjd
Item j lode thak for the same thakkyng xijd

northaw wod
Item ffor plaschyng and hedghyng ther lxv poll iiijs

at holdernes hows
Item half j dos' thak Rope ther and in other places vjd

Item j mason mendyng jeawnys govyls ther and at toppars hows with hys servar	xvjd
Item ij lode erth for the same wark	iiijd
Item ij lode ston for the same	iiijd
Item viij lode erth for govylls of dyverse howsys	xvjd
Item for warkmanschypp off the seyd govylls	xxijd
at Bullys howse	
Item iiij lode erth for a govyll ther	viijd
Item for makyng the seyd govyll	xd
at skargells	
Item splentyng and makyng a govell ther	xijd
Item v lode erth spent at hyksons hows	xd
Summa	xxviijs iijd

Summa lateris xxxs ijd ob
probatum est per me henricum wykys

fol 24

Ad hoc de compoto pro A° Regni Regis henrici vij xiiij°
Et hic est finis istius compoti

Reparacion at the hows in northwithom next the parsonage Beomond

In primis iij lode stobbull	vs
Item j thakkar and hys servar to the same stobbull	ijs iiijd
Summa	vijs iiijd

Reparacion at the cotag' ther Beamond

Item ij lode stobbull spent ther	ijs viijd
Item j thakkar to the same iij days and half	xvijd ob
Item hys servar iij days and half	xd ob
Item j mason and hys servar at the cotag' j day	viijd
Item j lode mortar for the same wark	ijd ob
Summa	vs xd ob

Reparacion at stretton at Robard skelyngtons hows - Beomond

Item j sklatter iij days	xviijd
Item straw to thak j hows	xijd
Item wattyll to the hows	jd
Item for j threschold	jd
at akyrlonds hows	
Item for strey to the thakkyng with the servyng a grete	vjs viijd
Item for thakkyng the dofcote hows	xijd
Item j thakkar on the insett hows iij days	xvd
Item an other thakkar other iij days	xvd
Item j thakkar j day	iiijd
Item for masonwark at the same hows	ijs vd
Item vj lode ston	ijs
Item v lode mortar	vijd

Item j sparr jd

Summa xviijs iijd

Summa istius partis xxxjs vd ob

Item the seyd Robard beomond Baylyff is allowyd hys fee thys yer xls

Summa lateris iij li xjs vd ob

Summa total off payments to the warden, hys confrater, the beydmen and wymen, annuall charges, cheff Rents, mercyments, costs off cowrts, casuall costys, dekays, Reparacions and baylyffs ffee thys yer is xlix li viijs jd ob qa

Summa superplusagij off the Rents thys yer to the incresyng off the stok thatt was dekayd and gon in arrerag' byfor xij li xiiijs iijd qa

[96]*et sic ex statutis nil vicario ex debito*

Summa finalis Remaynyng of the stok now incresyd xix li vijs ijd ob
probatum est per me henricum Wykys

[96] 'nothing is owed to the vicar'

fol 24v
[Account of John Taylor for the year 1499-1500]

Sequitur compotus quintus istius dom' et est de A° Regni Regis henrici vij xv°
her foloeth the vth accompt' off the state off thys almos hows accowntyd by the seyd john taylyor warden of thys seyd hows off j holl yer that is to say from the fest off Seynt myhell' in the yer off owr lord m[l] cccc° lxxxxix° unto the seyd fest off Seynt myhell in the yer off owr lord god m[l] vC Or els aftyr an other date from the fest of Seynt myhell in the xv yer off the Reygne off kyng harry the vij unto the fest of Seynt myhell in the xvj yer off the Reygne off the seyd kyng harry

In primis the seyd John taylyor warden chargeth hymself with the stok
Remaynyng as aperyth in the fote off hys last accowmpt' xix li vijs ijd ob
Item with the money Receyvyd off John colston off corby for the sale the second tyme off owr wod off Swynhawe for to encrese the stok xiiij li vjs viijd
Summa of the stok xxxiij li xiijs xd ob

Item the Rentale off Robard beomond owr baylyff as hyt aperyth by the boke off hys accompts for thys yer is the extent off lxij li iijs vd
Item the seyd warden Receyvyd of the seyd baylyff ffor mercyments of dyverse yers past as hytt aperyth by hys seyd accompt vijs viijd
Item off hym for a sklatt pytt in eston feld' iiijs
Summa of the lyflode lxij li xvs jd
Summa total off both togedyr the stok and the lyflode lxxxxvj li viijs xjd ob

of thys summa the warden dischargeth hymself by thes parcels foloyng
Mensis Octobris
Memorandum quod prima die admissus est Wyll's Umfrey et appositus ad numerum pauperum istius dom'
Item eodem die thomas Bentley habuit licenciam ut se absentaret per xiiij dies
Item payd to the beydmen ther wag' the iiij day vjs vd
Item payd to the beydmen the xj day vjs vd
[97]*Iterum Readvenit thomas Bentley*
Item payd to the beydmen the xviij day vijs
Item payd to the beydmen the xxv day vijs

Summa solucionis istius lateris xxvjs xd
probatum est per me h Wykys

[97] First day [of October] William Umfrey admitted; same day, Thomas Bentley had licence to be absent for 14 days; Bentley readmitted

fol 25

de Anno Regni Regis henrici vij xv° *compotus quintus*

Mensis Novembris	
Item payd to the beydmen the fyrst day	vijs
Item payd to the beydmen the viij day	vijs
Item payd to the beydmen the xv day	vijs
Item payd to the beydmen the xxij day	vijs
Item payd to the beydmen the xxix day	vijs
Mensis decembris	
Item payd to the beydmen the vj day	vijs
Item payd to the beydmen the xiij day	vijs
Item payd to the beydmen the xx day	vijs
Item payd to the beydmen the xxvij day	vijs
Item payd to my self and to my confrater owr quart' wag'	iij li
Mensis Januarij	
Item payd to the beydmen the iij day	vijs
Item payd to the beydmen the x day	vijs
Item payd to the beydmen the xvij day	vijs
Item payd to the beydmen the xxiiij day	vijs
Item payd to the beydmen the xxxj day	vijs
Mensis ffebruarij	
Item payd to the beydmen the vij day	vijs
Item payd to the beydmen the xiiij day	vijs
Item payd to the beydmen the xxj day	vijs
Item payd to the beydmen the xxviij day	vijs
Mensis Marcij	
Item payd to the beydmen the vj day	vijs
Item payd to the beydmen the xiij day	vijs
Item payd to the beydmen the xx day	vijs
Item payd to the beydmen the xxvij day	vijs
Item payd to my self and my confrater owr quart' wag'	iij li
Mensis Aprilis	
Item payd to the beydmen the iij day	vijs
Item payd to the beydmen the x day	vijs
Item payd to the beydmen the xvij day	vijs
Item payd to the beydmen the xxiiij day	vijs
Mensis maij	
Item payd to the beydmen the fyrst day	vijs
Item payd to the beydmen the viij day	vijs
Item payd to the beydmen the xv day	vijs
Item payd to the beydmen the xxij day	vijs
Item payd to the beydmen the xxix day	vijs

Summa lateris xvj li xvijs
probatum est per me henricum Wykys

fol 25v

Ad huc de compoto pro A° Regni Regis henrici vij xv° compotus quintus

Mensis Junij

Item payd to the beydmen the vth day	vijs
Item payd to the beydmen the xij day	vijs
Item payd to the beydmen the xix day	vijs
Item payd to the beydmen the xxvj day	vijs
Item payd to my self and to my confrater owr quart' wag'	iij li

Mensis Julij

Item payd to the beydmen the iij day	vijs
Md that thomas bentley had lycens for xiiij days	
Item payd to the beydmen the x day	vjs vd
[98]*Memd quod xiiij die mortuus est wyll's Umfrey huius dom' pauper*	
Item payd to the beydmen the xvij day	vs xd
Item payd to the beydmen the xxiiij day	vs xd
Item payd to the beydmen the xxxj day	vs xd

Mensis Augusti

Bentley cam nat ageyn at hys day to hym prefyxid J[de]o[99] etc	
Quia Relatum est pro certo quod mortuus est Ideo etc	
Item payd to the beydmen the vij day	vs xd
Item payd to the beydmen the xiiij day	vs xd
Item payd to the beydmen the xxj day	vs xd
Item payd to the beydmen the xxviij day	vs xd

Mensis Septembris

Item payd to the beydmen the iiij day	vs xd
[100]*Memd quod tertia die mortuus est Johannes cantyng huius domus pauper*	
Item sextus die mortuus est wyll's hesull istius domus pauper	
Item payd to the beydmen the xj day	iiijs viijd
Item payd to the beydmen the xviij day	iiijs viijd
Item payd to the beydmen the xxv day	iiijs viijd
Item payd to my self and my confrater owr quart' wag'	iij li
Summa istius part'	xj li xs xd

Summa solut' custod' et confratr'	xij li
Summa solut' pauperibus hoc Anno	xvij li xiiijs viijd
Summa utriusque solucionis	xxix li xiiijs viijd

---

[98] '14 July death of William Umfrey'

[99] 'Therefore etc; because it is said for certain that he is dead - therefore etc'

[100] '3 September John cantyng died; 6 September William Hesull died'

Annuall charges

Item payd to the parson off sent myhells for hys pencion of thys yer vjs viijd
Item for makyng off j m[l] kydds att wolfhows vs xd
Item for cariag' of the seyd kyds to the almos hows xs
Summa xxijs vjd

Summa lateris xij li xiiijs ijd
Probatum est per me h Wyk'

fol 26

Ad huc de compoto pro A° Regni Regis henrici vij xv° *compotus quintus*

Chef Rent' allowyd Robard Beomond in hys accompt'

In primis for owr tenements in stawnford to the kyng xxixs
Item for owr clossys on Bredcroft to the kyng j li peper pric' thys yer ijs iiijd
Item the hows at the mallere brygg to John wyk' ixd
Item the awngell to corpus Xti gylde xijd
Item the hows in seynt myhell parysch to seynt leonards vjd
Item the hows in sent marten parysch of thomas hondslow to John thorney iijs
Item ij howsys and j garden in the same parysch to the abbey off Boro ixd
Item the ferm att pylsyat to the same abbey ixs ijd ob qa
Item j part off j closs longyng to the same ferm hyerd of John thorney vd
Item the place in warmyngton to the abbey off Boro iiijs
Item the same place to the schyryves geld off northamton vjd
Item Bryans hows in eston to the kyng [101]xxd)
Item the same tenement to the charter hows in coventre ijs viijd)
Item the closse off John wrygts hows hyerd of the colleg' of tatursale xvjd)
Item the hows that John wrygt dwellyth in to the kyng jd and j li comyn iiijd)
Item the hows in Barnek to master vincent ixd
Item the ferm place at northluffnam to thomas Bassett iijs viijd
Item the seyd place to lord Sowch jd ob
Item the seyd place to the prior off Brooke iijd ob
Item the maner off Swafeld to lord grey ls
Item percroft closse in swafeld to s' thomas delalaund xijd
Item the hows in northwithom next the parsonage to s' thomas delaland vs
Item the hows in twyford to the seyd s' thomas xijd
Item the hows in Barham to the kyng jd
Item the seyd hows to therle off Westmorlamd ob
Item the hows in wylsthorp to Robard eylond j li comyn vd
Summa v li xixs xd qa

mercyments

Item for langdyk cowrt sewt for pylsyate viijd
Item for wyrthorp to the same cowrt iiijd
Item for northluffnam to dyverse lords xixd
Item for swafeld to lord greys cowrt at corby viijd

---

[101] no sub-total has been included with these items

Item for stretton to the kyngs cowrt vd
Item for horshyer to thystylton to boscheys cowrt for sowthwithom vijd
Summa iiijs iijd

Summa lateris vj li iiijs jd qa
probatum est per me henricum Wyk'

fol 26v

Ad huc de compoto pro A° *Regni Regis henrici vij xv* *compoto quintus*

dekays and abatements off certen Rents *in compoto* Rob beomond

In primis the hows at mallery bryg j yer xxs
Item j sklatt pytt in wyrthorp feld' vjs viijd
Item ij tenements in walcote xixs
Item the barn in skofgate vjs
Item Rent off owr ladys gyld howse in eston ijs
Item j hows at wirthorp j yer vjs viijd
Item j other hows ther half j yer iijs iiijd
Item j garden in seynt marten parysch toward the nonnys ijs
Item j hows in seynt marten parysch wher netylton dwelt half j yer vjs viijd
Item the hows in seynt petur parysch wher old Buk dwellyd xs
Item the hows next the vycar of al haloes xviijs vjd
[102]ffor Brandens wyf xtofer Bro pleg
Item the Rent of the awngell was abatyd pro A° R' R' henr' vij xiiij vjs viijd
Item the seyd Rent is abatyd thys yer A° R' R' henr' vij xv vjs viijd
Item Rent off iij acr' of medo at smale Bryg is abatyd thys yer vjd
Item the tennant of carlby is allowyd for the land that
John thorney holdeth viijd
Item the myln hows at northwithom abatyd vs iijd
Item ij cotags in the same town thys yer in dekey ij quart' xxd
Item an other cotag' ther in dekey j yer iijs iiijd
Item the hows next the parsonage is abatyd thys yer vs
Item Arnolds closse in Swafeld is abatyd pro A° R' R' henr' vij xiiij ijd
Item the seyd close is abatyd for thys yer present ijd
Item closse callyd hallyng ther is abatyd thys yer iiijd
Item the pastur' ther callyd hawkenyng abatyd iiijd
Item the pastur callyd hollyng is abatyd pro A° R' R' henr' vij xiiij iijd
Item the seyd pastur is abatyd in Rent pro A° R' R' henr' vij xv iijd
Item I ask allowance for the hows wher Bartylmew holm dweld in swafeld
for half yer for the whych wyllam holm hys son was sewerte afor
the warden (by syde the reparacion *ins*) vs
Item the hows in stawnford wher John Bene dwelt in the key
[i.e. in dekey] j quart' ijs vjd
Item the Rent of the chyrch Revys of northwithom in dekey ijd
Item the hows in sent myhell parysch in the key half yer xs

[102] in right-hand margin

Item John Joyner the tennant axeth allowance for vj yer every yer *ijs* whych he seyth m thomas stok promysyd hym to abate off the Rent off *xxs* - summa abatyd xijs

Summa off dekeys and batements viij li xxijd

Summa lateris viij li xxijd
probatum est per me henricum Wyks

fol 27

Ad huc de compoto pro A° Regni Regis henrici vij xv compotus quintus

cost' off owr cowrts swafeld and northwithom

In primis the wedynsday afor all halo day at swafeld xixd
Item for horshyer to the cowrt aftyr pasce the viij and ix day of maij viijd
Item the wedynsday aftyr the invencion of the crosse the same tyme costs of cowrt xviijd
Item the cowrt at northwithom opon all halo evyn iiijd
Item payd to herry tokey for kepyng thes cowrts hys fee thys yer xiijs iiijd
Item payd to the seyd herry for wrytyng the cowrt Rollys in parchment iijs iiijd

Summa xxs ixd

Casuall costs

In primis expenses to northwithom to spek with m delalaund for swynhaw the sale of hyt viijd
Item for horshyer to Barham with Robard beomond xxv day off febryarii ijd
Item expendyd at Swafeld when I delyverd hallyng closse to Alen toppar ijd
Item expendyd at wylsthorpe ([103]... *del*) in takyn pers knyyt to owr tennant ijd
Item for the halylofe for the barn in skofgate ijd
Item for horshyer to Barham to feche a stressyd kow' ijd
Item I expendyd at Barham goyng thyder dyverse tymys ijd

Summa xxd

ffor thalmoshows

Item j book hyllying for the book off accompts of Robard beomond jd
Item vij Rode poyntyng at almoshows vjs vd
Item iiij sem lym for the same poyntyng ijs viijd
Item ij lode sande viijd

Summa ixs xd

Reparacions in stawnford - By Robard beomond - Al halo parysch

Item sowderyng j guttar at cleypols schopp viijd
Item makyng off an entertes at the schop next viijd
Item makyng clene the hows ageyn the glover the tennant schuld com iiijd
Item j key to the barn lok in skofgate jd
Item for cariag' of old tymbur of the leynto in thomas wrygts hows to the barn ijd
Item for the halylofe for the same hows on trinite sonday iijd

---

[103] uncertain reading - 'hoehyh', perhaps horshyer?

Item payd to lessy for caryag off ij lode of the wardens tymbur to the water iiijd
Item for sowderyng the guttar at john thomas xijd
Item for cariag' off ston and mortar to John thomas oven ijs iiijd
Item for makyng an hedgh next the vycar off al halos xjd
Summa vjs ixd

Summa lateris xxxixs
probatum est per me henricum Wykys

fol 27v

Ad huc de compoto pro Anno Regni Regis henri' vij xv^{o} compotus quintus

Reparacion at the Aungell Beomond
Item payd to John wylson for poyntyng xvj Rode wark xiijs viijd
Item to the seyd John wylson sklatter for dyverse fawts mendyng
vij days ther ijs ixd
Item iij lode sande for the same poyntyng xijd
Item ij lode sklatt vs
Item cariag' off the seyd sklatt viijd
Item for x sem lyme to the same wark vjs viijd
Summa xxixs vd

Bredcroft Bemond
Item for thornys and hedhgyng of the closse ther ijs iiijd
Item j lode thornys and cariag' to kesten and schafton xd
[104]Summa iijs ijd

in seynt marten parysch Beomond
Item payd to wyllam wylys ffor makyng keys and mendyng lokks viijd
Item j wryght for drawyng in off j sparr ijd
Item to John wylson for vj Rode and half poyntyng at the fardest hows vs vd
Item the same John mendyng j gutter and dyverse other fawts
ther vij days ijs xjd
Item ij lode erth to the same hows vjd
Item j mason iij days and hys servar ij days xxjd
Item j lode sande iiijd
Item v sem lyme for the same poyntyng iijs iiijd
Item the halylof for the same hows jd
Item ij days of j thakker and hys server at netyltons that was xvjd
Summa xvjs vjd

Reparacion at pylsyate Beomond
Item iij lode sklatt vijs vjd
Item for cariag' off ij lode lyme to the same place xijd
Item x sem lyme for the same vjs viijd
Item ij lode sand viijd
Item for cariag' of the seyd iij lode sklatt xviijd

---

[104] in right-hand margin

Item iiij rode wark and j quart' new hyllyng on the grete Barn xxjs iijd
Item vj days wark of j sklatter mendyng fawyts iijs
Summa xljs vijd

Swaffeld Beomond
Item Richard campion was allowyd by the warden to the makyng of hys chymney vs
Item he was allowyd to the makyng off the florth over the hall iijs iiijd
Summa viijs iiijd

Summa lateris iiij li xixs
probatum est per me henricum Wyk'

fol 28

Ad huc de compoto pro Ao Regni Regis henr' vij xvo compotus quintus

Reparacion at wyrthorp Beomond
In primis iiij lode stobull viijs
Item for thakkyng the same xxd
Item hys servar xijd
Item iij lode stobull vjs
Item makyng off j wall bytwene the tenements in the yard viijd
Item j thakker vij days and hys servar as moch iiijs viijd
Item to denys the mason makyng j wall next kestens garden xvd
Item lath iijC to kestens chymney xd ob
Item hewgh douch for cariag' of tymbur from stawnford to the seyd chymney iijd
Item the seyd hewgh for viij lode ston to the chymney and the wall ijs
Item the seyd hew for iij lode mortar erth to the same vjd
Item denys the mason for ij days wark at the bak of the chymney xd
Item j days wark to fynysch hytt vd
Item for wrytwark of John depyng to the seyd chymney xvjd
Item for tymbur to kesten the tennant for the same chymney viijd
Item for lathyng off the same vjd
Item jC lath nayles jd qa
Item for mortar to dawb hytt with viijd
Summa xxxjs iiijd ob qa

Reparacion at Barham maad by the warden / allowyd Beomond
Item to Robard dey for ij lode Rye strey xvjd
Item to Robard bayard the thennant [sic] for j lode strey and half xxd
Item ij lode Rye strey of the same Robard iijs
Item vj bond thak Rope iijd
Item ij Rede shevys jd
Item j thakker ij days ~~xd~~ vjd
Item j servar ij days vjd
Item j thakker vj days xviijd
Item hys servar vj days xviijd
Item kesten of wyrthorp thakkyng iiij days xxd

Item hys servar iiij days xijd
Item thornys to hedgh the yard xijd
Summa xiiijs

Summa lateris xlvs iiijd ob qa
probatum est per me h Wyk'

fol 28v

Ad huc de compoto pro Ao Regni Regis henr' vij xv Compotus quintus et hic est finis

Reparacion at Bryans hows of eston Beomond
Item payd to john depyng carpent' of eston for mendyng the strete yat' xxijd
Item for cariag" of tymbur from stawnford for the said yat' ijd
Item for plats and naylys to the seyd yate viijd
Item to john wrygte for makyng the orchard yat' viijd
Item j lode erth jd
Summa iijs vd

At northluffnam / Beomond
Item j warkman to mend the well ij days xijd
Item j wrygt to mend the kyln ij days xijd
Item xij trasyns for the kylne and splentyng the same xxd
Summa iijs viijd

Reparacion at edward Bakers in Stanford / Beomond
Item j lode mortar erth iijd
Item payd to Richard Roes and Robard elys masons for mendyng the oven mowth and mendyng the wall of the cross hows in the yard ij days xxd
Summa xxiijd

Item the seyd Robard baylyff is allowyd for hys fee of thys yer xls
Summa lateris xlixs

Summa total off payments to the warden, hys confrater, the beydmen and women, annuall charges, chef Rents, mercyments, dekays and abatiments off Rents, costs off cowrts, casuall costs, reparacions, balyffs fee lvj li xvjs (vd *del*) iiijd

Summa off the superplusage off the Rents mercyments and strays toward the mendyng off the stok that was gon on Rerarges [arrears] afor v li xviijs
Summa Rema[n]yng off the stok at thys accowmpt xxxix li xijs vijd ob

probatum est per me h Wykys

fol 29
[Account of John Taylor for the year 1500-1501]

[105]Compotus sextus istius dom' elemosinarie factus per magistrum Johannem' taylyor custodem secundum eiusdem dom' et est de Anno Regni Regis henrici septimi decimo sexto

her foloeth the sext accompt' off thys almos hows maad Rekynd and accowntyd by John taylyor warden of the seyd hows ffor j holl yer that is to sey ffrom the fest of Seynt myhell tharchawngell in the yer off owr lord god xvC unto the seyd fest off the seyd seynt myhell in the yer off owr lord god xvCj. Or els aftyr an other date ffrom the fest off seynt myhell in the yer off the Reygne off kyng herry the vij[th] the xvj yer unto the seyd fest of seynt myhell in the yer off the Reygne off the seyd kyng herry the xvij[th] yer

In primis the seyd John taylyor chargeth hymself with the stok Remanyng as hytt aperyth in the foote off hys last accompt xxxix li xijs vijd ob
Summa off the stok xxxix li xijs vijd ob
Item the seyd John taylyor chargeth hymself with the Rentale off Robard beomond baylyff off the holl lyflode of thys almos hows whos charge is as hyt aperyth by the accowmpt off hym thys yer lxij li iijs vd
Item he Receyvyd off Robard Whythed for half j Rode sklatt pytt iiijs
Summa of the lyflode lxij li vijs vd
Summa off the stok and lyflode togedyr Cij li ob [*erasure*]

Off thys holl summa the seyd john taylyor axeth allowance and dyscharge off the supervisors off hys accompt by thes parcells foloyng

Mensis octobris
[106]Md quod xxix die mensis septembris mortuus est will's Bacon huius dom' pauper
In primis payd to the beydmen for her wag' the ij day iiijs jd
Item payd to the beydmen the ix day iiijs jd
Item payd to the beydmen the xvj day iiijs jd
Item payd to the beydmen the xxiij day iiijs jd
Item payd to the beydmen the xxx day iiijs jd

Mensis novembris
Item payd to the beydmen the vj day iiijs jd
Item payd to the beydmen the xiij day iiijs jd
Item payd to the beydmen the xx day iiijs jd
Item payd to the beydmen the xxvij day iiijs jd

Summa solucionis istius lateris xxxvjs ixd
probatum est per me henricum Wykys

---

[105] 'sixth account of this house rendered by John Taylor second warden in the 16th year of Henry VII'

[106] '29 September death of William Bacon'

fol 29v

De compoto pro Anno Regni Regis henrici vij xvj^o compotus sext'

Mensis decembris

Item payd to the beydmen the iiij day	iiijs jd
Item payd to the beydmen the xj day	iiijs jd
Item payd to the beydmen the xviiij day	iiijs jd
Item payd to the beydmen the xxv day	iiijs jd
Item payd to my confrater sir wyllam and to my self owr quart' wag'	iij li

Mensis Januarij

Item payd to the beydmen the fyrst day	iiijs jd
Item payd to the beydmen the viij day	iiijs jd
Item payd to the beydmen the xv day	iiijs jd
Item payd to the beydmen the xxij day	iiijs jd
Item payd to the beydmen the xxix day	iiijs jd

Mensis ffebruarij

[107]*Memod quod ultim' die Januarii admissus est Johannes stretton et appositus ad numerum pauperum istius domus*

Item payd to the beydmen v day	iiijs viijd
Item payd to the beydmen the xij day	iiijs viijd
Item payd to the beydmen the xix day	iiijs viijd
Item payd to the beydmen the xxvj day	iiijs viijd

mensis marcij

Item payd to the beydmen the v day	iiijs viijd
Item payd to the beydmen the xij day	iiijs viijd
Item payd to the beydmen the xix day	iiijs viijd
Item payd to the beydmen the xxvj day	iiijs viijd
Item payd to my confrater sir wyllam and to my self owr quart' wag'	iij li

mensis Aprilis

Item payd to the beydmen the ij day	iiijs viijd
Item payd to the beydmen the ix day	iiijs viijd
Item payd to the beydmen the xvj day	iiijs viijd
Item payd to the beydmen the xxiij day	iiijs viijd
Item payd to the beydmen the xxx day	iiijs viijd

mensis maij

Item payd to the beydmen the vij day	iiijs viijd
Item payd to the beydmen the xiiij day	iiijs viijd
Item payd to the beydmen the xxj day	iiijs viijd
Item payd to the beydmen the xxviij day	iiijs viijd

Suma lateris xj li xvjs jd
probatum est per me henricum Wyk'

---

107 'admission of John Stretton 31 January'

fol 30

De compoto pro A° Regni Regis henrici vij xvj°   compotus sextus

Mensis junij

Item payd to the beydmen the vth day iiijs viijd
Item payd to the beydmen the xij day iiijs viijd
Item payd to the beydmen the xix day iiijs viijd

[108]*Md xx die admissus est Johannes lynley et appositus ad numerum pauperum huius domus*

Item payd to the beydmen the xxvj day vs iijd
Item payd to my confrater and to myself owr quart' wag' iij li

Md xxvij die admissus est edmundus grenham et appositus ad numerum pauperum

Mensis Julij

Item payd to the beydmen the ij day vs xd
Item payd to the beydmen the ix day vs xd
Item payd to the beydmen the xvj day vs xd
Item payd to the beydmen the xxiij day vs xd
Item payd to the beydmen the xxx day vs xd

Mensis Augusti

Item payd to the beydmen the vj day vs xd
Item payd to the beydmen the xiij day vs xd
Item payd to the beydmen the xx day vs xd
Item payd to the beydmen the xxvij day vs xd

Mensis Septembris

Item payd to the beydmen the iij day vs xd
Item payd to the beydmen the x day vs xd
Item payd to the beydmen the xvij day vs xd
Item payd to the beydmen the xxiiij day vs xd
Item payd to my confrater and myself owr quart' wag' iij li

Summa istius part' x li xvs jd
Summa solut' custodi et confrat' xij li
Summa solut' pauperibus h° A° xij li vijs xjd
Summa utriusque xxiiij li vijs xjd

Annuall charges

In primis payd to the parson off seynt myhells in stawnford hys pencion xxj day of maij vjs iijd
Item payd for makyng j m^l^ kydds att wolfhows vs xd
Item for caryag' of the same kydds to thalmoshows xs
Summa xxijs vjd

Summa lateris xj li xvijs vijd
Probatum est per me h wyks

---

108 20 [June] John Lynley admitted; 27 [June] Edmund Grenham admitted

fol 30v

Ad huc de compoto pro Anno Regni Regis henrici vij xvj° compotus sextus

Chef Rents Allowyd Robard beomond

In primis for the tenements in stawnford to the kyng xxixs
Item for the clossis in Bredcroft to the kyng j li peper price thys yer ijs iiijd
Item the howse at the mallery brygge to John wyks ixd
Item the awngell to corpus Xti gylde in stawnford xijd
Item the hows in seynt myhell parysch to seynt leonards vjd
Item thomas hondsleys hows in sent marten parysch to John thorney iijs
Item ij howsys and j garden in the same parysch to the abbey off Boro' ixd
Item the ferm at pylesyate to the abbey of Boro' ixs ijd ob qa
Item part off j closs longyng to the same ferm hyerd of John thorney vd
Item the place at warmyngton to the abbey of Boro' iiijs
Item the same place to the scheryfs gelde vjd
Item the tenements in eston to dyverse lords vjs
Item the hows in Barnek to master vyncent ixd
Item the ferm at northluffnam to dyverse lords iiijs jd
Item the maner off swaffeld to lord grey ls
Item per'croft closs in swafeld to s' thomas delalaund xijd
Item the hows in twyford to s' thomas delalaund xijd
Item the hows next to the parsonage in northwithom to s' thomas delalaund vs
Item the hows in Barham to dyverse lords jd ob
Item the hows at Wylsthorp to Robard eylond j li comyn iijd

Summa v li xixs viijd qa

Casuall costs

In primis payd to thomas Reynold beydman for fechyng the cowrt Rollys from sowthluffnam jd
Item I Rewardyd thomas Bull when he browgt from John colston money for the sale off owr wod of Swynhaw the fyrst tyme ijd
Item I expendyd to northwithom to se wher schershaws yate schuld be maade in hys closs the xxvij day of marche iiijd
Item I Rewardyd John' misterton ffor evidence off northwithom and coynthorp viij day of maij viijd
Item expend to northwithom to s' thomas delalaund and to Swafeld for hewgh holm when cast owt the hey owt off alen toppars barn vjd
Item for mendyng of my sadell the same tyme ijd
Item ther was expendyd at sessions at Bylsfeld for the indytment off hewgh holm xix day off Julij xijd
Item I Rewardyd john mysterton the fyrst day off august xijd
Item I haf expendyd overseyng the lyflode thys yer and Reparacions in dyverse places os [as] stawnford wyrthorp eston stretton barnek barham and wylsthorp ijs

Summa vs xjd

Summa lateris vj li vs vijd qa
probatum est per me h Wyk'

fol 31

Ad huc de compoto pro A° Regni Regis henrici vij xvj° *compoto sextus*

Mercyments for sewts off cowrts

In primis payd for esseyng ['essoining'] at langdyk at myhelmes cowrt for pylsyate jd
Item for an essoyn at the same cowrt for wyrthorp jd
Item ffor mercyments at the cowrt after pasce viijd
Item an essoyn at wylsthorp jd
Item for dyverse cowrts at north luffnam xxd
Item for Swaffeld to lord greys cowrt at corby viijd
Item at stretton vd
Summa iijs viijd

Costs in kepyng owr cowrts swaffeld and northwithom *h[abe]o nil*

Dekays and abatments off Rents thys yer Beomond

In primis the tenement callyd the crane in seynt [Peter's] parysch xxvjs viijd
Item the hows in mallere Brygg xxs
Item j sklatt pytt in wyrthorp feld at Bulgate vjs viijd
Item ij tenements at walcote xixs
Item the barn in skofgate iiijs viijd
Rent of owr ladys gylde at eston ijs
Item at wyrthorp j hows iij quart' vs
Item the hows in Barham abatyd Rent thys yer xijd
Item j garden in seynt marten parysch thys yer goth with the hows of thomas hondlos ijs
Item the hows in seynt peter parysch wher old Buk dwelt dekey ixs
Item In of the awngell is abatyd Rent thys yer vjs viijd
Item john lytster hath abate off x acres arabyll for v yers passyd iiijs
Item the tennant off carlby is allowyd for land that john thorney hath viijd
Item the myln hows at northwithom abatyd Rent vs iiijd
Item ij cotags in the same town in the key [dekey] xxd
Item j cotag ther half j yer xxd
Item the closse callyd arnolds closse in Swafeld abatyd ijd
Item the closse callyd hallyng abatyd iiijd
Item the pasture callyd hawkeyng abatyd iiijd
Item the pasture callyd hollyngs falo and certen Ryggs or leys falo iiijs viijd
Item the hows in seynt myhell parysch in staunford j yer dekey xxs
Item the chyrch Revys off northwithom dekey ijd
Item john tenman abats off hys chef Rent for iij yer every yer *ijd ob*
Summa vijd ob
Summa of dekays and abatments vij li xxiijd ob

Summa lateris vij li vs vijd ob
Probatum est per me henricum Wykys

fol 31v

Ad huc de compoto pro A° Regni Regis henr' vij xvj° *compotus sextus*

Stuff bowyt for buyldyng for stoor Beomond

In primis vij payr dor bands xxd
Item j m[l] clowt nayle xvjd
Summa iijs

Reparacion at Swaffeld by a byll off arnold morton balyf depute undyr Robard beomond at Swafeld and therabowts

In primis jC Rede for Barnards hows ijs xd
Item for cariag' of the same xd
Item iij lode ledyngs off tymbur to the sayd hows viijd
Item j wrygt xv days at hys schopp hows viijs
Item for watyllyng the same hows and Ric' haks hows viijd
Item j dosen thak Rope to the same hows ixd
Item j thakkar to Barnard' hows and haks hows vij days *vd* j day Summa ijs xjd
Item j servar to hym *iijd* j day Summa xxjd
Item for drawar of thak vij days *ijd* j day Summa xiiijd
Item v lode straw to the same howsis *xijd* j lode Summa vs
Item j wrygt to alen toppar' hows *vd* j day Summa xd
Item ij hopys off yrn ijd
Item j mason to make j bench iijd
Item j mason j day at Robard coys hows vjd
Item xvj lode ston and mortar at Barnards and Robard coys ijs viijd
Item hewyng ij kybulls for borde vd
Item ij sawars sawyng the seyd kybulls ij days and half *vjd* j day Summa ijs jd
Item thomas stroxton was alloyd by the warden towards costs of hys kyln ijs
Item for makyng ij doors at the seyd thomas stroxtons hows vd
Summa xxxiijs xjd

Reparacion at north luffnam by a byll of the tennant Beomond

Item ij days wrygt wark xijd
Item viij sparrs xvjd
Item for Reede viijd
Item thak Rope iiijd
Item v lode thak vs
Item the thakkyng of the same iiijs
Item j sklatter iij days wark xviijd
Item j sem lyme in stonys from stawnford to the same xvjd
Item bord for the lovar xviijd
Item j wrygt makyng the same lovar vjd
Summa xvijs ijd

Summa lateris liiijs jd
probatum est per me henricum Wykys

fol 32

Ad huc de compoto pro A° R' R' henrici vij xvj°

Reparacions in seynt marten parysch Beomond

Item payd to john wylson sklatter and to hys servar for iiij days werk at the Roper' hows	iijs
Item the seyd sklatter for iiij days and hys servar as moche at hondslows hows	iijs
Summa	vjs

Reparacion at stretton by a byll of the tennant Allowyd by the warden Beomond

Item for cariag' off tymbur to a chymney at Robard Skelyngton		vjd
Item j manteltree for the same		xijd
Item tymbur bowgt of the tennant for the sam		xijd
Item to the carpentar for making of the seyd chymney		vijs iiijd
Item j mason j day		iiijd
Item iij dawbers iij days at *vjd* a day	Summa	iiijs vjd
Item j sem lyme and half in stonys caryd from Stawnford		ijs
Item for cariag' of the same		iiijd
Item j lode sande		ijd
Item j sklatter vij days *vjd* j day	Summa	iijs iiijd
Item j servar to hym v days *iiijd* j day	Summa	xxd
Item j carpenter to mend the gutter at the barn		iijd
Item j mason to mende the golf of the barn		iijd
Item iij sparrs of the tennant to the gutter		iijd
	Summa	xxijs xjd

Md that the tennant Robard Skelyngton gaf to the makyng of the chymney of hys cost xij lode erth with cariag' and all the lyttar to dawb bysyd hys labor so he is contentyd

Reparacion at john wrygts hows in eston by a byll of thes parcels Ro beomond

In primis for Rede to wattylyng off the barn	iijd
Item for thak Rope	ijd
Item for wrygtcraft	iiijd
Item j thakkar ij days	xd
Item j servar to the thakkar	iiijd
Item for strey to the thakkyng	xxd
Item thakkyng j gutter at the seyd hows	xijd
Item for ij threschholds	iiijd
Summa	iiijs (xijd *del*) xjd

Reparacion at fox hows at eston   Beomond
Item ij masons to mend the garden wall   ijs iiijd
Item ij lode ston for the same   iiijd
Summa ijs viijd

Summa lateris xxxvjs vjd
Probatum est per me h Wykys

fol 32v

*Ad huc de compoto pro A^o^ Regni Regis henrici vij xvj^o^*
her foleth certen Reparacions maade and overseyne by me jhon taylyor' warden and they are putt in the accompts off Robard beomond for hys dyscharge

Reparacion at Barham by thes parcels
In primis j lode strey off Robard dey of the same town   xviijd
Item j lode of olde hey of Robard bayard the tennant   xiiijd
Item ij lode stobull off john ffoldygton   ijs viijd
Item ij lode stobull off Robard bayard   ijs vjd
Item j lode barley strey and Rye strey   xiiijd
Item for barley strey off wyllam foldyngton   ijd
Item v bonch thak Rope   iijd ob
Item j thakkar vj days   ijs vjd
Item j servar vj days   iijs iiijd
Item j wrygt to mend the gate hows   xiiijd ob
Item for tymbur to the same wark   iijd
Item for j manger   iijd
Item j mydyll dor for the entre   iiijd
Item for mendyng off the dawb wall toward the garden   iijd
Summa xvijs viijd

Reparacion at the wall' of the barn yard in skofgate
Item ij sklatters half j day   vd
Item j server them half j day   ijd
Item for iij lode erth   ixd
Item j mason v days and half   ijs iijd ob
Item j laborer iiij days and half   xvd ob
Item iij lode ston from owr bakyate   iijd
Item iij Rodewark off j mason   iijs
Item ij days wark off j mason and mor'   viijd
Item for mendyng off j soo to ber' in water   iijd
Summa xs iiijd

Reparacion off the hows of john thomas next master elmes
Item j sem lyme   viijd
Item j sklatter iij days and half   xviijd
Summa ijs ijd

Reparacions at eston at Bryans hows
Item payd to ij masons for makyng a drye ston wall' toward the felde syde
ijs viijd

Summa lateris xxxijs xd
Probatum est per me henricum Wykys

fol 33

Ad huc de compoto pro A° R' R' henrici vij xvj° compotus sextus

Reparacion at Brawnstons howse in peter parysch
In primis j stapull ob
Item j peyr dor bands for the kyln hows dor jd ob
Item ij sem lyme xvjd
Item ij sklatters iij days ijs vjd
Item j servar to them iij days xijd
Item ij lode stobull ffom yngthorp iijs iiijd
Item iiij lode stobull ffom tekyngcote vs iiijd
Item j thakkar v days xxd
Item ij lode erth to Rygg withall vd
Item for Beryng water from the west wellys and drawyng thak viijd
Item for xiij crests spent ther and in other places xiijd
Summa xxs xd

Reparacion at edward bakers in all halo parysch
Item for makyng the garden dor ijd
Item j stapull to the same jd
Item Robard beomond allowyd the tennant in hys Rent for thornys to the hedgh' xxd
Item ij werkmen for to make the hedg in the garden vijd
Item iiij sem lyme spent ther and at the next hows ijs viijd
Item j lode sand iiijd
Item j sklatter j day vd
Item ij sklatters v days iijs viijd
Item j servar iij days and half xiijd
Item j wryght leyng in of j threschold at hys Bakhows dor' iijd
Item for clensyng the gutter bytwene both howsys aftyr the sklatters jd
Summa xjs

Reparacion at the lytyll closse in Bredcroft
Item j wrygt to make j threschold ijd
Item ij masons ij days to sett up the dor and mend the wallys xxd
Item servar to them ij days viijd
Item j stapull to the dor ob
Summa ijs vjd ob

Summa lateris xxxiiijs iiijd ob
Probatum est per me h Wyk'

fol 33v

Ad huc de compoto pro A° R' R' henrici vij xvj Compotus sextus

Reparacion at wylllam Bakers in sent peters parysch

In primis iij sem lyme and half	ijs iiijd
Item j sklatter iiij days	xxd
Item j servar iiij days	xvjd
Item for sand bowt off thomas keston	ijd
Item j sklatter ij days	xd
Item j servar ij days	viijd
Item j sklatter j day	vd
Item j servar j day	iiijd
Item ij wrygts drawyng in ij balks in the bakhows	xijd
Item for cariag' off the seyd balks and other tymbur	ijd
Item j mason to mend the swyncote	vd
Item j lode mortar for the same wark	iijd
Item j plommar to mend the gutter off the chymney	iiijd
Summa	ixs xjd

Reparacion at the cotage in wyrthorpe

Item ij lode stobull	iijs jd
Item ij lode barley strey	ijs iiijd
Item ij lode stobull	iijs
Item ij lode stobull	iijs
Item keston the thakkar vij days wark	ijs xjd
Item hys servar vij days	xxjd
Item v days wark off hym and hys servar stoppyd in hys Rent	iijs iiijd
Item j wrygt to make ij payr' dor darnys and j dor	vjd
Item for naylys to the seyd dor	jd
Item for caryag off the seyd dor and darnys to wyrthorp	ijd
Item sawyng off Bords and leghys for the same dor	xvd
Summa	xxjs viijd

Reparacion at the sygne off the crane

Item j sem lyme	viijd
Item j lode mortar	iijd
Item ij masons ij days makyng up a withdrawgt in the hye chambyr	xxd
Item j servar to them j day and half	vjd
Item j sklatter to mend fawts j day and half	xijd ob
Item j servar to hym j day	iiijd
Item j carpentar j day	vd
Summa	iiijs xd ob

Summa lateris xxxvjs vd ob

Probatum est per me h Wyk'

fol 34

Ad huc de compoto pro Aº Regni Regis henr' vij xvjº　*compotus sextus*

Reparacion at Barnek

In primis for cariag' off tymbur to undersett ij howsys the stabull and j chambyr vijd
Item john wrygt and hygen ij carpentars for to undersett the howsys ijs
Item iiij sem lyme and iij stryk iijs iiijd
Item vj crests vjd
Item for cariag' off lyme sklatt and crests vijd
Item j wrygt to mak a dorr for the stabull vd
Item payd to Robard Bryce the mason for j days wark at the corn chambyr vjd
Item to Rychard uffyngton mason j day vjd
Item to john gee mason off Barnek j day vd
Item j laborer to Rydd ston and mortar v days xxd
Item xij lode mortar ijs
Item ij lode sand iijd
Item j skottyll to ber in ston jd ob
Item ij grete stapulls for the stabull dor jd ob
Item ij masons iij days ijs viijd
Item iiij masons half j day xd
Item iiij masons ij days iijs iiijd
Item ij servars ij days viijd
Item ij masons half day vd
Item j servar to them half day ijd
Item for ij gret dor bands off yrn for the grete cart gate and the yard dor viijd
Item for xxij li led of the whych part was spent ther in settyng off hoks vjd
Item ij masons j day and half xvd ob
Item j servar to them j day and half vjd
Item j sklatter ij days xd
Item ij sklatters iij days and half ijs xjd
Item j servar to them iiij days xvjd
Item ij sklatters iiij days iijs iiijd
Item j servar iiij days xvjd
Item j bonch of lath and mor' vijd
Item payd to the sklatter for sklatt pynnys iiijd ob
Item to john wrygt and john hygen carpentars for drawyng off iij balks in the corn chawmbyr and in the kychyn xd
Item ij masons ij days and half ijs jd
Item j servar to them ij days and half xd

Summa xxxviijs vjd

Summa lateris xxxviijs vjd
probatum est per me henricum Wykys

fol 34v

Ad huc de compoto pro A° R' R' henrici vij xvj compotus sextus et hic est finis istius compoti

Reparacion at wylsthorp

In primis for makyng off vj wyndows iiijd
Item for hoks and bands to them ijd
Item ij sklatters for mendyng the dofcote xxjd
Item vj stryk lyme for the same mendyng vjd
Item payd to a wrygt ffor wark ther xiiijd
Item for iijC ffen thak ffor the barn ijs
Item for cariag' off the same xijd
Item to a thakkar vj days xviijd
Item for iiij lode strey iiijs
Item for cariag' off sklatt lym and tymbur viijd
Item v lode erth to Rygg with the howsys vd
Item for mendyng the cope off the wall xd

Summa xvjs vijd

Item payd to a tennant for sowderyng the gutter at greswods hows in all halo parysch and the gutter off cleypolls schopp and making off vij li sowdyr xjd
Item I john taylyor warden bowgt off yong cordale of eston for stor' off byldyng of the lyflode iij Rode bord and a quarter with the cariag' metyng and cowchyng in owr barn xxvjs ijd
Item for j pece ledd jd ob
Item I allowyd wyllam skarboro off north luffnam for iij days sklattyng that he payd to yong Robard whythed off eston hym and hys servar A° Regni Regis henrici vij xv° ijs
Item Robard beomond baylyff is allowyd in hys rekenyng for hys tymbur in owr barn of Skofgate that he bowgt off john ley to be stor for the lyflode xxxs
Item the seyd Robard beomond baylyf is allowyd for hys fee off thys yer xls

Summa iiij li xixs ijd ob

Summa lateris v li xvs ixd ob

Summa total off payments to the warden hys confrater, the beydmen and beydwymen, annuall charges, chef Rents, casuall costs, mercyments, dekays and abatments of Rents, Reparacions, thyngs bowgt and and [sic] allowyd for stor of hows for byldyng and baylyffs ffee lvj li xs ijd qa

Summa off the superplusage off Rents of the lyflode thys yer to perform the stok that was gon in arrerages and dekey byfor' v li xvijs ijd ob qa

et nil vicario ex debito

Summa finalis Remaynyng of the stok of thys hows at thys tyme whych stok with ...[109] at thys present accompt Remaynyth in the hands of Robard beomond baylyff of hys arrerag' de A° R' R' henrici vij xv and xvj xlv li ixs xd qa

---

[109] text hidden in the binding

Arrerag' Robart beomond de A° R' R' henrici vij xv° xiiij li xiijs ijd ob qa
Arrerag' Robart beomond de A° Regni Regis hen' vij xvj° xxxij li ijs iijd qa
Summa total off hys arrerag' xlvj li xvs vjd

probatum est per me henricum Wyk'

fol 35
[blank]

fol 35v

[Account of John Taylor 1501-2; in this year, Taylor came from Oxford to the Hospital full-time]

Compotus septimus istius dom' elemosinarie factus per me johannem taylor custodem secundem eiusdem dom'

her foloweth the vij^th accompt' off the state off thys almos for j holl yer that is to sey from the fest off seynt myhell thearchaungell in the yer off owr lord god xvCj unto the fest of seynt myhell in the yer off owr lord god xvCij Or els aftyr an other dat' ffrom the fest off seynt myhell in the (Reygne *del*) xvij yer of the Reygne off kyng harry the vij^th unto the seyd fest of seynt myhell in the xviij yer of the Reygne off the same kyng

In primis the stok off thys almos remaynyth in the hands of Robard beomond late baylyff[110] as hytt aperyth in the fote of the last accompt' xlv li ixs xd qa
Item the Rentale off thys almos hows thys yer is lxij li xvs xd ob

Summa total off the stok and extent of the lyflode cviij li vs viijd ob qa

Of thys summa the seyd john taylyor dischargeth hymself by thes parcells foloyng

Mensis octobris

Item payd to the beydmen and wymen for j wek' wag' the fyrst day	vs xd
Item payd to the beydmen the viij day	vs xd
Item payd to the beydmen the xv day	vs xd
Item payd to the beydmen the xxij [sic]	vs xd
Item payd to the beydmen the xxix day	vs xd
Mensis novembris	
Item payd to the beydmen the v day	vs xd
Item payd to the beydmen the xij day	vs xd
Item payd to the beydmen the xix day	vs xd
Item payd to the beydmen the xxvj day	vs xd
Mensis decembris	
Item payd to the beydmen the iij day	vs xd
Item payd to the beydmen the x day	vs xd

Summa solucionum istius lateris iij li iiijs ijd
probatum est per me h Wykys

fol 36

de compoto pro A^o Regni Regis henrici vij xvij^o compotus septimus

Item payd to the beydmen the xvij day off december	vs xd
Item payd to the beydmen the xxiiij day	vs xd

110 Beomond has been dismissed as bailiff.

Item payd to the beydmen the xxxj day vs xd
Item payd to my confrater and to myself owr quart' wag' iij li

Mensis januarii
Item payd to the beydmen the vij day vs xd
Item payd to the beydmen the xiiij day vs xd
Item payd to the beydmen the xxj day vs xd
Item payd to the beydmen the xxviij day vs xd

Mensis februarii
Item payd to the beydmen the iiij day vs xd
Item payd to the beydmen the xj day vs xd
Item payd to the beydmen the xviij day vs xd
Item payd to the beydmen the xxv day vs xd

Mensis marcii
Item payd to the beydmen the iiij day vs xd
Item payd to the beydmen the xj day vs xd
Item payd to the beydmen the xviij day vs xd
Item payd to the beydmen the xxv day vs xd
Item payd to my confrater and to myself owr quart' wag' iij li

Mensis aprilis
Item payd to the beydmen the fyrst day vs xd
Item payd to the beydmen the viij day vs xd
Item payd to the beydmen the xv day vs xd
Item payd to the beydmen the xxij day .
vs xd
Item payd to the beydmen the xxix day vs xd

Mensis maii
Item payd to the beydmen the vj day vs xd
[111]*Memo quod vij° die admissus est johannes midylton et appositus ad numerum pauperis istius domus*
Item payd to the beydmen the xiij day vjs vd
Item payd to the beydmen the xx day vjs vd
Item payd to the beydmen the xxvij day vjs vd

Summa istius lateris xiij li xxjd
probatum est per me henricum Wykys

fol 36v

de compoto pro Anno Regni Regis henrici vij xvij° compotus septimus
mensis junii

Item payd to the beydmen the iij day vjs vd
Item payd to the beydmen the x day vjs vd
Item payd to the beydmen the xvij day vjs vd
Item payd to the beydmen the xxiiij day vjs vd

[111] admission of John Midylton

Item payd to my confrater and to my self owr quart' wag' iij li

mensis julii
Item payd to the beydmen the fyrst day vjs vd
Item payd to the beydmen the viij day vjs vd
Item payd to the beydmen the xv day vjs vd
Item payd to the beydmen the xxij day vjs vd
Item payd to the beydmen the xxix day vjs vd

mensis augusti
Item payd to the beydmen the v day vjs vd
Item payd to the beydmen the xij day vjs vd
Item payd to the beydmen the xix day vjs vd
Item payd to the beydmen the xxvj day vjs vd

mensis septembris
Item payd to the beydmen the ij day vjs vd
Item payd to the beydmen the ix day vjs vd
Item payd to the beydmen the xvj day vjs vd
Item payd to the beydmen the xxiij day vjs vd
Item payd to the beydmen the xxx day vjs vd
Item payd to my confrater s' wyllam hawkyn and to myself owr quart' wag' iij li
Summa istius partis xj li xvs vjd

Summa soluta custodi et suo confratri hoc A° xij li
Summa solut' pauperibus hoc A° xvj li xvijd
Summa utriusque solucionis xxviij li xvijd

Annuall charges
Item payd to the parson off seynt myhels in staunford hys pencion vjs viijd
Item for makyng off j m[l] kydds at wolfhows wode vs xd
Item for cariag' of the same kydds to the almos hows xs
Summa xxijs vjd

Summa lateris xij li xviijs
probatum est per me henricum Wyk'

fol 37

de compoto pro A° Regni Regis henrici vij xvij compotus septimus

Chef Rents to dyverse lords
In primis for owr tenements in stawnford to the kyng by yer xxixs
Item for the clossys in Bredcroft to the kyng j li peper pric' thys yer ijs viijd
Item the howse at mallere brygg to john wyk' ixd
Item tenement of the awngell to the gyld of corpus Xti in stanford xijd
Item the hows in seynt myhel parysch to the cell' off seynt leonard in stanford vjd
Item the hows of thomas hondslow in seynt marten parysch to john thorney thys yer payd bot [but] ixd

Item the tenement of owrs in the same parysch on the est syde)
next the chyrch oweth chefe [rent] to the abbay of Boro iijd)
Item owr tenement in the same parysch next the seyd) summa
tenement to thabbay of Boro' iiijd) ixd
Item j garden off owrs in the same parysch toward the)
nonnys of stanford to the seyd abbay ijd)
Item the ferm at pylsyate to the seyd abbey of Boro ixs ijd ob
Item certen land of the seyd ferm inclosed hyerd of john thorney vd
Item the tenement at warmyngton to the abbey of peterboro' iiijs
Item the same tenement payth to the scheryfs yeld of northamton vjd
Item the hows in eston off Bryans stokley chef to the kyng xxd)
Item the seyd place to the charterhows in coventre ijs viijd)
Item the closs of john wrygts hows hyerd of the colleg' of tatersale xvjd)
Item the hows of john wrygt chef to the kyng *jd* and j li comyn summa iiijd)
Summa vjs
Item the hows in Barnek to master vincent of Barnek ixd
Item the ferm' at north luffnam to thomas Bassett iijs viijd)
Item the seyd ferm' to lord sowch jd ob) Summa
Item the seyd ferm to the prior of Brooke iijd ob) iiijs jd
Item the maner off swaffeld aforetyme to lord grey now gyven to
hys servaunts[112] ls
Item j close in the same town callyd per' croft to s' thomas delalaund xijd
Item the hows in twyford to s' thomas delalaund xijd
Item the hows in northwithom next the parsonag' to s' thomas delalaund vs
Item the closse in coynthorp payth thys yer to the scheryfs torn iiijd ob
Item hows in Barham to the kyng jd
Item the seyd hows to the erle off westmorland ob
Item the hows at wylsthorp to Robard eylond j li comyn iijd
Item the hows (off Robard akyrlond *ins*) in stretton for certen land in the
feld payth to the bellys off stretton chyrch by yer *xijd* so for the last yer
and thys yer ijs

Summa lateris for chef Rents thys yer vj li jd ob
probatum est per me h Wykys

fol 37v

de compoto pro Anno Regni Regis henrici vij xvij° compotus vij°

Tenement' in dekay

In primis the hows in seynt peter parysch callyd the crane xxvjs viijd
Item j tenement in the same parisch wher Brawnston dwellyd j quarter ijs vjd
Item j hows in al halo parysch at the mallere Brygg xxs
Item j schopp in the schop bothys that john cleypoll hadd xxs

[112] Taylor is writing at the end of the year in which Christopher Browne took a distraint from the Hospital tenants in Swayfield for this rent which Browne claimed should have been paid to him; hence the careful wording of this entry. See folio 38b

Item j tenement in the same parysch next the vycarag' (half j yer and half quart' *del*)	xijs vjd
Item the barn in skoftgate in seynt clement parysch	iiijs iiijd
Item the hows in seynt myhell parysch that john joyner had j yer	xxs
Item the garden toward the nonnys in seynt marten parisch thys yer leyd to thomas hondsley hows	ijs
Item viij acres land in the est feld of staunford lay ley	iiijs
Item j tenement in wyrthorp where the taylyor dwellyd half j yer	iijs iiijd
Item j sklatt pytt ther buttyng on bullgate	vjs viijd
Item owr ladys Rent in eston	ijs
Item ij tenements in walcott	xixs
Item the mylnhows at north withom	xs
Item the chef Rent of Robard walton	ijd ob
Item the chef rent of john tenman	ijd ob
Item the chef rent of the chyrch Revys off northwithom	ijd
Item the hows of john thomas on wolrow in all halo parysch half j quart'	ijs vjd
Item the pastur in swafeld callyd hawkeryng (falo thys yer *del*)	xxd
Item the closs off coynthorp	iijs
Item j cotag' in northwithom j quart'	xd
Item j cotag' ther half j quart'	vd
Summa off dekays	viij li ijs

Abatments off Rents

In primis ij clossys in Bredcroft with the medo plott by hytt	vjs iiijd
Item the awngell in seynt mary parysch	vjs viijd
Item the tenement in Barham	ijs
Item the cotag in swafeld that was Brent	xxd
Item the hows thas [sic] was Brent callyd tollys howse	vs
Item the closse callyd hallyng in swafeld	iiijd
Item the closse callyd arnolds closse	ijd
Item iij acres medo at smale Brygg of stawnford	xijd
Item j pastur in swafeld callyd hollyng	ijd
Item j pastur callyd lytylyng	xjd
Item the tenement in north withom next the parsonag'	xijd
Item the land (to wyllam Baker *ins*) of the pyngulfeld and the west feld in stanford	xijd
Summa	xxvjs iijd

Summa lateris ix li viijs iijd
Probatum est per me henricus wykys

fol 38b

[small piece of paper inserted and bound in before fol 38]

Memorandum yat Christofer[113] tok a dysstresse at swafelld for ye cheyff rent at owr ladeys dey be for crystemes wass twell mond' and so kepp hyt to a sennyt after ca[n]dylmes' to ye gret peyn of my tennands and to ye undoyng of ye cattell therfor I had gret trobyll and becynes [busyness] with all and cost me gret labur and charg' as folowyht heyr after. Item fyrst tym hyt was taken I went to swafeld and callyd ye tennands togeder for confortyng yem hyt cost me apon yem vjd

fol 38a

de compoto pro Anno Regni Regis henrici vij xvij° compotus vij'

Mercyments

Item for northluffnam to the cowrt off the prior off broke vd)
Item for essoyn at the kyngs lete jd) Summa
Item for j fyne for the cowrt Baron off the kyng ther xijd) xviijd
Item for ij essoyns at stretton cowrt ijd
Item for lord greys cowrt at corby viijd
Summa ijs iiijd

Costs off owr cowrts kepyng at swafeld and northwithom thys yer - *h[abe]o nil*

Casuall costs

In primis the haly lofe for the hows at mallery Brygg xxij day of december iijd
Item the halylofe for the hows next the vycar of all halos xxij day of Maii iijd
Item the halylofe for the hows in seynt myhel parysch xxiiij day of julii ijd
Item the halylofe for the corner hows on wolrow the last day of julii iijd
Item the halylofe for the barn in skofgate xxv day of march ijd
Item the byndyng of the boke off statut' off master nycolas tryggs wrytyng xd
Item for byndyng off j dyryge book of the chapell of thys almos hows vjd
Item for wrytyng off the statut' in iij partys vjs viijd
Item for parchmen and velom to the same wrytyng viijd
Item payd to j skryvener for mendyng the old porthose[114] in thys chappell ijs
Item I payd to the clerk of the cownseyll off my ladys for j lettur to master thomas Grymysby for the distrayne takyn in the closse of coynthorp iiij day of maij viijd
Item I expendyd at colyweston the same tyme jd
Item payd to the clark of the seyd cownsell for wrytyng the second lettur to the seyd thomas grymmysbe xijd
Item I expendyd at colyweston the same tyme jd
Item for j crowper to myn sadell and mendyng the same sadell iijd ob
Item I payd to john mysterton for the closse in coynthorp xxvj day of december xxiiijs iiijd

---

[113] this was Christopher Browne; this dispute is mentioned in the suit between the gild and the Hospital

[114] perhaps for *porteous* a breviary

Item I payd to thomas Reynold beydman for goyng with the seyd john mysterton to grantham for certen evydence the same tyme xijd
Item for j boke hyllyng for the boke off accompts jd
Item I Rewarded Arnold morton off swafeld for hys labors in gaderyng off owr rents and overseyng Reparacions for thys howse xs
Item I john taylyor warden haf expendyd thys(yer *ins*) in overseyng the lyflode and Reparacions and gaderyng Rents iiijs
Summa liijs iijd ob

Summa lateris lvs vijd ob
Probatum est per me h wykys

fol 38av

de compoto pro Anno Regni Regis henrici vij xvij° compoto septimus

off thyng' bowght for the stor off the hows

In primis j Rode borde bowgt off john whythed off eston pric' vijs iijd
Item lxxxxiiij fote off Bord of the same man xxjd
Item xviij bonch hart[115] lath vjs ijd
Item vij bonch sapp lath xiiijd
Item iij m[l] and half off sklatt bowgt at Wyrthorpp pytts xiijs viijd
Item for cariag' off the same ijs
Item ij m[l] sklatt off yong Robard Whythed of eston viijs jd
Item for cariag' of the same xvjd
Item j m[l] sklatt bowgt at colyweston pytts off john haydon of wyrthorp iijs vd
Item for cariag' off the same to eston vjd
Item j pekax to dygg withall xijd
Item viij skottylls to putt in naylys xijd
Item x m[l] lath nayls viijs iiijd
Item vj lokkys xvjd
Item iij m[l] clowt nayls iiijs
Item vij m[l] clowt nayls viijs ijd
Item for makyng off j schort leddyr off myn own wod jd
Item for j other schort leddyr ijd
Item for j ij hand [two-handed] sawe xvd
Item for iij wedhys off yrn ixd
Item j ladyll off yrn to melt in led ijd
Item ij lode sand (wyllam Baker *ins*) for sklatts in tyme off nede viijd
Item xij lode sand leyd in owr barn off skofgate ijs ijd
Item xlij crests iijs
Item for cariag' (wyllam Baker *ins*) off iij lode fre ston from the crane to the almoshows vjd
Summa iij li xvijs xjd

[115] heart lath, the top quality from the heart of the tree, sap lath from the outer branches

Reparacion at the Aungell

Item vj sem lyme and half — iiijs vjd

Item payd to yowng Robard whythed for iij Rode wark and half and j quart' new hyllyng wark — xviijs ixd

Item j lode sand besyde owr sand of the almoshows — iiijd

Item j sklatter with hys servar ij days and half mendyng fawts — ijs jd

Item for iiij crests — iiijd

Item for cariag' awey of Ramell aftyr the sklatters had don — viijd

Item payd to one tennant ther for mendyng off dyverse gutters bysyde iij li sowdyr spent off owr own — xiiijd

Summa xxvijs xd

Summa lateris v li vs ixd

Probatum est per me h Wyk'

fol 39

De compoto pro Anno Regni Regis henrici vij xvij° compotus septimus

Reparacion at the sygne off the crane in seynt peter parysch

In primis j pyn off yrn to the grete yatt on the strete syd — ijd

Item j wrygte callyd hygen to mend the seyd yat' — xijd

Item ij lode ston from wyrthorp — viijd

Item viij lode mortar erth owt wyllam Bakers yard — viijd

Item to Bacon off seynt peter parysch for cariag' off x lode ston from Bredcroft — ijs vjd

Item to the seyd bacon for iiij lode ston caryage from owr feld yate — viijd

Item to wyllam baker owr tennant for ij lode ston from owr bak yate — iiijd

Item to the seyd wyllam Baker for xij lode ston from Bredcroft — iijs

Item for dyggyng the seyd ston — vijd

Item to the seyd wyllam Baker for cariag' off xxxiiij lode ston and mortar — viijs iijd

Item for dyggyng off ston — xijd

Item ij masons iiij days *vd* j day — Summa iijs iiijd

Item ij servars to them iiij days *iijd* j day — Summa ijs

Item j wrygt to make ij peyr dors darnys — viijd

Item abbott the carpentar to mend the grete yat' toward the cowrt and dyverse other thyngs v days and half — ijs iijd ob

Item j lapp off yrn to the seyd yate — jd ob

Item for sawyng off leghys ffor dyverse dorrs — xd

Item j Rope to draw watyr — jd

Item for mendyng off j schovell — jd

Item for hoopyng j soo — jd ob

Item iij masons vj days — vijs vjd

Item ij laborers vj days — iijs

Item iij masons iij days — iijs ixd

Item ij servers iij days — xviijd

Item j mason to fynysch the chymney and gresyngs iiij days — xxd

Item j servar to hym iiij days xijd
Item for dawbyng and pargettyng vij days ijs xjd
Item j laborer to helf [sic] hym vij days xxjd
Item ij sem lym' and half to pargett with xxd
Item for yelo sand thatt was golyns the tennant [sum missing]
Item payd to john hygen the carpentar for hys bargeyn agreyte to make iiij schopp wyndows leyng off somertre and trasyngs abof ij peyntes and iiij dors xs
Item j somertre bowgt off the parson off petur' vs xd
Item for sklattyng the seyd peyntes (xvjd *del*) iijs ixd
Item ij sem lyme to the seyd sklattyng xvjd
Item for j crest jd
Item iiij peyr geanows for the schopp wyndows xvijd

Summa lateris iij li xvs vjd ob
probatum est per me henricum Wykys

fol 39v

Ad huc de compoto pro A° Regni Regis henrici vij xvij° *compotus septimus*

Item j lode sand for the sklattyng off the seyd peynteshys iiijd
Item for wollyng Ropys for the masons and sklatters ijd
Item for cariag' (wyllam Baker *ins*) off iij lode plaster from the almos [sic] to the crane vjd
Item I bowgt iij lode plaster for the florth over the schoppe viijs viijd
Item iij lode plaster ageyn vijs vjd
Item for wod to born [burn] the plaster bowgt of wyllam Baker ijs
Item the wod thatt the tennant Golyn left in the hows [no sum]
Item ij lode wod off myn owen from the almoshows [no sum]
Item jC Reede for the plaster florth with the cariag' iijs iiijd
Item to the plasterar for burnyng betyng syftyng schotyng the florth over the schopp and entre xxij days xjs
Item j laborer to help hym xxij days vijs iiijd
Item j other servar to hym when he schott the florth v days xvijd
Item iij lode mortar for the syde walls in the entre ixd
Item ij plats of yrn to ley undyr the grete yate iiijd
Item for mendyng off the grynde off yrn ijd
Item j lode ston to fynysch the wall in the entre iijd
Item for sawyng off trasyngs ijs
Item j mason to fynysch the wall in the entre and pykyng owt stonys for to undyrsett the hows and pykyng owt stonys wher the (*deletion*) (trasyng *ins*) schuld lyg over the entre vj days ijs vjd
Item j laborer to help hym and serve hym the seyd vj days xviijd
Item for bem fyllyng' bytwene the trasyngs to the mason and hys servar payd viijd

Item ij laborers to brek down the wall toward the weysyde over the schop wyndows xd
Item vj lode mortar to mak up the seyd wall ageyn xviijd
Item half j sem lym to sett the coynys off the schopp wyndows iiijd
Item to sherwyn the mason for ij days wark at the seyd wall xijd
Item ij grete hoks and ij grete stapulls for the schopp wyndows viijd
Item payd to denys the mason for v days wark at the wall over the wyndows ijs vjd
Item to Denys felo the mason j days work vjd
Item to henley and john hostelar ij laborer to serve the masons v days iijs iiijd
Item for j lok and j key delyverd to Robard cave the tennant iiijd
Item half j sem lyme to pargett the schopp iiijd
Item j lode stobull to thak the hows in the yard xviijd
Item for mendyng lokks and keys iiijd

Summa istius part' iij li iijs vijd

Summa total off the Reparacion of the crane vj li xixs jd ob

Summa lateris iij li iijs vijd
Probatum est per me h Wyk'

fol 40

Ad hoc de compoto pro A° Regni Regis henrico vij xvij° compotus septimus

Reparacion at wyllam Baker hows in seynt peter parysch
In primis iij lode mortar erth for the garden wall xijd
Item for cariag' off mortar erth owt off the garden that was the mud wall vjd
Item for iij lode ston ffrom wyrthorp xijd
Item xxviij lode ston ffrom the dofcote in Bredcroft vijs
Item for dyggyng and castyng owt the seyd ston xijd
Item for ij lode ston caryd ffrom owr feld yate iiijd
Item ij masons makyng the seyd garden wall iiij days iijs iiijd
Item ij laborers iij days xxjd
Item j mason to undyrpyn the garden dor jd
Item j wrygt to mend the garden dor and the gyle hows dowr xd

Item at the same hows Reparacion aftyr the gret water[116]
In primis for gadyryng up the ston in the yard and the strete skatyrd abrode ijd
Item j wrygt to make ageyn the garden dor and darnys ijd
Item iij lode morter for to make the wall at the garden yate ixd
Item iij masons to make the seyd wall j day and half ijs iijd
Item ij servars to them j day and half xijd
Item j wrygt to mende the grete yate at the strete syde and the swyncote dor and the hall dor where Brawnston dwellyd ixd

---

[116] This flooding of the Welland seems to have occurred in 1501-2. For the great flood of 1499-1500, see M K Jones 1986 Lady Margaret Beaufort, the royal council and an early Fenland drainage scheme, *Lincolnshire History and Archaeology* vol 21 p 14; another flood is recorded in TNA SC6/1115/9

Item j pyn off yrn to the seyd grete yate ijd
Item payd to Reynold lokkey sklatter for mendyng the evys off the stabull vjd
Item half j sem lyme to the same sklattyng iiijd
Item to the seyd sklatter for mendyng the pentes on the weysyde iijd
Item for clensyng the comen sewer that was wrekkyd
bytwene hys and jaksons iiijd

Summa xxiijs vjd

Reparacion (at the awngell *del*) at the stabell at the almoshows
In primis viij (sem lyme and half *del*) (lode mortar *ins*) ijs
Item iiij lode ston xijd
Item j mason and hys servar ij days xxd
Item wrygtwark makyng the hows and florth over the stabull iiijs vd
Item for j Rode new sklattyng iiijs vjd
Item ij sem lyme and half to the same xxd
Item for dawbyng and Rokkyng iijs ixd
Item for iiij crests iiijd
Item for pavyng the stabull vjd

Summa xixs xd

Summa lateris xliijs iiijd
Probatum est per me henricum wykys

fol 40v

Ad huc de compoto pro Anno regni regis henrici vij xvij compotus septimus

Reparacions at the almoshows
In primis ffor sowderyng the gutter at the wardens chawmbyr
and the ledys off the chapell att dyverse tymys xvjd
Item for j key to the dor thatt was bytwene the kychyn
and the beydwomens hall iijd
Item j wrygt to mak j dor overthwart the entre off the warden
and hys confrater vijd

Summa ijs ijd

Reparacion at edward Bakers in all halo parysch
Item for glasyng off hys hall wyndow xxd
Item j wrygt to make j wyndow to the same and j dorr to
hys corn' schawmbyr vjd
Item j wrygt to mend hys swyncot dor viijd
Item j mason to mend dyverse jeawmys there iijd
Item ij mason to make j manger at the the [sic] hows by yond the
bakhows and pavyng the seyd hows and undyrpynnyng the stabull
in the garden iij days ijs vjd
Item j servar to theym ij days vjd
Item j lode ston ffrom wyrthorp pytts to the seyd pavyng iiijd
Item ij lode mortar erth for the manger and the seyd undyrpynnyng vjd

Item j (part off *ins*) lode stobull for the stabull in the garden vijd
Item a thakkar for the same stobull and hys servar viijd
Summa viijs ijd

Reparacion at the hows next the vycar off all halos
Item ij wrygts to mak and mend dors and wyndows and to undyrsett the florth in the gyle hows j day and half xviijd
Item ij masons to undyrpyn the hows within next the garden ij days xxd
Item ij laborers to Ryd the grownd and to serve the masons ij days xiiijd
Item ij lode ston for the same wark vjd
Item ffor pavyng off the yard and the entre ijs viijd
Item j hesp and ij stapulls for the hows next the garden jd
Item ij laborers to mak evyn the florth in the seyd hows and dawbyng the manger botom in the long stabull xd
Item for havyng awey the dong in the yard and the chawmbyrs and clensyng the gutter bytwene bothe howsys xijd
Summa ixs vd

Summa lateris xixs ixd

Summa total off payments to the warden, hys confrater, the beydmen the beydwymen, annuall charges, chef Rents, dekays, abatments off Rents, mercyments, Casuall costs, off thyngs bowgt for stor off hows, Reparacions thys yer is lxij li xvs xd ob

Summa in superplusag' off the Rents *h[abe]o nil*
Summa finalis Remaynyng of the stok xlv li ixs xd qa the whych summa Remaynyth in the hands off Robard beomond late beyng bayllyff off arrerags off hys accompts as hytt apperyth by the booke off hys accompts pro A° R' R' henr' vij xv° - xiij li xiijs ijd ob qa. Item de A° R' R' henr' vij xvj° arrerag' xxxij li ijs iijd qa

Summa of both arrerag' xlvj li xvs vjd ([117]*et sic debet in ultra summa Remanentum in le stok* xxvs vijd ob qa *del*) *Solut est in* [sic]
probatum est per me henricum Wyk'

---

[117] 'and so he owes in the further total remaining in the stock £25 0s 7¾d; payment is in [incomplete]'

fol 41

[Account of John Taylor for the year 1502-3; this is his longest and most detailed account as he threw himself into the role of warden]

per A° Regni Regis henr' vij xviij°

Compotus octavus de statu istius dom' elemosinarie factus per me johannem taylyor secundum custodem euisdem dom'

Her foleth the viij accompt' of the stat' off thys almos hows ffor j holl yer that is to sey from the fest off seynt myhell the archawngell in the yer off owr lord god xvCij unto the fest off the seyd seynt myhell in the yer off owr lord god xvCiij Or else aftyr another date, ffrom the fest off seynt myhell in the xviij yer off the Reygne off kyng herry the vijth unto the fest off the seyd sent myhell in the xix yer off the Reygn of the same kyng

In primis the stok afor rehercyd of thys hows Remaynyth in the hands off Robard beomond as aperyth in the fote off the last accompt xlv li ixs xd qa
Item ther was borod off all halo gylde afortyme[118] xx li
Summa off the stok and borod money lxv li ixs xd qa
Item the Rentale and the extent of the lyflod thys yer is lxij li xvs ijd ob
Item Rec' for mercyments and perquesyts off owr cowrts thys yer xxijd
Summa off the lyflode and mercyments lxij li xvijs ob
Summa total off both togedyr the stok borod money and the Rentale Cxxviij li vjs xd ob qa

Off thys summa the seyd john taylyor dischargeth hymself by thes parcels foloyng

Mensis octobris

In primis payd to the beydmen and wymen for wag' of j weke endyd the vij day vjs vd
Item payd to the beydmen the xiiij day vjs vd
Item payd to the beydmen the xxj day vjs vd
Item payd to the beydmen the xxviij day vjs vd

Mensis novembris

Item payd to the beydmen the iiij day vjs vd
Item payd to the beydmen the xj day vjs vd
Item payd to the beydmen the xviij day vjs vd
Item payd to the beydmen the xxv day vjs vd

Summa solucio' istius lateris ljs iiijd
probatum est per me henricum Wyk'

118 this is the sum involved in the law suit between the gild of All Saints and the Hospital

fol 41v

de compoto pro A^o R' R' henrici vij xviij^o compotus octavus

Mensis decembris
Item payd to the beydmen the ij day vjs vd
Item payd to the beydmen the ix day vjs vd
Item payd to the beydmen the xvj day vjs vd
Item payd to the beydmen the xxiij day vjs vd
Item payd to the beydmen the xxx day vjs vd
Item payd to my self and my confrater owr quart' wag' iij li

Mensis Januarii
Item payd to the beydmen the vj day vjs vd
Memorandum quod elizabeth huntley una de mulieribus pauperibus istius [119]*domus mortua est viij die Januarij*
Item payd to the beydmen the xiij day vs xd
Item payd to the beydmen the xx day vs xd
Item payd to the beydmen the xxvij day vs xd

Mensis ffebruarii
Item payd to the beydmen the iij day vs xd
Item payd to the beydmen the x day vs xd
Item payd to the beydmen the xvij day vs xd
Item payd to the beydmen the xxiiij day vs xd

Mensis marcii
Item payd to the beydmen the iij day vs xd
Item payd to the beydmen the x day vs xd
Item payd to the beydmen the xvij day vs xd
Item payd to the beydmen the xxiiij day vs xd
Item payd to the beydmen the xxxj day vs xd
Item payd to my self and my confrater owr quart' wag' iij li

Mensis Aprilis
Item payd to the beydmen the vij day vs xd
Item payd to the beydmen the xiiij day vs xd
Item payd to the beydmen the xxj day vs xd
Item payd to the beydmen the xxviij day vs xd

Mensis Maii
Item payd to the beydmen the v day vs xd
Item payd to the beydmen the xij day vs xd
Item payd to the beydmen the xix day vs xd
Item payd to the beydmen the xxvj day vs xd

Summa lateris xiij li xvs ijd
Probatum est per me h Wyk'

---

[119] 'Elizabeth Huntley one of the women paupers died 8 January

fol 42

de compoto pro Anno Regni Regis henrici vij xviij° compotus octavus

Mensis Junij
Item payd to the beydmen the ij day vs xd
Item payd to the beydmen the ix day vs xd
Item payd to the beydmen the xvj day vs xd
Item payd to the beydmen the xxiij day vs xd
Item payd to the beydmen the xxx day vs xd
Item payd to my self and my confrater for owr quart' wag' iij li

Mensis Julii
Item payd to the beydmen the vij day vs xd
Item payd to the beydmen the xiiij day vs xd
Item payd to the beydmen the xxj day vs xd
Item payd to the beydmen the xxviij day vs xd

Mensis Augusti
Item payd to the beydmen the iiij day vs xd
Item payd to the beydmen the xj day vs xd
Item payd to the beydmen the xviij day vs xd
Item payd to the beydmen the xxv day vs xd

Mensis Septembris
Item payd to the beydmen the fyrst day vs xd
Memorandum that the ij day dyede john Borgoyn beydman of thys hows
Item payd to the beydmen the viij day vs (xd *del*) iijd
Item payd to the beydmen the xv day vs iijd
Item payd to the beydmen the xxij day vs iijd
Item payd to the beydmen the xxix day vs iijd
Item payd to my self and my confrater owr quart' wag' iij li
Summa isstius part' xj li ijs viijd
Summa soluc' costodi et confrater xij li
Summa soluc' pauperibus hoc A° xv li ixs ijd
Summa utriusque solucionis xxvij li ixs ijd

Annuall charges
Item payd to s' thomas forster parson of seynt myhels in stawnford
for the pencion of thys hows vjs viijd
Item for makyng off j m[l] kydds at Wolfhows vs xd
Item for cariag' off the same kydds to the almos hows xs
Summa xxijs vjd

Summa lateris xij li vs ijd
Probatum est per me henricum Wykys

fol 42v

de compoto pro A^o Regni Regis henrici vij xviij^o compotus octavus

Chef Rents to dyverse lord'

In primis ffor owr tenements in stawnford to the kyng by yer xxixs
Item for owr clossys in bredcroft to the kyng by yer j li peper price thys yer ijs
Item the hows at the mallere brygg in All halo parysch to John Wyks ixd
Item the tenement callyd the Awngell to the gyld off corpus Xti xijd
[120]Item the hows in seynt myhell parysch payeth to the cell off seynt leonard vjd
Item the of [sic] thomas hondslo in seynt marten parysch to
john thorney off carlby iijs
Item j garden toward the nonnys in the same parysch in the hold
of thomas hondslo (to Boro abbey *ins*) ijd
Item the hows in the same parysch that john dowse dwellyth in
to the abbey off peterboro iijd
Item the hows of netyltons in the same parysch to the abbey of boro iiijd
Item the ferm at pylsyate to (Bro *del*) Boro abbey ixs ijd ob qa
Item land in a closse of the seyd ferm hyerd off john thorney vd
Item the tenement at Warmyngton to the abbey off peterboro iiijs
Item the same tenement payth to the scherefs tern' of northamptonschyr vjd
Item the hows at eston off Bryan stoksley to the kyng xxd)
Item the seyd hows to the charter hows in coventre ijs viijd)
Item the hows of john wrygts to the kyng jd and j li comyn summa iiijd)
Item the closse of the same hows hyerd off the collag' off tatersale xvjd)
[121]Summa vjs
Item the hows in bernak to master Vincent of the same town ixd
Item the ferm at northluffnam to thomas Bassett iijs viijd)
Item the same ferm to lord sowch jd ob)
Item the seyd ferm to the prior off Broke iiijd ob) Summa iiijs jd
Item the maner off swafeld gyffyth now to lord grey servaunts ls
Item j closs in the same town callyd per'croft to s' thomas delalaund xijd
Item the hows in twyford to s' thomas delalaund xijd
Item the hows in northwithom next the parsonag to s' thomas delalaund vs
Item the hows in Barham to the kyng jd
Item the seyd hows to the erle off westmorland ob
Item the hows in wylsthorp to Robard eylond j li comyn iiijd
Item Robert (Skelyngtons *del*) (Akyrlond' *ins*) hows in stretton to
the bellys off stretton church xijd
Item the closse in coynthorp payth to the scherefs torn iiijd ob
Item the seyd closse chefyth to Master Grymmysbe of Skotylthorp [no sum]
Summa off chef Rents thys yer vj li ixd ob qa

---

[120] this line has been inserted

[121] this and the next sub-total are in the right-hand margin against the bracketed items

Abatments off Rents thys yer

In primis off the awngell	vjs viijd
Item of the barn in skofgate	iiijs iiijd
Item of the clossys in bredcroft with the medo plott	vjs iiijd
Item of the xj acres in the est feld in staunford	ijs xd
Item of the xxij acres in the mydyl feld	
(xix acres and iij Rodes lay falo *ins*)	ixs xd ob
Item of the ix acres (and half *ins*) in the pyngull feld	iijd
Item off the xij acres in the west feld (an acres and half abatyd *ins*)	ixd
Item of the tenement in stretton where acr'lond dwelt	xijd
Item of the tenement in north withom next the parsonag	ijs vjd
Item of the tenement in barham	xvjd

[122]*vide Residu' folio sequ'*

[123]Summa xliijs ijd ob (xiijs ijd ob *del*) (xxxiijs ijd ob *del*)

Summa istius part' xxxvs xd ob

Summa lateris (xv *del*) vij li xvjs viijd qa

probatum est per me h Wyk'

fol 43

de compoto pro Anno Regni Regis henrici vij xviij compotus octavus

Abatment' off Rent'

Item the myln hows in northwithhom for the fyrst half yer	ijs viijd
Item the cheff Rent off john tenman off Steynby	ijd ob
Item the hows in Swaffeld callyd tollys hows late brent	vs
Item the cotag' that was brent in the same towne	xxd
Item j lytyll closse ther callyd arnolds closse	ijd
Item the pastur callyd hawkenyng in swafeld	jd
Summa istius part'	ixs ixd ob
Summa (total' *ins*) off the abatments off Rents thys yer	xlvs viijd

Dekays

In primis the schopp in all halo parysh that john cleypoll had	xviijs iiijd
Item the hows next the vycar off all halos	xviijs
Item the hows at the mallere brygg wher the clark off all halos	
dwellyth j quart'	vs
Item the hows in seynt myhell parysch j yer	xixs vijd
Item the tenement in seynt petur parysch where old Bukk	
dwellyd the fyrst quart'	ijs vjd
Item the hows in seynt marten parysch where the Roper	
dwelt j quarter	iijs iiijd
Item j garden towards the nonnys in the same parysch now joynyd to thomas	
hondslo hows	ijs

122 'see the rest on the following page' - in right-hand margin

123 there are two deleted sub-totals in right-hand margin

Item j sklatt pytt in eston felds bysyde wyrthorp Buttyng on bulgate vjs viijd
Item Rent assyse off owr ladys gylde hows in eston ijs
Item ij tenements in walcote xixs
Item the myln hows in northwithom thys last half yer vjs
Item the chef Rent off the chyrch Revys in northwithom ijd
Item the chef Rent off Robard Walton ijd ob
Item the pastur in swafeld callyd hollyng thys yer falo xxd
Item the pasture in swafeld callyd lytylling thys yer falo xijd
Item certen off the lxxxx leys in the feld callyd broken land
thys yer falo ijs viijd
Item the closse in coynthorp lyeth vacant with the land that
longyth therto [no sum]
Summa off dekays v li viijs jd ob

Merceyments ffor sewt off cowrt to dyverse lords
In primis to the kyngs cowrt at Staunford [no sum]
Item to the kyngs cowrt at eston [no sum]
Item to the kyngs cowrt att langdyk for owr land in Borosokyn
(for thes ij yers *ins*) ijs
Item for northluffnam to the prior of brooke (essoyn and mercyments *ins*) vijd
Item for the kyngs lete ther (essoyne and mercyments *ins*) vijd
Item ffor j ffyn to the kyng ffor hys cowrt Baron ther xijd
Item to the kyngs cowrt at Stretton ffor ij essoyns ijd
Item to my lady boschers[124] cowrt at thystelton for Sowthwithom [no sum]
Item to lord greys cowrt at corby for the maner off Swafeld viijd
Item to Robard eylonds cowrt att wylsthorpe [no sum]
Summa vs

Summa lateris vj li ijs xjd
probatum est per me henricum wykys

fol 43v

Ad huc de compoto pro Anno Regni Regis henrici vij xviij^{o} compotus octavus

costys in kepyng off owr cowrts att swaffeld and northwithom
In primis I the warden expendyd goyng to the cowrt at swafeld
the vj and vij days off october vjd
Item for costs off cowrt kept ther the viij day off october ijs ijd
Item for horshyer to the cowrt at northwithom the ix day off october vjd
Item for costs in kepyng owr cowrt ther the same day xxd
Item I Rewardyd the steward for kepyng thes ij cowrts ijs
Item I expendyd goyng to swaffeld cowrt the xix the xx
the xxj day off aprill viijd
Item for costs in kepyng the cowrt ther the same tyme ijs vd
Item I Rewardyd the steward for kepyng thys cowrt xijd
Summa off costs off cowrt xs xjd

---

[124] Busshey, see VCH *Rutland* ii pp155-6

Casuall costys thys yer

In primis for papur iiijd

Item the halylofe for the hows at the mallere brygg xix day of november iijd

Item the halylofe for the hows in seynt myhell parysch v day off march ijd

Item payd to john mysterton ffor accquietans off all maner maters and accions past vjs viijd

Item for Red wax to the sealyng off the seyd accquietaunce jd

Item I Rewarded hym an other tyme viijd

Item I expendyd opon hym at the awngell when he browgt evydence ijd

Item I expendyd at john golyns hows when I brak the indenture bytwene hym and the almoshows jd

Item for makyng the tapurs off wax opon the awter in the chappell off the almoshows xvjd

Item for horshyer to gretham to speke with hyr that was hyksons wyffe off carlby for to bye hyr hows and land in carlby that joynyth opon owr hows xviij day off junii vjd

Item I expendyd ther the same day opon me and mydylton[125] beydman (iiijd *del*) vd

Item the halylofe for the schopp that cleypoll hyred in all halo parysch vj day off august iijd

[126]Summa off casuall costys xs xjd

Expenses in gaderyng up the Rent and overseyng the lyflode off thys almoshows and the Reparacions

In primis I Rewardyd Arnold morton for gaderyng Rents off Swaffeld coynthorp northwithom Sowthwithom twyford gunby Sewstern Steynby wolsthorp and other hys labors overseyng Reparacions xs

Item for hys gown the last yer and thys yer iijs (iiijd *del*) iijd

Item I john taylyor warden haf expendyd in gaderyng the Rents and overseyng the lyflode and dyverse Reparacions thys yer as hyt aperyth by a byll off my expens' vjs viijd

Summa xxs

Summa lateris xljs xd
probatum est per me h Wykys

fol 44

Ad huc de compoto pro Anno Regni Regis henrici vij xviij° *compotus octavus*

off thyngs bowgt ffor stor off hows

In primis ij payr geamaws vijd

Item j henglok ijd

Item j lode playster ijs xjd

Item j lytyll peyr bonds ffor wyndows and hoks jd

[125] alias John Bendslow bedesman

[126] A substantial space has been left before the total of these casual costs, as if there were more to be copied up.

Item for sawyng leghys and evysbord viijd

Item j m^{l} sklatt off yong cordall off eston iiijs

Item to hewe douch for cariag' off the same to the almos hows viijd

Item v old dor bands ijd ob

Item ffor tymbur bord and evysbord bowgt off john scharps wife of seynt johns parysche xxs

Item payd to wyllam Baker for cariag' of the same to the barn vjd

Item j m^{l} sklatt off the seyd agnes scharpe john scharps wyffe iiijs viijd

Item to arnold morton for cariag' off the same to the almoshows iiijd

Item to arnold for cariag' off olde sklatts ffrom edward Bakers dor jd

Item bogt of agnes scharpe j so to ber in water vd

Item off hyr j schovell iiijd

Item off hyr a whelebaro xd

Item off thomas andrew beydman j schovell iijd

Item off jarves cowpar j soo to ber in water xd

Item off john stanley off carlby vij skaffold hyrdylls xxjd

Item for makyng off ij keys for ij loks bowgt off old [sic] iiijd

Item ij Ryddells and j syffe iiijd

Item iij mortar bollys and hopyng off them vjd

Item half C grete naylys ffor grete yat iiijd

Item half m^{l} grete spykyngs iijs iiijd

Item j grete wyndull to putt in naylys iijd

Item jC and x crestys vijs viijd

Item j m^{l} hart lath off yong cordale off eston iiijs ijd

Item ij m^{l} sap lathe off the seyd cordale iiijs ijd

Item j bord kebull bowgt off john holm off Swaffeld xjd

Item (to Arnold *del*) for cariag' off the same from Swafeld to stawnford vjd

Item for hewyng the same kebull vjd

Item payd in exchawnge for j grete balk at Swafeld iiijd

Item for cariag' of the seyd balk from Swafeld xd

Item for hewyng the same balk iiijd

Item for cariag' off the same balk to the barn when he was hewyn jd

Item j bord kebull bowgt off Arnold morton off Swafeld xvijd

Item for cariag' off the seyd kebull xjd

Item for hewyng the same kebull vjd

Item cariag' off tymbur that was exchawnged with campion of Swafeld xd

Item john hygen for hewyng the seyd tymbur ij days and half xvd

Item for tymbur bowgt off john wrygt off eston xvij cowpyll spars xx sawyn trasyngs iiij stod loggys ij brase loggys v balks iiij wall plats ij planks and j pelor logg xxjs iiijd

Item payd to hew douch of eston for cariag' of the seyd tymbur to the barn v lode xxd

Item payd to Robard newton sawar and john geffreyson sawer for sawyng the bord kebull that was bowgt off john holm and that kebull that was bowgt off Arnold and the tymbur that I had off campion and the iiij stod loggys and ij brase loggys and the pelor logg bowgt off john wrygte viij days viijs
Item for cariag' off the seyd sawyn tymbur to the barn vjd
Summa istius part' v li iijd ob

Summa lateris v li iijd ob
probatum est per me henricum Wykys

fol 44v

compotus octavus
Ad huc de compoto pro Anno Regni Regis henrici septimi decimo octavo
off thyngs bowgt for stor off hows

Item payd to hewgh douch ffor cariag' off j long leddyr pece	)	
ffrom eston [to] stawnford	iiijd)	
Item to john hygen for hewyng the seyd leddyr pece	vjd)	
Item for sawyng the seyd leddyr pece	vjd)	Summa
Item to john hygen for makyng the seyd leddyr	vjd)	ijs vd
Item for j clasp off yrn to mend a frett in the same leddyr	vjd)	
Item for cariag' off the seyd leddyr to the almos hows	jd)	

Item for j Roope to draw watyr in tyme off neede for buyldyng xd
Item for mendyng off the cheynys off the bokett thatt was at the well off the almoshows ijd
Item to john henley and Robard yats for cowchyng up off tymbur in the barnvjd
Summa istius part' iijs xjd
Summa (total *ins*) off thyngs bowgt for stor off hows v li iiijs ijd ob

Reparacion at Stawnford at the hows next mallere brygg in all halo parysch
In primis ij keys on to the hall dor an other to the bak yate iiijd
Item to wyllam mason of seynt clement parysch for undyrpynnyng dyverse threscholds and dawbyng up the dor beneyth the well j day and half vijd ob
Item the seyd wyllam to mend the walls toward the lane off the mallere aftyr the grete water xvjd
Item j lode ston to the same mendyng (payd to wyllam Baker *ins*) iijd
Item the seyd wyllam Baker for j lode mortar erth to the same iijd
Item to john hygen carpentar for mendyng the pale vj days iijs
Item to wyllam baker for j lode ston for to mend the growndwark of [*del*] the seyd pale iijd
Item to wyllam baker for ij lode mortar to the same growndwark vjd
Item john denys mason and hys felo makyng the same growndwark j day xijd
[127]Item john henley and john hosteler ij servars to the seyd masons j day viijd

[127] left hand marginal note 'Stawnford'

Item to john hygen carpentar for wrygtwark mendyng the well v days ijs vjd
Item to cutberd moor laborer to clense the howsys and the yard
aftyr the grete water vjd
(Item for j Rope to drawe water in tyme off nee *del*)
Item wyllam mason and hys felo to mend the cope wall abowt yard
j day and half xviijd
Item j servar to them j day iiijd
Item to wyllam Baker for ij lode mortar to the seyd copyng vjd
Item to john hygen carpenter for drawyng in off ij trasyngs in the florth
that was new plastyrd and mendyng the lytyll thakkyd stabull j day vjd
Item j lode playster to mend the florth ijs viijd
Item to harry playsterer off okham for bornyng betyng syftyng
Redyng and schotyng the seyd florth vj days iijs
Item hys laborrar to help hym vj days ijs
Item on other laborer to help ber water and to serve when he
schott the florth iijd
Item for makyng j trap dor hespys and stapulls to the seyd chawmbyr iiijd
Summa xxijs iijd ob

Summa lateris xxvjs ijd ob
Probatum est per me henricum wykys

fol 45

Ad huc compoto pro Anno Regni Regis henrici vij xviij° *compotus octavus*

Stawnford

Reparacion at edward Bakers in all halo parysch
Item for sawyng off planks for the stabull in the yard toward the garden xviijd
Item john hygen and john wrygt for plankyng the seyd stabull and
mendyng the florth for hys whete xvjd
Item to wyllam mason off seynt clement parysch for settyng
off j fornas for hys pan xjd
Item payd to john henley for goyng myne erand to speke with
the prior off fynshed for to hafe awey the Ramell in edward bakers yard jd
Item payd to wyllam Baker for cariag' off the seyd Ramell that was part
off the leynto thatt felle down part off the priors hows that fell down xd
Summa iiijs viijd

Reparacion at the hows next the vycar off all halos
In primis for clensyng the withdrawgt in the chawmbyr to john hemylden viijd
Item payd to john henley laborer to rensak the fowndacion off the old kyln and
castyng off the mortar erth that cam owt off edward Bakers yard iiij days xvjd
Item payd to john denys and thomas sayer ij masons makyng up the
wallys of the kyln iiij days and half iiijs vjd
Item ij servars to them iiij days and half john henley and Robard brewster iijs
Item I expendyd opon the warkmen ther jd
Item for cariag' off iiij lode ston from Robard cavys hows to the seyd kiln iiijd

Item to wyllam baker for ij lode mortar to the seyd kyln	vjd
Item to arnold morton for cariag' off a bem and trasyngs from swafeld to the seyd kyln	xxd
Item for hewyng the seyd tymbur	xijd
[128]Item to John Smyth for cariag' off the tymbur to the water[129]	iijd
Item to wyllam baker for cariag' off the seyd tymbur from the water	ijd
Item for sawyng off the seyd tymbur for trasyngs to the kyln	xjd
Item for wrygt ware [sic] abowt the seyd kyln	iiijd
Item for wrygt wark to john hygen and Robard clerk for mendyng the parlar dor the chawmbyr dor settyng in ij pelors in the chawmbyr wyndow and me[n]dyng other wyndows the spens dor the schop dor (and mendyng the garner *ins*) the space off j day	xijd
Item to harry west carpentar for makyng the partycion in the entre j day (with hys prentes *ins*)	vijd
Item allowyd bassyll laxton that schuld be tennant for tymbur to the seyd particion	vjd
Item payd to john henley for brekyng down the old particion and clensyng the gutter betwene both howsys mendyng the chymney in the hall and undyr pynnyng the wallys in the yard iij days	xijd
Item to wyllam mason for lathyng and dawbyng at the seyd particion j day	vjd
Item to the seyd wyllam and john henley for dawbyng the particion j day	xd
Item half sem lyme to pargett the particion	iiijd
Item wyllam mason and john henley for dawbyng the garner j day	xd
Item to wyllam Baker for j lode mortar to the seyd dawbyng	iijd
Item wyllam mason and john henley for makyng dyverse jeawmys and undyr pynnyng the wallys in the wod yard j day	xd
Item the seyd wyllam and henley for brekyng up a fre ston dor in the hall bytwene both howsys	xd
Item ij masons to stop up the dor ageyn ij days	ijs
Item john henley to serve them ij days	viijd
Item to wyllam Baker for cariag' off iij lode ston off Robard cavys from the bocherow to the same wark	vjd
Item to wyllam Baker for ij lode mortar to the seyd wark	vjd
Item for half j sem lyne to pargett the wallys	iiijd
Item to john henley for havyng away the Ramell of the kyln off the dawbyng and mason wark	vjd
Item for iij keys to the wykett the schope dor and the parlar dor	vjd
Item j dor band to the chawmbyr dor	jd
Item v keys to the iiij chawmbyr dor' and the gyle hows dor	xd

[128] 'Stawnford' in left-hand margin

[129] presumably to the river Welland but whether for seasoning the timber in the river or relating to river-borne transport is not clear.

Item for glasyng a lytyll wyndow at the grese hede iiijd
(Item for gret lathys to the kyln. Item for lathyng off the kyln Summa *del*)
Summa xxviijs vjd

Summa lateris xxxiijs ijd
Probatum est per me h Wykys

fol 45v

Ad huc de compoto pro Anno Regni Regis henrici vij xviij compotus octavus

Stawnford

Reparacion at the the [sic] hows on wolrow of john thomas in All halo parysch and at hys oven

Item to wyllam mason off seynt clement parysch to mend in plaster wark dyverse holys broken in the schopp and in the entre iij days xviijd
Item to mend hys oven ij lode walcot ston with the cariag' and hyeryng john henley twys to go for hytt xxijd
Item to wyllam baker for iij lode mortar ixd
Item to wyllam baker for cariag' off ij lode ston from the dofcote in bredcroft vjd
Item to john denys and wyllam scherwyn ij masons for makyng the seyd oven iij days and half iijs vjd
Item j servar to them iij days and half xiiijd
Item j sem lyme for to temper the mortar for the oven viijd
Item to john hygen carpentar for wrygt wark to make a Rofe for the owen [sic] j day vjd
Item to Rawlyn lokkey off wyrthorp sklatter in coveryng the seyd oven (iij *del*) and the hows end mendyng and the swyncote mendyng iij days and half xxd
Item j sem lyme to the same sklattyng viijd
Item to wyllam Baker for cariag' awey off ij lode Ramell aftyr the sklatter and masons had don iiijd
Summa xiijs jd

Staunford

Reparacion at the hows next master wyllam elmys

In primis payd to herry west and hys felo ij carpentars for makyng off j pentes and j hach at the hall dor ij days wark ijs
Item to john colyn off eston for sklattyng the seyd pentes xvd
Item for half j sem lym to the seyd sklattyng iiijd
Item to john hemeldon for clensyng the seage vijd
Item to wyllam mason off seynt clement parysch for mendyng the florths (ij days *ins*) xd
Summa vs

Stawnford

Reparacion at the sygne off the crane in seynt petur parysch at the wall toward the castell

Item to john henley for Ryddyng off ston and mortar and dygyng the fundacion aftyr the wall was fallen havyng awey the Ramell and the mukk aftyr the thak hows was fallen down iij days and half xiiijd
Item to john denys mason to mak the wall ij days xijd
Item to Robard brewster hys servar ij days viijd
Item to john denys mason and thomas Sar off weteryng mason iij days and half iijs vjd
Item to Robard brewster ther servar iij days and half xiiijd
Item to wyllam Baker for cariag' off v lode ston from the dofcote in Bredcroft xvd
Item to the seyd wyllam Baker ffor iiij lode mortar to the seyd wall xijd
Item to john henley for to dygg ston at the dofcote for the seyd wall iiij days xiiijd
Summa xs xjd

Reparacion at bredcroft at the gret closse

Item ij masons off okham to stop up the old dor in the est end and to mak a new dor in the myddys off the wall xxd
Item ij servars to dygg ston and to serve the masons ij days xiiijd
(Item j wrygt to mend the dor *del*)
Item to Robard yatt laborer for dyggyng the fundacion and Rensakyng the ston iij days and half xd ob
(Item to wyllam Baker for havyng awey the Ramell of the dofcote lode *del*)
Summa iijs viijd ob

Summa lateris xxxijs viijd ob
Probatum est per me henricum wykys
(*Summa lateris* del)

fol 46

Ad huc de compoto A° Regni Regis henrici vij xviij° *compotus octavus*

Staunford

Reparacion at the hows in Seynt myhell parysch

Item payd to wyllam hynkley for cariag' off a grete pece of tymbur from the barn to mend the govell off the seyd hows ijd
Item to john hygen and harry laxton ij carpentars for leyng off the seyd pece and settyng in dyverse stodds in the west govell off the hyest chawmbyr xviijd
Item to john henley for cariag' off the plaster off the seyd govell to the almos hows iijd
Item to the sere [seyd?] henley for takyng down the old leynto in the yard iijd
Item to hym for Ryddyng the ston and mortar of the wall that fell down over the fornas iijd

Item payd to john denys mason for makyng the seyd wall over
the fornas ij days and half xvd
Item to Robard brewster hys servar ij days and half xd
Item to wyllam baker for iiij lode mortar to the same wall xijd
Item to wyllam mason of seynt clement parysch ffor stoppyng up a
blynd chymney in the chambyr and mendyng the harthys off other
ij chymneys iij days xviijd
Item for xij tyle stonys to the same mendyng jd
Item to john henley hys servar iij days xijd
Item to wyllam Baker for cariag' off iij lode ston to the same wark
from owr feld yate vjd
Item for ij stryk lyme to pargett with all ijd
Item to the seyd wyllam baker for cariag' off (iij *ins*) lode old plaster
from the seyd hows to the almos hows vjd
Item payd for ij lode new plaster vs iiijd
Item ffor wod to born the seyd plaster ijs
Item payd to harry plasterar off okham for bornyng betyng syftyng the
seyd playster makyng the panys in the seyd west govell Redyng and
schotyng the florth over the hall and the kychen and mendyng in
plaster wark dyverse fawgts in the chawmbyrs xv days and half vijs ixd
Item to hys servar to help hym to serve all thes xv days and half vs ijd
Item to cutberd mor laborer to help to bete plaster and ber plaster
and watter v days xviijd
Item to Robard alenson laborer to help when he schott the florth j day iiijd
Summa xxxjs iiijd

Stawnford Reparacion at the almos hows
Item to john denys rhe mason for removyng off the dor off the beydmens
garden ij days and half xvd
Item to Robard brewster hys servar ij days and half xd
Item to the plommar of seynt andrew parysch for mendyng the
spowt toward the wey syde xijd
Summa iijs jd

Summa lateris xxxiiijs vd
Probatum est per me henricum Wykys

fol 46v

Ad huc de compoto pro A° R' R' henrici vij xviij compotus octavus

Staunford

Reparacion at the awngell
In primis payd to dyverse laborers for Ryddyng the ston and mortar
and tymbur off the brew hows thatt ffell down at mydlent ijs xd
Item payd to Bacon of Seynt peter parysch for vj lode ston to the
walls of the seyd hows ijs
Item to the seyd Bacon ffor x lode mortar erth to the same iijs iiijd

Item to the seyd Bacon for cariag' off old tymbur from the seyd awngell to the almos hows and off the new Rofe aftyr hytt was framyde to the seyd awngell xjd
Item for wrygtwark makyng the seyd Rofe a grete to john hygen and john wrygt carpentars vjs iiijd
Item payd to ij masons off ufford for making the wallys v days wark vs
Item ij laborers to serve them v days iijs
Item for ij m[l] sklatt and half with the cariag' of the same for the Rofe xijs ijd
Item for tymbur to make the seyd Rofe bowrt by the carpenter john hyggen at Belmysthorp viijs jd
Item vj sem lyme (and half *del*) to the sklattyng iiijs
Item for cariag' off sand from the barn by the hands off laborers for defawt of j cart xvd
Item payd to Rawlyn lokkey off wyrthorp and pers polver off the same town for sklattyng wark off the seyd hows iij Rode wark xiijs vjd
Item the seyd ij masons to furr up the govells and fynysch the wallys when the sklatters had don j day xijd
Item j server to them j day iiijd
Item to Rawlyn lokkey sklatter for mendyng dyverse other fawyts ther iiij days ijs
Item for half j sem lyme to the same mendyng iiijd
Item ij wrygts john hygen and john wrygt to mend a gresyng foote vjd
Item ffor clensyng off the gutter bytwene the awngell and the Bull off the Ramell that was left off the fallyng off the hows (iiii laborers iiij days *ins*) vjd
Item to dyverse laborers to cary awey the Ramell owt off the yard aftyr the wark was don v days ijs iiijd
Item to john Smyth Baker for cariag' off iiij lode Ramell owt of the same viijd
Item the tennant was allowyd toward the losse of a maschfatt thatt was Broken with the fall off the hows xijd
Item I payd to harry plasterar off okham for mendyng dyverse holys in the chawmbyrs specially in the grete chawmbyr ij days wark xijd
Item to hys laborer to serve hym ij days viijd
Item to hew smyth for yrn wark and settyng up the sygne of thawngell ijs
Summa iij li xvjs vijd

probatum est per me h Wyk'

fol 47

Ad huc de compoto pro A° R' R' henrici vij xviij compotus octavus
Stawnford

Reparacion at the hows in seynd marten parysch ther as the Roper dwellyd last yer wher the myllar john dowse dwellyth now thys yer
In primis for thak to thak the gy hows in the yard toward the garden ijs iijd
Item to kesten of wyrthorp thakkar for thakkyng off the same xijd
Item to john denys the mason for makyng a wall of the hows that is now the myll hows iijs iiijd

Item to john hygen carpentar for makyng a new dor and dornys to
the seyd hows vjd
Item to the smyth of seynt mary parysch for j peyr hoks to the seyd dor ijd
Summa vijs iijd

Stawnford

Reparacion at the hows in seynt marten parysch where netylton the mason dwellyth

In primis payd to john hygen and herry laxton ij carpentars for undyrsettyng the hows syde toward the garden with cariag' off tymbur for the same wark xiijd
Item payd to john denys the mason for makyng the wall off the seyd hows syde agrete by the Rode sqwar pric' the Rode aftyr *vd ob* j fote viijs iijd the [*del*] wark conteyning j Rode and half summa total xijs iiijd ob
Item to hewgh douch off eston for xv lode ston to the same wall vs
Item for laborers in having in the seyd ston vjd
Item for mortar to the seyd wark ijs
Item expendyd opon the masons ther when they wrowgt jd
Item to the seyd mason to make the heynyng walls at both ends of
the wall j day vjd
Item to hys servar Robard brewster j day to serve hym iiijd
Item for cariag' off skaffold hyrdyls to the same wark ijd
Item to john hygen carpenter for drawyng in off ij balks in the
seyd hows j day vjd
Item to john henley and other folk to help hym to lyft the balks vd
Item to (the seyd *del*) wyllam Baker for cariag' of the seyd ij balks
from the barn ijd
Item for tymbur to mak taylefete to the seyd hows xijd
Item to john hygen and Robard clerk ij carpentars to make the seyd
taylefete and settyng in off them and the evys bord j day and half xviijd
Item for cariag' off the seyd taylfete evys bord and sklatt from
the almos hows ijd
Item to Rawlyn lokkey sklatter mendyng the seyd hows vj days iijs
Item to hys servar iij days xijd
Item for j sem lyme to the same wark xijd
Item to john hygen carpenter for makyng j dor in her brewhows vjd
Item ffor j peyr hoks and new bands to the seyd dor ijd
Item john denys mason and wyllam scherwyn mason for settyng in
the seyd dor and bem fyllyng the chawmbyr abofe j day ijd
Item Robard brewster ther servar j day iiijd
Item for mendyng off the hedgh iiijd
Summa xxxiijs jd ob

Summa lateris xls iiijd ob
probatum est per me henricum Wyk'

fol 47v

Ad huc de compoto pro Anno Regni Regis henrici vij xviij° compotus octavus

Reparacion at pylsyate

In primis payd to John geoy off bernak mason and wyllam mason of seynt clement parysch in stawnford for ij days wark at the govell off the grete barn xxd
Item j servar to them ij days viijd
Item to the tennant for ij lode mortar to the same wark iiijd
Item for j sem lyme from stawnford to the same wark viijd
Item for cariag' off lyntels to the same wark jd
Item to Robard caryngton off ufford mason to mend the wall toward the feld syde xxd
Item peyd to the tennant waren for cariag' off iiij lode ston from whypps pytt off Bernak viijd
Item payd to the seyd whypp off bernak for the seyd iiij lode ston viijd
Item to the tennant for ij lode mortar to the seyd wall iiijd
Item to the seyd Robard caryington for mendyng dyverse coynys and the oven mowth xd
Item to wyllam mason off seynt clements parysch for mendyng the wall undyr the evys off the long barn toward the yard syde and the wall off the same toward the wey syde ij days xijd
Item to john henley to serve the seyd mason ij days viijd
Item Robard Kesten off wyrthorp for thakkyng the ij barnys and sewyng iiij days xxd
Item j servar to hym iiij days xijd
Item j servar to hym when he sewyd iij days ixd
Item for cariag' off Reed to the same thakkyng jd
Item j half dos[en] thak Rope viijd
Item for j lode stobull from tekyngcote xviijd
Item iij lode stobull from Burley ijs vijd
Item to the tennant for iij lode mortar to Rygg with all vjd
Item to yong hamulden off wyrthorp ffor half thowsand sklatt to mend dyverse fawts ther ijs
Item to the tennant waren for cariag' off the seyd sklatt from wyrthrop to pylsyate vjd
Item to Rawlen lokkey off wyrthorp sklatter for mendyng the grete barn end ij days xijd
Item j servar to hym j day iiijd
Item to the seyd Rawlyn lokkey for ij Rode and half poyntyng of the kyln hows ijs iijd ob
Item to the seyd Rawlyn for j Rode and half poyntyng off the hall toward the hye wey xvjd ob
Item for iij sem lyme and half from stawnford to the seyd wark ijs iiijd
Item to the tennant for cariag' off the seyd lyme from stawnford vd

[130]Item for sande ijd
Item to John Smyth Baker for cariag' off j balk to mend the long thakkyd barn and j standard bord' leghys and naylys for dyverse dorrs iiijd
Item to john hygen and john wrygt ij carpentars for drawyng in the seyd balk in the seyd long barn and makyng j dor in the entre off the garrett yate, makyng the garden dor, mendyng the feld yate by the long barn syde j day and half xviijd
Item for j peyr off hoks to john tyard for the seyd feld yate ijd

Summa lateris xxxs vd
probatum est per me h wyk'
(*Summa lateris* del)

fol 48

Ad huc de compoto pro Anno Regni Regis henrici vij xviij° compotus octavus

Reparacion at eston

At Bryans hows

In primis Rawlyn lokkey sklatter for vj days wark iijs)
Item hys servar iiij days xvjd)
Item ij sem lyme and half to the same wark xxd)
Item for cariag' of the lyme from stawnford ijd)
Item to hew douch for j lode sand iiijd)
Item for a mason allowyd the tennant for mendyng the)
corner off the kyln hows viijd) [131]Summa
Item for j stolp to the feld yate ijd) xjs vd
Item for wrygt wark mendyng the feld yate iiijd)
Item to wyllym yvys mason mendyng the oven mowth)
and other fawts ther he and hys prentes j day xd)
Item to Robard Russell hys servar j day iiijd)
Item to the tennant for j ston for the oven mowthe iiijd)
Item to john denys and wyllam scherwyn masons mendyng the (feld *del*) wall toward the feld j day xd
Item Robard brewster ther servar j day iijd
Item wyllyam scherwyn by hymself ther j day vd
Item Robard brewster to serve hym the same day iijd
Item to heugh douch for iij lode ston to the same wall vjd

At fox hows callyd the dowry

Item j lode sand spent ther and at other plac' bowgt off hew douch iiijd)
Item to Rawlyn lokkey sklatter for poyntyng ther j day vjd)
Item j sem lyme with cariag' ffrom stawnford ixd)
Item to hew douch for ij lode stobull for the barn ijs viijd)
Item to kesten of wyrthorp to thak the same iij days xvd)
Item hys servar iij days ixd)

[130] this line is written at the end of the previous line

[131] in right-hand margin

Item j servar when he Ryggyd ij days vjd)
Item for thak Rope iiijd)
Item for mortar to Rygg with all ijd)
Item to ij masons scherwyn and denys to mend the)
garden wall bytwene hym and Bryans (iij days *ins*) ijs vjd)
Item j servar to them iij days Robard brewster ixd)
Item for ston to the same j lode ijd)
[132]Item vj lode mortar xijd)
Item for a laborer Ryddyng the ston off the seyd (wall *ins*) viijd)
[133]Summa xijs iiijd

At the carvers hows
Item ij lode stobbull of hew douche ijs viijd)
Item to kesten off wyrthorp to thak the same iij days xvd)
Item hys servar iij days ixd)
Item to j pec' of tymbur off yong cordale to mak a)
plaster florth over the hall vs vijd)
Item allowyd the tennant the carver toward makyng of the seyd florth xijs)
Item for mortar to Rygg withall to the thakkar ijd)
Item j lode stobull off hew douch xvjd)
Item the thakkar off belmsthorp for the same stobbull ij days xd)
Item j servar to hym ij days *iijd ob* j day vijd)
Summa xxvs ijd

Summa lateris xlviijs xjd
Probatum est per me henricum Wykys

fol 48v

Ad huc de compoto pro A° R' R' henrici vij xviij compotus octavus
Reparacion at Eston

Att the cotag' next the carver where wyllyam yvys dwellyth
Item to (hew douch *del*) (john elys son *ins*) off eston for ij lode stobull iijs
Item to kesten for thakkyng the same on the strete syde
iij days and half xvijd ob
Item hys servar iij days and half xd ob
Item an other lode off hew douch xviijd
Item kesten and hys servar for the same xijd
Item for mortar to Rygg withall ijd
Item j lode stobbull off hew douch xvjd
Item the thakkar off belmysthorp to thak hytt ij days xd
Item j servar to the thakker ij days vijd
Summa xs ixd[134]

---

[132] This line inserted at the end of the previous line

[133] in right-hand margin

[134] in right-hand margin

At john wrygts hows
Item the tennant was allowyd for mendyng the wall toward the closse of tatersale | vjd
Item Rawlyn lokkey sklatter j day | vjd
Item to wyllyam yvys mason and hys prentes for mendyng the wall toward whytwell ij days | ijs vjd
Item to Robard Russell ther servar iij days | xijd
Item to hew douch for iiij lode ston to the same wall | viijd
Item for vij lode mortar | xiiijd
Item for strey to mend the evys of the hows | [no sum]
Item to a thakkar for the same mendyng | [no sum]
Item to wyllyam yvys mason and hys prentes for takyng down the chymney topp j day | xd
Item to the seyd wyllyam and hys prentes to sett up the chymney ageyn ij days | xxd
Item to Robard Russell ther servar ij days | viijd
Item for ij lode ston for the same chymney | iiijd
Item for ij lode mortar to the same | iiijd
Item to hew douch for cariag" off skaffold hyrdylls from stanford to the same wark | ijd
Item to old hawkyn sklatter for mendyng the hows aftyr makyng of the chymney iij days | xviijd
Item for j sem lyme and half to the same mendyng | xijd
Item for cariag' of the seyd lyme and sand | iiijd
Item for cariag' off Reede from stawnford to mend the long hows | ijd
Item allowyd john wrygte the tennant in hys departing for j speer at the tabull ende of the particion in the entre and a lytyll mylk hows in the celar and bords on the gresyngs in the same hows and ij lokks | ijs

Summa xvs iiijd[135]

Summa lateris xxvjs jd
(*Summa lateris* del)
probatum est per me h Wyk'

fol 49

Ad huc compoto per Anno Regni Regis henrici vij xviij^o compotus octavus

Reparacion at warmyngton
Item payd to john elys the mason for mendyng the jealmys off the hall iiij days | xijd
Item j lode ston from owndell pytts to the same wark | viijd
Item to the seyd john elys for makyng erth wark at the kyln | xvjd
Item to the seyd John for underpynnyng off the malt hows viij days | ijs
Item for ij lode ston for the same wark | xvjd
Item ffor Reede and thak Rope with the cariag' | iijs

---

[135] in right-hand margin

Item j thakkar vj days iijs
Item vij lode straw bowgt by Robard beomond off [sic] vs xd
Item for of [sic] vj lode of the seyd straw xijd
Item ij servars to the seyd thakkar vj days *vjd* j day iijs
Item payd to Robard eton carpentar by Robard beomond for makyng the malt hows the whych payment I allowyd Robard beomond in hys accowmpts *de Anno R' R' henr'* vij xv° and Rekynd with hym in *anno R 'R' henr'* vij xviij the xxiiij day of decembar[136] amongst other Receyts vjs viijd
I allowyd Robard person the tennant for payng to the seyd Robard eton for makyng the seyd malt hows viijd
Item to the seyd tennant allowyd for the same cawse ijs viijd
Item for dawbyng and splentyng the wall off the malt hows vs iiijd
Item for hooks and hengels xijd
Item for mendyng off the sewstern in the malt hows xijd
Item for mendyng off the oven xvjd
Item for makyng off a mud wall at the malt hows ende vjd
Item for j dorr to the seyd malt hows (xd *del*) viijd
Item for j lode straw to thakk the seyd malt hows xd
Item for thakkyng off the same straw xd
Item payd to a carpentar for settyng in off vj stodds and ij brasys in the seyd malt hows xd
Item for splentyng open the kyln viijd
Item for nayle to the seyd splentyng ijd
Item for ix trasyngs to mend the chawmbyr florth vjd
Item for wrygt wark off the same florth and Rokkyng off the same vjd
Item payd to a mason for drawyng off the govell at the hall ende for hys Bargeyn agreyte ijs xd
Item for makyng the yate for commyng in off a cart at the strete syde iiijd
Item for vart nayls to the seyd yate ijd
Item I payd to the tennant for iij lode straw to thak the howsys ijs vjd
Item for Reede to the hows ende [no sum]
Item for thak Rope to the same
Item to the thakkar on the hall end aftyr drawyng off the govell
Item for a balk to the barn xd
Item for wrygt wark drawyng in the balk xvjd
Item for a walplate vd
Item for j growndsell to the barn iiijd
Item wrygt wark drawing in the walplate and leyng in the seyd growndsell and settyng in off vj stodds vd
Item for leyng in of an other growndsell at the barn end and settyng in iij stodds vd
Item for dawbyng the barn iiijd

---

[136] this sum was in Beomond's account for 1499-1500 but was not accounted for until 24 December 1502; it does not appear in Taylor's account for 1499-1500 above. Accounts were apparently drawn up on Christmas Eve.

Item for a walplate at the hall ende vijd
Item for leyng in the wall plate and iij spars vjd
Item ij lode ston for the govell iiijd
Item the cariag" at the tennant' cost[137]
Item for masyn wark at the same govell[138] xvijd

Summa lateris lixs jd
probatum est per me henricum Wykys

fol 49v

Ad huc de compoto pro A° Regni Regis henrici vij xviij° compotus octavus

Reparacion at northluffnam

Item skarboro the tennant was allowyd for makyng off j wall at skulthorp in A° R' R' henr' vij xvij° [1501-2] xiijd
Item for j peyr off hengels to a dorr ijd
Item ffor dykyng and hedghyng of a grownd by the nete gate v akers and j Roode in lenghth pric' j acr' lenghth *xiiijd* and the Roode lenghth *iiijd* summa vjs ijd
Summa vijs vd

Reparacion at stretton at Skelyngtons hows

Item for watyllwand xijd
Item for schreddyng the same iiijd
Item for wattyllyng the nett hows syde viijd
Item for iij lode strey to the thakkyng off the hows iijs jd
Item j thakkar on the same hows iij days xvd
Item ij servars to hym iij days xviijd
Item ij lode mortar to Rygg with all vjd
Item allowyd the tennant Robard skelyngton for tymbur to the particion in the selar xijd
Item for bords to mak certen dorrs viijd
Item for j peyr off gresyngs in the selar iiijd
Item for ij new lokks with ij keys viijd
Item for ij stapulls ijd
Item for j key for the lok on the hall dor ijd
Item for x stryk lyme xd
Item j sklatter to mend the chambyr and the barn ij days xijd
Item j servar to hym ij days vjd
[139]Summa xiijs viijd

[137] It may be that the items for which no sums are given are those for which the tenant was responsible.

[138] there is no *summa* for the repairs at Warmington

[139] this *summa* and the next are in the right hand margin, not below the entries

At the hows that akerlond dwelt in
In primis vij trasyngs for a chawmbyr florth bowgt off Robard Skelyngton xijd
Item to a carpentar for leyng off the seyd trasyngs iijd
Item for ij lode plaster for the florth vs iijd
Item j lode wod to born' the plaster xvjd
Item for cariag' of Rede lath and nayle for the florth ijd
Item to herry plasterar of okham for makyng the florth
vj days *vd* j day summa ijs vjd
Item hys servar vj days xviijd
Item j servar to ber water and plaster when he schott the florth j day iijd
Item for candyll lygt to wyrk withal jd
Summa xijs jd

Summa lateris xxxiijs ijd
probatum est per me henricum wykys

fol 50

Ad huc de compoto pro A° Regni Regis henrici vij xviij° *compotus octavus*
Reparacion at northwithom - at wyllam scherschaws
In primis to a sklatter ffor poyntyng on the hall ix Rode viijs iijd
Item vij sem lyme to the same with cariag' from swafeld vs ijd
Item for ij lode sand to the same poyntyng xijd
Item the tennant wyllam scherschaw is allowyd for makyng off
a stabull dor and mendyng off hys barn dorrs ijs
Summa xvjs vd

Reparacion at the hows next the parsonage in the same town
Item for fellyng off xxx sparrs and other tymbur for the kyln' hows
that was brent xijd
Item for cariag' off the same from swynhaw wod ixd
Item for wrygt wark off the same hows vs iijd
Item a wrygt to mend other fawts vd
Item a mason to mend fawts ther half j day ijd ob
Item a mason to make a gutter thoro the entre xxjd
Item iiij lode ston for the same gutter xiijd
Item ij lode mortar for the mason and the thakkar vd
Item iij lode stobull for the kyln' hows vs
Item j dosen Rede schevys for the same vjd
Item for Redyng off the same hows vjd
Item j thakkar to the same hows iij days xvd
Item hys servar iij days ixd
Item j drawer off thak iij days vjd
(Item j thakkar on the barn j day and half vijd ob *del*)
(Item hys servar j day and half iiijd ob *del*)
Item for fellyng off thornys at swynhaw vijd ob
Item for cariag' off the seyd thornys xxd

Item for hedghyng the seyd thornys abowt the hows a man
iij days and half xd ob
Item j wrygt to mak the manger and plank the stabull
and mendyng the yat iij days wark xvd
Summa xxiijs viijd ob

At the cotag'
Item j thakkar j day and half vijd ob
Item j servar to hym j day and half iiijd ob

Summa lateris xljs jd ob
probatum est per me henricum Wykys

fol 50v

Ad huc de compoto pro A° Regni Regis henrici vij xviij° compoto octavus

Reparacion at wolsthorpe by syde northwithom
Item for brekyng off j wall iiijd
Item a mason to mak the wall iiijs vjd
Item viij lode mortar to the seyd wall xvjd
Item ij dosen thak Rope and half xxd
Item for wrygt wark ijd
Item j lode thak with cariag' xxd
Item for thakkyng the same thakk ixd
Item lxxx schevys off Reede xxjd
Item for cariag' of the same xd
Item ij laborers to tak down the hows vjd
Item for cariag' off tymbur from Swynhaw to the seyd hows xijd
Item nycolas wrygt and john cotrell for v days wark and half
makyng the hows vs vjd
Item for Reedyng the hows j day vjd
Item for ij laborers to draw thak and serve the thakkar
ij days and half *vijd* j day Summa xvijd ob
Item j thakkar to thak the seyd barn iij days xviijd
Item iij lode stobbull pric' j lode *xvjd* Summa iiijs
Item j lode mortar to Rygg withal ijd ob
Item to a carpentar ffor makyng the barn dorrs vd
Item for cariag' of the same dorrs from Swafeld to Wolsthorp ijd
Summa xxviijs iijd

Reparacion at swynhaw wode
Item for hedghyng the labor off a man xxiiij days
and half *iijd* j day summa vjs jd ob

Reparacion at northaw wod
Item for hedghyng the north syde lxiiij poll pric' the poll *ob qa* Summa iiijs
Item for hedghyng the sowthsyde xxiij poll pric' the poll *ob qa* Summa xvijd

Reparacion at the closse at coynthorp
Item for hedghyng the seyd closse lxx poll pric' the poll *jd* Summa vs xd

Summa lateris xlvs vijd ob
probatum est per me henricum Wykys

fol 51

Ad huc de compoto pro A° R' R' henrici vij xviij° *compotus octavus*

Reparacion at swafeld

At Arnolds hows
Item for cariag' off peyr gresyngs, bords naylys and dor bands from stawnford to swafeld viijd
Item the seyd arnold was allowyd in hys accompts de A° R' R' hen' xvij° [1501-2] for certen Reparacions don by the cost of the seyd arnold whych Reparacions schuld hafe ben maade by bartylmew holm that was baylyf and tennant ther *A° Regni Regis henrici* vij xv° [1499-1500] wyllam holm (the son of *del*) off gorinschester the son of the seyd Bartylmew being pledgh both for hys Rent *vs* and hys Reparacion iijs xjd
Item j mason j day vd
Item j lode mortar ijd
Item for ij keys for ij lokks iiijd
Item to a carpentar for makyng a speer at the bench end ijd
[140]Summa vs [*erasure*] viijd

At Barnards hows
Item for brekyng down off hys wall off hys schopp ij days vjd
Item for cariag' off ston to the same wall ijs
Item for makyng up the same wall v Rode wark vs

At ffabions hows
Item for sklattyng the dofcote ijs vd ob
Item j sem lyme and half to the same xijd
Item for sand to the same jd

At Robard coys hows
Item iij lode mortar to a wall syde vjd
Item for splentyng the seyd wall iijd
Item for dawbyng the wall ixd
Item j mason j day (at hys kyln hows wall *ins*) vd
Item hys servar j day iijd
Item j lode mortar to the same wark ijd
Item j wrygt to mend trescholds and the standard off hys barn dor iijd
Summa ijs vijd

[140] this and the following sub-totals are in right-hand margin

At jenett holms the wedos hows

Item for splentyng off a govell	iiijd
Item ij dawbers j day	viijd
Item j servar to them j day	iijd
Item iij lode mortar	vjd

At Margarett Janys hows

Item a carpentar to mak a treschold	ijd

Summa lateris xxjs ijd ob
probatum est per me henricum Wykys

fol 51v

Ad huc de compoto pro Anno Regni Regis henrici vij xviij° compotus octavus

Reparacion at Swafeld

At Roger Speds hows

Item iij lode mortar	vjd
Item for splentyng off j govell	iiijd
Item ij dawbers j day	viijd
Item j servar to them j day	iijd
	Summa xxjd

At thomas stroxtons

Item to wynpeny the mason for settyng in off a window with hys server	xiiijd
Item a carpentar to make a threschold (at thomas stroxton *del*) at the stabull dor	ijd
Item j wrygt to mend the chawmbyr j day	vjd
Item iij lode mortar	vjd
Item for splentyng off a govell	iiijd
Item ij dawbers j day	viijd
Item j servar to them j day	iijd
Item I payd to hygen and john wrygt for makyng a window j day	xijd
Item for ij payr bands and hoks for the same wyndow	iiijd
	Summa iiijs xjd

At Bullys hows

Item j mason v days and half	ijs iijd ob
Item hys servar iiij days and half *iijd* j day	summa xiijd ob
Item vj lode mortar to the same wall	vjd
Item j wrygt to mak a payr dor darnys	iijd
	Summa iiijs ijd

At hakks hows

Item j wrygte to mend dorrs and wyndows j day	vjd

At alen toppar barn

Item for cariag' off iiij lode ston	viijd
Item xij lode mortar	ijs
Item a mortar boll	ijd

Item to wynpeny the mason iiij days and half ijs iijd
Item ij other masons iiij days and half iijs ixd
Item j servar to them iiij days and half xviijd
Item j wrygte to mend the barn dor j day vjd
Summa xs xd

Summa lateris xxijs ijd

Summa total off payments to the warden / hys confrater / to the beydmen and beydwomen / annuall charges / chef Rents/ abatments off Rents / dekays / mercyments for sewte of cowrts / costs of kepyng off owr cowrts / casuall costs/ expenses in gaderyng the Rents / off thyngs bowgt for stor off buyldyng/ and Reparacions in dyverse place lxxxiij li viijs ixd qa
Summa in superplusag' off the Rents thys yer *h[abe]o nil*
Summa Remaynyng off the stok xliiij li xviijs jd ob
Off thys stor Remaynyth in the hand' off Robard beomond at thys accowmpt' off hys arrerag' afor Rehersyd to the summa off xliiij li xvs vjd

probatum est per me henricyn Wyk'

fol 52
[The following two pages belong to the account for this year, although the account has been totalled]

Ad huc de compoto pro Anno Regni Regis henrici vij xviij° compotus octavus
Reparacion at bernak
In primis payd to Robard caryngton off ufford mason for hys bargeyn agreyte to mak an oven in the kychyn he to fynde stuff and warkmanschypp vijs
Item to ij masons off ufford for undyrsettyng the seyd kychyn whyll they toke down the wall iiijd
Item to the seyd ij masons for theyr bargeyne agrete to mak up the wall ageyn viijs
Item allowyd to the tennant ffor xvj lode morter to the same wall ijs viijd
Item payd to the tennant for cariag' off skaffold hyrdyls (to stawnford *ins*) and other tymbur that was left ther of (the last *ins*) buyldyng (last yer *del*) (anno RR henrici vij xvj° *ins*) [1500-1] iijd
Item payd to john hyggen and john wrygt for drawyng in a balk in the kychyn over the oven vjd
Item to old hamulden off wyrthorp sklatter for mending the evys of the seyd kychyn xxd
Item for half sem lyme to the same mendyng (be syde the cariag' from stawnford *ins*) iiijd
Item ij laborers to tak down the porch of the barn to mak the swyncote on of them ij days the tother iij days and half *iiijd* j day summa xxijd
Item to wyllam Ryk off casterton mason and wyllam scherwyn of stawnford mason for makyng of the wallys off the swyncote and ij partycions bytwen them agrete iijs viijd

Item to hygen and john wrygte off Ryall for makyng iij swyncote dorrs
(and iij peyr hoks and bands to them - *viijd ins*) xvd
Item to the seyd wrygts for makyng the Rofe of the swyncote
j day and half xviijd
Item to john denys mason and (wyllam sch *del*) thomas sar of weteryng mason
for leyng brode stonys in the swyncote bottom and furryng up the govells
of the swyncote aftyr the wrygts j day xijd
Item to Robard brewster ther servar j day iiijd
Item to the tennant for j lode erth to the same furryng ijd
Item to the tennant for cariag' off tymbur brode ston and old sklatt
that was off a swyncote at walcote xijd
Item to the seyd tennant for cariag' off tymbur from stawnford for the seyd
swyncote and j balk for the barn and bords and legbys and naylys
for the barn dor vjd
Item to old hawkyn off eston for di[m] thowsand sklatt to
the seyd swyncote ijs vjd
Item to hewgh douch of eston for cariag' of the seyd sklatt
from eston pytts to barnek vjd
Item for cariag' off lath and Rede from stawnford payd to the tennant ijd
Item to the seyd old hawkyn for sklattyng the seyd swyncote
j rode except o[ne] quarter iiijs iiijd ob
Item for ij sem lyme to the seyd sklattyng
(with the cariag' to the tennant *ins*) xvjd jd [sic]
Item for sand to the same allowyd the tennant ijd
Item to john hygen and john wrygt for mendyng off j principall
copull that was broken in the barn vjd
Item to the tennant for cariag' off tymbur from stawnford to
the seyd mending iijd
Item to the seyd john hygen and john wrygt for drawyng in off a balk in the
barn and makyng the yat' of the barn all new and the stabull dor iij days iijs
Item payd to hew smyth off Stawnford for ij catts off yrn ij hopys
ij plats of yrn to pyk' off yrn for the seyd barn dor xvijd
Item to john denys mason and thomas sar mason for making
off a botras at the grete barn dor syde iij days iijs
Item to Robard brewster ther servar iij days xijd
Item for ij sem lyme to the seyd botras xvjd
Item for cariag' of the seyd lyme from stawnford ijd
Item to the tennant for cariag' of sklatt from pylsyate to the seyd swyncote iijd
Item to a thakkar for thakkyng the barn syde wher the porch stode ij days viijd
Item j servar to the seyd thakkar ij days vjd
Item for strey to the seyd thakkyng xxd
Item for thak Rope jd
Item the tennant is allowyd toward the the [sic] thakkyng off
all other howsys iijs iiijd

(*Summa later* del) *Summa lateris* lviijs xjd ob
probatum est per me henricum Wykys

fol 52v

Ad huc de compoto pro Aº Regni Regis henrici vij xviijº compotus octavus

Reparacion at wylsthorp

In primis payd to john hygen carpentar for stayng the grete barn and drawyng in a balk in the chawmbyr and other wark in the same hows vs jd
Item to the seyd hygen carpentar for makyng the tymbur wark off a chymney in the hall vs jd
Item for a manteltre to the seyd chymney xijd
Item for ston from clypsam pytts to the growndwark off the chymney with the cariag' of the same xxd
Item for mortar to the same wark iiijd
Item payd to warwyk the mason for makyng the seyd grownd wark ijs viijd
Item allowyd the tennant for cariag' off tymbur from stawnford for the seyd chymney vjd
Item for lyttar and dawbyng of the chymney at the tennants cost [no sum]
Item for (the *del*) half m[l] brykk to make the topp off the chymney iiijs jd
Item the tennant for cariag' of the same [no sum]
Item for mason wark of the seyd brykk (ij masons ij days *ins*) ijs
[141]Item j servar to them ij days iiijd
Item for j sem lyme to the same makyng viijd
Item to the seyd warwyk mason for undyrpynnyng the wall on the stretesyde and mendyng the hall wyndow toward the yard syde iijs iiijd
Item to a mason for mendyng the coyn off the long wall toward the felde syde and undyrpynnyng the growndwark off the cart yat' vjd
Item j thakkar on the long nett hows viij days *iiijd* j day summa ijs viijd
Item j servar to hym viij days *iijd* j day summa ijs
Item j servar to hym when he Ryggyd ij days vjd
Item bowgt off the tennant strey to the seyd thakkyng vjs viijd
Item for mortar erth to Rygg withall at the tennants cost [no sum]
Summa xxxixs jd

Reparacions at wyrthorp

Item payd to kesten the tennant for mendyng and dawbyng the entre in hys hows ijd
Item to hym for makyng off a bench in the hows next hym iijd
Item to john denys mason and wyllam scherwyn for making a wall on the feld syde iiij days iiijs
Item Robard brewster ther servar iiij days xvjd
Item to hew douch for j lode ston to the same wark iijd
Item for mendyng off j lok of the hall dor wher kesten dwelt jd
Summa vjs jd

Summa lateris xlvs ijd
probatum est per me henricum Wyk

[141] this entry is made at the end of the previous line of text

fol 53

[Although the heading of this account is for a full year from Michaelmas to Michaelmas, in fact this account only ran from Michaelmas 1503 to February 1504 when Taylor left the Hospital]

compotus ix'

[142]*Compotus nonus de statu istius domus elemosinarie Willielmi Brown in stawnford inceptus per me Johannem taylyor predictum et divina favente clemencia per me terminandum pro uno anno integre administracionis mee videlicet a festo sancti michaelis in A° Regni Regis henrici vij xix° usque ad festum sancti michaelis in A° Regni Regis [sic]; vel serim aliud dat' a festo sancti michaelis in A° domini incarnacionis millessimo quingentessimo tercio usque ad festum sancti michaelis in Anno dom m° quingentessimo quarto*

In primis the stok of thys hows Remaynyth as aperyth in the fote off my last accompts (in the hands of Robart beomond late baylyff *del*) xliiij li xviijs jd ob
Item off money Rec' off m thomas hykham parson off seynt peturs and Syr harry wyks by the commaundment off master elmes by byll indendyd vj li
Item off money Rec ffor wod solde at swafeld by arnold[143] vs
Item off j asch at pylsyate (xxd *del*) iijs iiijd
Item Receyvyd off dyverse tennants thys yer as aperyth by a byll v li viijs iijd ob
Summa off Recepts (the *del*) charge lvj li xiiijs jd [sic]
Item the Rentale conteynyng the extent off the lyflode thys yer [144](lxij li vs vjd ob *del*)

[145]Summa off ye charge off M' John taylyor at hys departyng from ye bedhouse lvj li xiijs ixd
Summa total off [sic]

Off thys summa the seyd John taylyor dyschargeth hymself by thes parcells foloyng

Mensis octobris

In primis payd to the beydmen and wymen for ther wek' wag' endyd the vj day vs iijd
Item payd to the beydmen the xiij day vs iijd
Item payd to the beydmen the xx day vs iijd

---

[142] 'Ninth account of Browne's Hospital begun by me John Taylor and by divine clemency finished for one whole year of my administration from Michaelmas 19 Henry VII until Michaelmas [year missing], alternatively from Michaelmas 1503 to Michaelmas 1504'. Taylor presumed that Sharpe his successor would complete the annual account.

[143] marginal note: 'wode solde'

[144] sum heavily scored through

[145] This sentence and the accompanying deletions and corrections have been made by John Taylor but at a different time, in a larger script and in a blacker ink; he has gone over the account subsequently to make changes.

Item payd to the beydmen the xxvij day vs iijd

Mensis Novembris
Item payd to the beydmen the iij day vs iijd
Item payd to the beydmen the x day vs iijd
Item payd to the beydmen the xvij day vs iijd
Item payd to the beydmen the xxiiij day vs iijd

Mensis decembris
Item payd to the beydmen the fyrst day vs iijd
Item payd to the beydmen the viij day vs iijd
Item payd to the beydmen the xv day vs iijd
Item payd to the beydmen the xxij day vs iijd
Item payd to the beydmen the xxix day vs iijd
Item payd to s' wyllam hawkyn my confrater and to myself owr quart' wag' iij li

Summa lateris vj li viijs iijd
probatum est per me henricum Wykys

fol 53v

A° Regni Regis henrici vij xix° *compotus ix'*

Mensis Januarii
Item payd to the beydmen for ther wag' the v day vs iijd
Item payd to the beydmen the xij day vs iijd
Item payd to the beydmen the xix day vs iijd
Item payd to the beydmen the xxvj day vs iijd

Mensis ffebruarii
Item payd to the beydmen the ij day vs iijd
memorandum that the iij day off ffebruarij I payd to my self
my half quart' wag' xvjs viijd
Summa soluc' custod' confratr' et pauperibus viij li xjs ijd

cassuall costs
In primis ffor the halylofe ffor ye barn in skofgat' xv day off october ijd
Item ye halylof for ye hows in seynt myhell parysch xx day of October ijd
Item an essoyn at langdyk cowrt post fest mychael jd
ffor makyng off v endenturs bytwene the almoshows and v dyverse
tennants xxd ffor Red wax to seale ye seyd endenturs iijd
ffor j reward to john stanley off carlby ffor bowndyng off owr lande
ther and hys hys[sic] gud wyll in purchasyng certen lond ther xxjd
ffor cariag' off certen stuff as skaffold hyrdyls boords studds baros
ffrom the almoshows to the barn off skofgate iiijd
ffor expens' in gaderyng the Rent off thys yer afor rehersyd iiijd
ffor expens' of a man to go to aylton to spek with arnold morton
aftyr he was atachud to know whethyr hyt wer he or natt iiijd
ffor expens' at swafeld when I arrestyd hys goods and let' the land,
with the Reward to ye man that went with me iij days space xviijd

Summa off casuall costs vjs vijd

costs off cowrts at swafeld

ffor horse hyer thydyr the viij and ix day off november	viijd
Item expendyd ther	iiijd
Item for ye dyner at ye cowrt kepyng	ijs vijd
Item ffor ye stewards ffee kepyng the sayd cowrt	xijd
Summa	iiijs vijd
[146]Summa off casuall costs	xjs ijd

Item payd to john Colyn of eston ffo j m^l sklatt	iijs viijd
Item to hew douch of eston ffor cariag' off ye same from eston to the almos hows	viijd
Stor	iiijs iijd

Reparacion at eston

Item payd toward the makyng off a swyncote at John cordals	iijs iiijd
reparacion	xxixs ixd

Summa lateris iij li xxjd

[147]*probata sunt et omnia predicta approbata sunt per me henricum Wykys*

[146] this and the following two sub-totals are in the right-hand margin

[147] this is a final probate of all the above accounts by Henry Wykes.

[The account of William Sharpe the new warden for the remainder of the year 1503-4 is missing and also the accounts for the years 1504-5 and 1505-6. There are no signs that folios are missing.
The account for this year was written by Sharpe, at first leisurely but later in a hurry; he then revisited several of his totals and made changes in a hurry. A number of the totals have been corrected or written by the auditors, see folio 68v]

fol 54
[Account of William Sharpe for the year 1506-7]

Anno r' r' henrici septimi xxiij°   Compotus xij

Here foloythe the xij accompt off the state off thys almesehouse and by me Willam Sharpp warden the iiijth accompth for on hoyle yer yat ys [to] sey from the fest off sanct michell tharchangell in the xxij yer off the regn off kynge henry the vij to the same fest in the xxiij yer off the regn off the same kyng undur thys forme

In primis the stoke off the last accompth ys	lxviij li (xvs vijd *del*) vs
Item thextenth of owr lyflood thys yer	lxij li vs vjd ob
Item receved for aschese [ashes] at swafelde	vjs viijd
Summa total off my charge ys thys yer	(vj^{xx} xj li vijs xd ob *del*)
	vj^{xx} xj li vijs ijd ob

By thys parcells foloyng I discharge my selff to ye bedfolke

In primis the forth day off october	vs xd)	
Item the x day	vs xd)	xxiijs iiijd
Item the xvij day	vs xd)	
Item the xxiiij day	vs xd)	
November		
In primis ye iiij day	vs xd)	
Item the ix day	vs xd)	xxixs ijd
Item the xvij day	vs xd)	
Item the xxiiij day	vs xd)	
Item the xxx day	vs xd)	
December		
In primis the vj day	vs xd)	
Item the xij day	vs xd)	xxiijs iiijd
Item the xix day	vs xd)	
Item the xxvj day	vs xd)	
Item to my brothur and me	iij li	

Summa pagine iij li xvs viijd

fol 54v

Januarius		
In primis the iiij^{r} day	vs xd)	
Item the x day	vs xd)	
[148]*In ipsa septimana moritur Thomas Sleng pauper*)		xxijs ijd
Item the xviij day	vs iijd)	
Item the xxvj day	vs iijd)	
Februarius		
In primis the ij^{d} day	vs iijd)	
In the viij day	vs iijd)	xxjs
Item the xiiij day	vs iijd)	
Item the xxij day	vs iijd)	
Marcius		
In primis the iij^{d} day	vs iijd)	
Item the x day	vs iijd)	
Item the xv day	vs iijd)	xxvjs iijd
Item the xxiij day	vs iijd)	
Item the xxx day	vs iijd)	
Item to my confrater and me	iij li	
Aprilis		
In primis the iiij day	vs iijd)	
Item the xj day	vs iijd)	xxjs
Item the xiij day	vs iijd)	
Item the xxiiij day	vs iijd)	
Maius		
Item in primis the iij day	vs iijd)	
Item the x day	vs iijd)	
Item the xvij day	vs iijd)	xxvjs iijd
Item the xxiiij day	vs iijd)	
Item the xxx day	vs iijd)	

Summa pagine v li xvjs viijd

[148] 'In this week Thomas Sleng pauper died'

fol 55

Junius

In primis the iiij day	vs iijd)	
Item the xij day	vs iijd)	xxjs
Item the xix day	vs iijd)	
Item the xxvj day	vs iijd)	
Item to my confrater and to me		iij li

Julius

Item in primis the ij[d] day	vs iijd)	
Item the ix day	vs iijd)	xxvjs iijd
Item the xvj day	vs iijd)	
Item the xxiij day	vs iijd)	
Item the xxix day	vs iijd)	

Augustus

In primis the vij day	vs iijd)	
Item the xiiij day	vs iijd)	
[149] *In ipsa septimana admissus est Johannes Perkyn pauper*	)	xxijs ijd
Item the xxj day	vs xd)	
Item the xxviij day	vs xd)	

September

In primis ye iiij[r] day	vs xd)	
Item the xj day	vs xd)	
Item the xviij day	vs xd)	xxixs ijd
Item the xxiiij day	vs xd)	
Item the xxx day	vs xd)	
Item to my confrater and me		iij li
Summa total stipendij custod' confrat' et pauper' hoc anno est		xxvj li xjs jd

Summa pagine iiij li xviijs vijd

fol 55v

Annuall charges

In primis to the parson off sanct' michelys ffor hys pencion	vjs viijd)
Item in expenses ffor owr ffownders dyryge	vjs viijd)
Item allowyd ffor gyffyng off owr tenantys drynke	)
when yei [they] come	vjs viijd)
Item to ye bayle [bailiff] allowyd	xls)
Item to maister brekdenall ffor hys ffee	xs)
Item to mayster Archer ffor hys ffee	vjs viijd)
	[150]iij li xvjs viijd

[149] 'In this week John Parkyn admitted'

[150] this and the following sub-totals are all in the right-hand margin

Abatmentys and dekeys

In primis in all halow paroche the schoppys in the tenur)
off John bacheler abatyd xs)
Item abatyd ffrom xs to viijs in ye tenur off ye pardoner)
and in dekey iij quarters vjs)
Item abatyd in Rychard Tymyng' howse by yere iiijs)
Item dekeyd hollyd ye place wher wytbred schall dwell xxs)
Item dekeyd holly ye place next ye vycar off all halowys xxs) vij li
Item dekeyd iij quarters in ye howse by John bacheler vijs vjd) xiiijs
Item debatyd in (ye *ins*) Clerkys howse off all halow paroche vjs viijd) ijd
Item dekeyd fully ye place wher Wyllam baker dwellyd xxvjs viijd)
Item dekeyd on quarter in ye crane vjs viijd)
Item debatyd in ye angell in Sanct' Mary paroche xls)
Item debatyd in ye howse wher John paynter dwellys in)
Sanct' Mychelys parysche vjs viijd)

Summa pagine xj li xs xd

fol 56

Item debatyd in Skoffgate in ye handys off (ye *ins*) parson
off Sanct' Mychel xijd
Item debatyd ffully ye garden place in Sanct' Martyn parische ijs
Item debatyd ye howse wher ye wever dwellyth
in Sanct' Martyn parosche iijs iiijd
Item debatyd in bredcroffth with hys pertenyngys [151]vs (vjs viijd *del*)
Item debatyd in owr land thys yer in Stanfford ffeld xs
Item debatyd the iij acrese at small bryg' ffor owr horse viijs
[Summa] xxxjs
debatyd and dekeyd in Stanfford ix li xvs ijd

Item dekayd in Worthorp in the towne xxiijs
Item dekayd a sklat pytte thys ij yer xiijs iiijd
Item dekayd in eston ffor a golve[152] longyn to ye gyld howse off our lady ijs
Item dekayd in Walcot xvs viijd
Item debatyd in Stretton in the cotage xijd
Item debatyd in george penbery howse yis iiij yer ijs every yer viijs
Item dekeyd ffully ye mylner howse in north wyttham xijs
Item dekeyd contropp thys ij yer vjs
Item John Tenman payd noo cheff renth yis iij yer xiiijd
Item in the ffalloys brodryng and le lytleyng in swaffeld ffeld iiijs
[153] (v li xijs vjd *del*) iiij li vjs ijd

---

[151] some of these corrections are done in a different hand which may be that of another person or the same accountant at a different time. In this case, the sub-total in the right-hand margin has not been amended.

[152] a 'govell' (i.e. gable), see fol 79

Cheff rents

Off the cheffe rents now alloode except thyes foloyng
Item in primis to thomas stokes ffor halff ye cheff rente off swafeld vs)
Item to ye abbot off peturborogh ffor Warmyngton iiijs) ixs

Summa pagine (vij li xiijs vjd *del*)
(vjj li xijs vjd *del*) vj li vjs ijd

fol 56v

Suet off Cowrt

Item in primis ffor twyse syuyng[154] at Cutbert Cowrt in Stanford ijd)
Item onys syuyng at ye kynges cowrth in stanfford jd)
Item onys syuyd [155] and onys mercyd at Eston vijd)
Item mercyd at landych ffor all boroo sokn xijd)
Item ffor owr ffyne at northluffnam to ye kyngys cowrth baron xijd) vs iiijd
Item to ye grete cowrth ffor syuyng and mercymentys vijd)
Item to ye grete leetys ffor ye prior off broke vijd)
Item at Stretton ffor syuyng and mercymentys vijd)
Item at Thystulton ffor ij tymys of assuyng ijd)
Item to maister Eylond ffor Wylsthropp vijd)

Store off howse

In primis ffor a m off vj^{d} nayle vs)
Item ffor m m m off iiij^{d} nayle xs)
Item ffor v^{m} off lathe nayle iijs)
Item to John cordall ffor iij rood off bord xxs)
Item ffor lathe iij^{m} iiij^{d} a bunche xs)
Item to ij sawers vij days *xd* a day vs xd)
Item to abbot ye wryte [wright] ffor chyppyng of)
tymber x days iijs iiijd)
Item to ye same wryte ffor makyng ye sege yat' and ye)
gardyn yat and to bord my chambur xxd) iij li xviijs ixd
Item ffor caryyng off ye bord and lathe iij lodys xvd)
Item ffor iiij lood off playster *ijs iiijd* a lood ixs iiijd)
Item ffor parchyments xiiijd)
Item ffor pauper all thys yere xijd)
Item ffor enke all yis yere vjd)
Item to John holme off swaffeld ffor iiij quarter off lyme)
in the stonys not slekkyd vs iiijd)
Item ffor gethurryng off iiij lood off sand and ffor)
caryyng yeroff xvjd)

Summa pagine iiij li iiijs jd

---

153 this and following sub-totals in right-hand margin

154 this word which occurs several times in slightly different forms looks as if it should be 'fynyng', but I am sure that it is meant to be 'syuyng' i.e. 'suing'

155 or 'fynyd'

fol 57

Expensys and casuall costys

In primis in expensys at Car[l]bey when whe toke seision off ye place	
at the dener all thyngys accompth [accomplished]	ijs
Item a Reward to heugt turner off ColyWeston	xxd
Item ffor makyng an oblygacion off ye seyd hug' and John barret	
off okam to perform ye bargyn off Eltham thyng	xijd
Item for makyng ye dede off Alic' hykson in hyr wedoo hode	viijd
Item ffor makyng off a Relese to ye sam dede	viijd
Item ffor makyng off a relese owt off ye ffeiffers handes	viijd
Item ffor a dede made after the sayd alic' was John barrets wyffe	viijd
Item ffor a Relese off ye same	viijd
Item payd ffor the Eltham Thyng in Carlby to the sayd Jhon barret	
and Alec' hys wyffe	iij li vjs viijd
Item expens' at okam when the ded' wer seiled	[156]xijd

Summa pagine iij li (xiiijs *del*) xvs viijd

fol 57v

[The first journey by the warden William Sharpe and his man Roger Sharpe to London to attend the king's court; almost certainly from Tuesday 3 November to Monday 21 December 1506; the decree of the court would then have been delivered on Friday 18 December]

Expenses goyng to london at all halos tyde

[157]**In primis** at hoggerstond	iiijd)	In die mertis
Item at aukonbery	iiijd)	viijd
Item at baldok	vjd)	in die mercurie
Item at hat ffeld	xiiijd)	xxd
Item at london all the day	viijd)	In die iuvis
Item to ye botmen to grene wyche	iiijd)	xijd
Item in expenses	viijd)	in die veneris
Item to the botmen	vd)	xixd
Item in wyne	vd)	
Item in ale	jd)	
Item to owr brekffast	ijd)	In die sabati
Item wythe master Archer at owr dener	iiijd)	xijd
Item at Westmynster	ijd)	
Item ffor owr suppar ye same nygth	iiijd)	
In primis to a botman to grene weche	iiijd)	In die do^ca^
Item to a botman to ffery hus to london	iiijd)	2^e^ septi^e^
Item to owr suppar ye same nyght	iiijd)	xxijd

156 this figure and the correction made in the next line were entered in a different hand, i.e. later.

157 I have highighted the first entry for each day to help the reader; in the original the days are marked in the right-hand margin by brackets. See Appendix V

Item ffor collys in to owr chambur	iiijd)	
Item ffor bred ale and chese	ijd)	
Item ffor owr brekfaste	ijd)	
Item for owr horse bred and lyvery v days beffore	xxd)	
Item to owr dener ye same day at greneweche	iiijd)	In die lune
Item in ale at after noon	jd)	iijs vjd
Item to owr suppar ye same nyght	iiijd)	
Item in Rynyche wyne ye same day	ijd)	
Item in horse mete	vijd)	
Item ffor owr fyre att grenweche	ijd)	
In primis at owr brekffaste	iijd)	
Item ffor shoyng off owr horse	vjd)	
Item ffor owr dener ye same day	iiijd)	In die mert'
Item in ale at after noon	jd)	xxd
Item ffor owr suppar ye same nyght	iiijd)	
Item in ale and fyre ye same nyght	ijd)	

Summa pagine xijs xjd

fol 58

In primis ffor my manys bord[158]	iiijd)	In die mercurie
Item ffor owr horse mete tuesday and wednesday	xiiijd)	xviijd
Item at owr brekffaste	iijd)	
Item ffor fferyyng down to grenweche	iiijd)	
Item ffor owr dener yat day	iiijd)	In die iuvis
Item in wyne that day	ijd)	ijs ijd ob
Item in fferyyng upp' to london	iiijd)	
Item ffor owr suppar	iiijd)	
Item ffor owr horse yat day	vd ob)	
In primis ffor fferyyng to Whestmynster	jd)	
Item in drynke theyr	ob)	In die veneris
Item at owr dener that same day	iiijd)	xijd
Item ffor drynke at after noon	jd)	
Item ffor owr horse that same day	vd ob)	
Item ffor owr bregfaste	ijd)	
Item at Whansbryge[159] at owr dener	iiijd)	In die sabati
Item ffor my horse yat day	vjd)	xviijd ob
Item at after noon in ale	jd)	
Item at owr supper	iiijd)	
Item ffor owr beddys at Wansbryng	jd ob)	

158 on this and the following Wednesdays, the warden fasted but he paid for the meals of his man

159 unidentified; see Appendix V

In primis ffor owr dener	iiijd)	In die doca
Item to master dean servand in wyne	iiijd)	[160]2e septie
Item at supper the same day	iiijd)	xvjd
Item ffor owr horse yat day	iiijd)	
In primis ffor owr brekfaste	iijd)	
Item at owr dener that day	iiijd)	In die lune
Item to s' john husey in wyne	viijd)	ijs vijd
Item to owr supper that day	iiijd)	

Summa pagine xs ijd

fol 58v

In primis ffor owr brekffast	ijd)	
Item at london ffor owr dener	iiijd)	In die mertis
Item ffor owr horse monday and tuysday and at	)	xvijd
Wansbryge in ye morning	vijd)	
Item ffor owr supper at London yat nyght	iiijd)	
Md. yat owr horse went to lyvery iijd day and nygth		
In primis ffor my manys brekfast	jd)	In die mercurie
Item ffor hys dener	ijd)	vd ob
Item ffor hys supper	ijd)	
Item ffor my bred that day	ob)	
Item ffor owr brekffaste	iijd)	In die iuvis
Item at Westmonester	jd)	xvjd
Item at owr denerse	iiijd)	
Item at ye wyne with maister bygot	iiijd)	
Item at owr supperse	iiijd)	
In primis to the botmen	jd)	
Item at Westmynster in ale	jd)	In die veneris
Item down to london to ye botmen	jd)	xjd
Item ffor owr dener that day	vjd)	
Item in ale at after noon	ijd)	
Item ffor brekfast	ijd)	
Item ffor owr feryyng to grenweche	iiijd)	In die sabati
Item ffor owr dener that day	iijd)	xviijd
Item in ale at afternoon	jd)	
Item ffor feryyng upp' to london	iiijd)	
Item ffor owr supper that day	iiijd)	
In primis ffor owr dener	iiijd)	In doca 4e
Item in wyne with maister breknall	iiijd)	septie
Item at owr supper	iiijd)	xijd

Summa pagine vjs vijd ob

[160] this should be the third week, not the second

fol 59

In primis ffor owr brekffast	ijd)	
Item ffor fferyyng to Rychemownth	vjd)	In die lune
Item ffor owr deners yat day	iijd)	xxjd
Item to maister dean off ye kyngs chappell in wyne	)	
ye same day	iiijd)	
Item ffor suppar yat nyght	iiijd)	
Item ffor owr beddys at rychemownth	ijd)	
In primis ffor owr brekffasts	ijd)	
Item ffor owr dener	iiijd)	In die mert'
Item ffor fferyyng down to london	vjd)	xvijd
Item in ale ye same tyme	jd)	
Item ffor owr supparys	iiijd)	
In primis ffor my manys dener	ijd)	In die
Item ffor hys drynkyng	jd)	mercurie
Item ffor hys supper	ijd)	vd ob
Item ffor my selff in bred yat day	ob)	
In primis at owr brekffast	iijd)	
Item ffor fferyyng to grenwech	iiijd)	In die iuvis
Item ffor owr dener yat day	iiijd)	xxjd
Item ffor fferyyng to london	iiijd)	
Item ffor drynke	ijd)	
Item ffor owr suppars	iiijd)	
In primis in ale	jd)	In die veneris
Item at owr dener	vjd)	ixd
Item ffor drynk at after noon	ijd)	
Item ffor drynkyng	ob)	
Item at owr dener	iiijd)	In die sabati
Item ffor drynkyng at after noon	ijd)	vjd ob

Summa pagine vjs viijd

fol 59v

Item in primis ffor owr denere	iiijd)	In die do[a]
Item at after noon in ale	jd)	quinte septi'
Item ffor owr supper	iiijd)	xxxd ijs [sic]
Item ffor ij li off candull	iiijd ob)	
Item in ffagoattys ther and xx nygthys beffore	xd ob)	
In primis ffor owr brekffaste	iijd)	In lune
Item ffor owr horse lyvery xij days beffore	iijs)	viijs jd
Item in horse bred thoo xij days	xijd)	
Item expensys allowyd roger Sharpe[161] ffrom	)	
london to stanfford	iijs iiijd)	

---

[161] Roger Sharpe his companion may have been a relative; he was sent back to Stamford, presumably for instructions

Item ffor my dener	ijd)	
Item ffor drynkyng at after noon	jd)	
Item ffor supper ye same nyght	ijd)	
Item ffor ale in to my chamber	jd)	
In primis ffor my brekfast	ijd)	
Item ffor fferyyng down to grewyche [sic]	ijd)	In die mertis
Item ffor my dener	ijd)	xviijd
Item in Wyne to master dean servandys	iiijd)	
Item in Wyne to S' John dygby and to m' bygot	iiijd)	
Item ffor fferyyng upp' to london	ijd)	
Item ffor my supper	ijd)	
Item ffor bred to my selff	ob)	In die mercurie
Item to m Rychard sutton in Wyne	ijd)	iiijd ob
Item to doctor hatfield in Wyne	ijd)	
In primis at my brekfast	ijd)	
Item ffor fferyyng down to grenwyche	ijd)	
Item at my dener	ijd)	In die iuvis
Item in ale at after noon	jd)	xvd
Item to s' John husey in wyne	iiijd)	
Item ffor fferyyng upp to london	ijd)	
Item ffor my suppar	ijd)	

Summa pagine xiijs ijd ob

fol 60

In primis ffor ale	ob)	In die veneris
Item at my dener	iijd)	vd ob
Item in ale at after noon	ijd)	
In primis at brekffast	jd)	
Item ffor fferyyng upp' to Westmenster	ob)	
Item in ale at Westmenyster	jd)	In die sabati
Item ffor fferyyng down to london	ob)	xiijd
Item at my dener	ijd)	
Item in ale yat day	jd)	
Item at suppar	ijd)	
Item ffor candull that weke	jd ob)	
Item ffor ffyre that weke	iijd ob)	
In primis at my dener	ijd)	In die doca
Item in Wyne that day	iijd)	sexte septi'
Item at my suppar	ijd)	ijs
Item for my horse lyvery vj days beffore	ixd)	
Item for horse bred vj days	vjd)	
Item ffor to ye hosteler for dressyng hym	ijd)	

[162]*In ipsa die venit Rogerus a stanfford*

---

[162] Roger Sharpe returned from Stamford

In primis ffor (owr *ins*) brekffast	ijd)	
Item ffor fferyyng down to grenweche	iiijd)	
Item ffor owr dener	iiijd)	In die lune
Item in ale the same day	ijd)	xxd
Item ffor fferyyng upp' to london	iiijd)	
Item ffor owr suppers	iiijd)	
In primis at owr brekffast	iijd)	
Item ffor fferyyng to Westmonyster	jd)	
Item in ale at Westmynster	ob)	In die mertis
Item ffor fferyyng down to london	ob)	xiiijd
Item at owr dener with maister Archer	iiijd)	
Item in ale at after noon	jd)	
Item at suppar yat nygth	iiijd)	

Summa pagine vjs iiijd ob

fol 60v

In primis in ale	jd ob)	
Item ffor fferyyng down to grenweche	iiijd)	In die mercurie
Item ffor my manys dener	ijd)	xjd ob
Item ffor fferyyng upp' to london	iiijd)	
Item in bred and ale at evyn	jd)	
In primis at owr brekffast	iijd)	
Item ffor fferyyng down to grenweche	iiijd)	
Item at owr dener theyr	iiijd)	In die iuvis
Item in Wyne that day	iiijd)	xxiijd
Item ffor fferyyng upp' to london	iiijd)	
Item ffor owr suppars	iiijd)	
In primis ffor ale	ob)	
Item ffor fferyyng upp' to Westmynster	jd)	
Item ffor ale at Westmynster	jd)	In die veneris
Item ffor fferyyng ffrom Westmynster	jd)	xd
Item at owr dener with maister Archer	vjd)	
Item in drynke at nygth	ob)	
In primis at brekffast	jd ob)	
Item ffor fferyyng upp' to Westmynster	jd)	
Item ffor brekyn owr ffast ther wyth mayster	)	
bygottys clerkys	ijd)	In die sabati
Item ffor fferyyng down to london	jd)	xix[d] ob
Item at owr dener	iiijd)	
Item in ale at after noon	jd)	
Item at owr suppar	iiijd)	
Item ffor candull that weke	jd ob)	
Item ffor ffyre that weke	iijd ob)	
Item ffor owr dener	iiijd)	In die doca sept'
Item in Wyne at after at noon [sic]	iiijd)	septimane

Item at owr suppers yat day	iiijd)	(xiijd xviiijd ob *del*)
Item in bred and drynke to owr chambur	jd)	xixd ob

Summa pagine vjs xjd ob

fol 61

In primis ffor owr brekffast	ijd)	
Item ffor fferyyng down to grenweche	iiijd)	
Item at owr dener that day	iiijd)	In die lune
Item ffor fferyyng upp' to london	iiijd)	xiijd
Item at owr suppars	iiijd)	
Item ffor ale to owr chamber	jd)	
In primis at owr brekffast	ijd ob)	
Item ffor fferyyng down to grenweche	iiijd)	
Item at owr dener that day	iijd)	In die mertis
Item ffor fferyyng upp' to london	vjd)	xxd
Item at owr suppar	iiijd)	
Item ffor ale to owr chambur	jd ob)	
In primis in ale to my man	ob)	
Item fferyyng down to grenweche	iiijd)	In die mercurie
Item ffor my mannys dener theyr	ijd)	xvd ob
Item ffor fferyyng upp' to london	viijd)	
Item in bred and ale at evyn	jd)	
In primis at brekffast	iijd)	
Item ffor fferyyng to grenweche	iiijd)	
Item at owr deners	iiijd)	In die iuvis
Item in Wyne at after noon	iiijd)	ijs
Item ffor fferyyng upp' to london	iiijd)	
Item at owr suppers that nygth	iiijd)	
Item in ale to owr chambur	jd)	
In primis in ale	ob)	
Item ffor fferyyng upp' to Westmynster	ijd)	In die veneris
Item in ale at Westmynster	ob)	xvijd
Item at owr deners that day	iiijd)	

Md yat uppon yat day ye kynkys honorabull councell gaff centenc' and (end *del*) mad an End by twyxth ye bedehowse and ye gyld off all alows for all maters as hyt apperythe in the decree

Summa pagine vijs vd ob

fol 61v

Item the same tyme to ye kynkes cownsell in Wyne	iiijd)	xd *que ex alter*
Item ffor ye copy off the decree	iiijd)	*latere*
Item in drynkyng at nyght	ijd)	
In primis in drynk	jd)	
Item ffor schoyng off owr horse	vjd)	

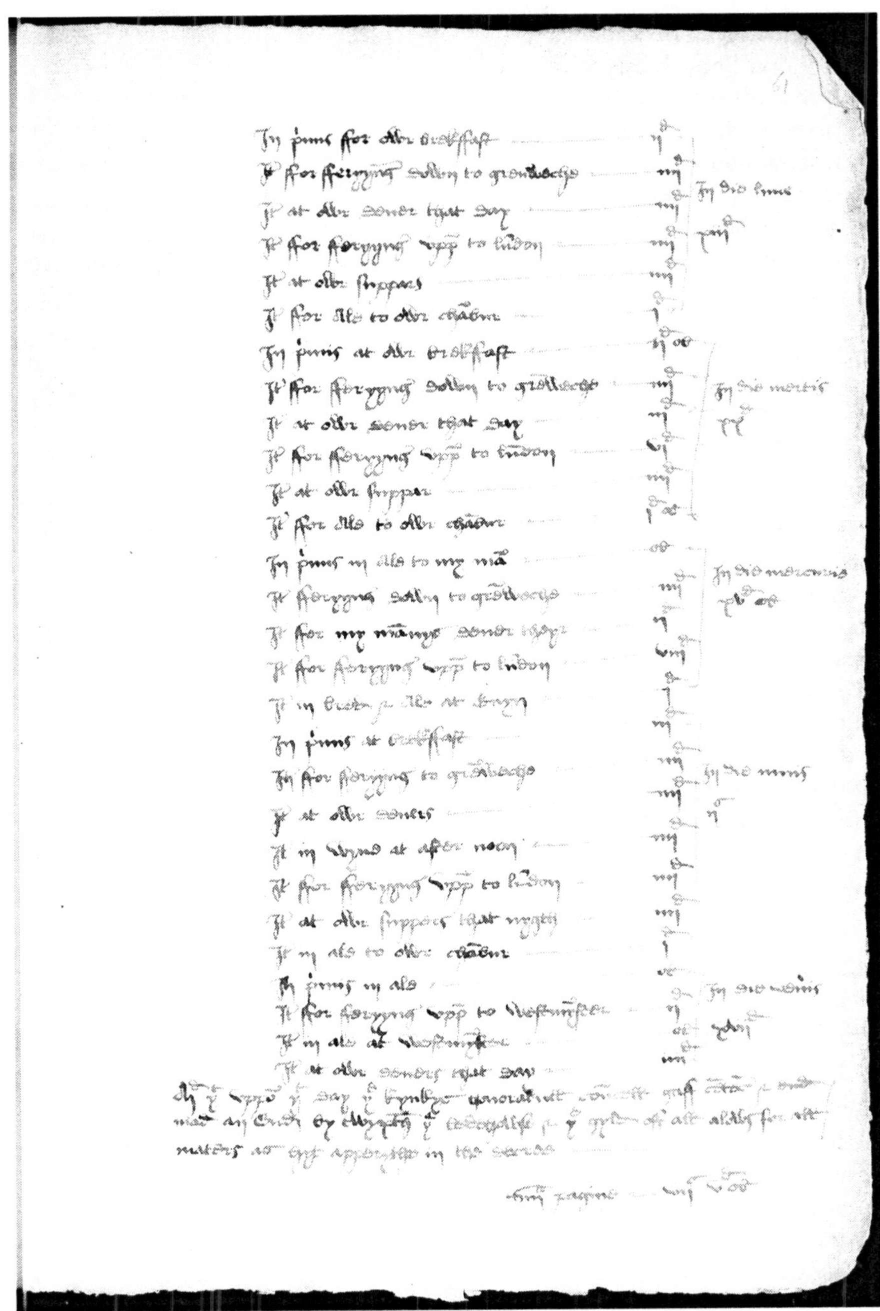

Folio 61 in William Sharpe's neat hand before it deteriorated: it describes the last few days of his stay in London and the decree of the king's council (bottom): note the fasting on Wednesday (Bodleian Libraries, University of Oxford).

Item ffor mendyng off sadullys iijd) In die sabati
Item ffor owr horse lyvery xij days iijs) vijs
Item ffor owr horse bred thoo days xvjd)
Item ffor owr dener yat day at london iiijd)
Item ffor candull yat weke jd ob)
Item ffor fyre that weke iijd ob)
Item at hatffelld all nyght xvd)
In primis at baldoke at betyng vijd) In die do[ca]
Item at bykules wade at betyng vjd) ijs iijd
Item at sanct evys all nygth xiiijd)
In primis at stelton betyng vijd) In die lune
Item at stamford betyng vjd) xiijd

Summa pagine xs iiijd
Summa total huius iteneris iiij li vjd

Expensys goyng to s' John husy at sleford at after crystomes
In primis ye ffyrst nygth at owr resupper iijd)
Item in Wyne ye same tyme iijd)
Item at brekffast the morn after ijd) xijs vjd
Item at Resupper all yat Evyn ijd)
Item in Wyne ijd)
Item to s' John husey ffor a newyerys gyffth a crown)
gyltyd and ameld valuerd xs)
Item ffor ye brekffast the morn after ijd)
Item ffor my horse thoys days xiiijd)
Item to the hosteler ffor dythtyng hym ijd)

Summa pagine xxijs xd

fol 62

Expensys goyng to lyddyngton and to M breknall at after crystomes
In primis at lyddyngton betyng iijd)
Item at Eston wher M breknall dwellyth iiijd) vijd

Expenses to my lord off boroo at after crystomes
Item at my suppar ijd)
Item ffor my horse all that nygth iiijd) viijd
Item in Ale when j whent from thens ijd)
In primis ffor wyne to s' John husey at after crystomese
when he was at M Rathclyffys viijd

Item in expensys when ye aldreman and ye honest men off ye town)
off stanfford whas at takyng off off ye loke off owr pantrey dore vjd)
Item in Wyne to M alderman and M Rathclyff iiijd)
Item to Wyllyam Smythe ffor drawyng off ye loke ijd) ijs iiijd
Item to M Lacy sum [?] ffor makyng off an enventory off ye goods)
belongyng to ye gyld off all halows wyth in the bedehowse iiijd)

Expenses rydyng to lydyngton to speke wyth ye abbot and Maister Breknall at cycientes[163]

In primis at lydyngton	ijd)	
Item at Eston all nygth	viijd)	xiiijd
Item at lydyngton in the mornyng	iiijd)	

[The second journey to London to attend the court; since midsummer day was 24 June, the journey started on either Tuesday 22 June 1507 or Tuesday 29 June and ended 6 or 13 July]

Expenses goyng to london at medsomer terme when Mayster brown callyd hus uppe with a pryvy sigell

[164]**In primis** at owr betyng	viijd)	In die mertis
Item at huntygton at owr betyng	vijd)	ijs vijd
Item at reloston all yat nygth	xvjd)	
In primis at Ware at owr betyng	vjd)	
Item at Waltam at owr betyng	viijd)	In die mercurie
Item at london at owr beddys all yat nygth	xvd)	ijs vd

Summa pagine [165](viijs ixd *del*) ixs jd

fol 62v

In primis at owr brekffast	ijd)	
Item ffor fferyyng down to grenweche	iiijd)	In die iuvis
Item at owr dener yat day	iiijd)	xviijd
Item ffor fferyyng upp' to london	iiijd)	
Item ffor owr suppar yat day	iiijd)	
In primis at owr drynkyng	ob)	
Item at owr fferyyng to Westmynster	ijd)	
Item to ye clarke off ye synet ffor my entrese	ijs)	In die veneris
Item ffor a new copy off ye decree	ijs)	vjs iiijd ob
Item at owr dener that day	iiijd)	
Item to M deane off ye kyngys chapell in Wyne	iiijd)	
Item to pygot servand ffor wrytyng off my answer	)	
to ye seyll[166] off complaynth	xijd)	
Item to Mayster pygott in Wyne	iiijd)	
Item ffor drynke at after noon	ijd)	

[163] sessions

[164] I have emphasised the first words of each day to help the reader to identify the days of the visit. The journey was done in a rush but the summer days allowed for more riding each day than the November days.

[165] total corrected by Sharpe later or by auditors

[166] perhaps [privy] seal of complaint, or an error for 'beyll' (bill) of complaint; see p47 above

In primis ffor owr brekffast	iijd)	
Item fferyyng upp' to Rychemonth	viijd)	
Item at owr dener yat day	iiijd)	In die sabati
Item in Wyne to s' john husey servandys	iiijd)	ijs iiijd
Item at owr suppars yat nygth	iiijd)	
Item ffor owr beddys at Rychemonth	iiijd)	
Item ffor ale in to owr chamber	jd)	
In primis at owr dener	iiijd)	In die do^{ca}
Item in Wyne at after noon	iijd)	xvjd
Item at owr suppar yat nygth	iiijd)	
Item ffor ale in to owr chambur	jd)	
Item ffor owr beddys	iiijd)	
In primis at owr brekffast	iijd)	
Item ffor fferyyng down to london	viijd)	In die lune
Item in ale in the botte	jd)	xxijd
Item at owr dener and suppar	viijd)	
Item in Wyne at london	ijd)	

Summa pagine xiijs iiijd ob

fol 63

In primis ffor owr brekffast	iijd)	
Item ffor fferyyng down to greneweche	iiijd)	In die mertis
Item ffor owr dener	iiijd)	(xx *del*) xixd
Item ffor fferyyng upp' to london	iiijd)	
Item at owr suppar yat nygth	iiijd)	
In primis ffor drynke	jd)	In die mercurie
Item fferyyng to Westmynster	ijd)	xiijd
Item at owr dener yat day	vjd)	
Item in ale at after noon	ijd)	
Item to my servand to see ye Wache	ijd)	
In primis at owr dener	iiijd)	In die iuvis
Item in Wyne at owr dener	ijd)	xvjd
Item to master Archer in Wyne	iiijd)	
Item ffor owr supper	vjd)	
In primis at owr drynkyng	jd)	In die veneris
Item fferyyng down to grenweche	iiijd)	xvjd
Item at owr dener theyr	iiijd)	
Item in Wyne theyr	ijd)	
Item ffor fferyyng upp' to london	iiijd)	
Item in ale at owr bedgat	jd)	
In primis at owr brekffast	ijd)	In die sabati
Item fferyyng upp' to Westmynster	ijd)	viijs
Item in ale at Westmynster	ijd)	

M[d] [167]yat day I Whas dismyst ffrom ye kyngs (cowrt *del*) councell and M Archer admytted my attorney

Item payd to ye clerke of ye councell (from *del*) ffor my dyssmyssyon	ijs)
Item to maister Archer to be my attorney yer	xxd)
Item ffor (owr *ins*) dener that day	vjd)
Item ffor owr horse thoo x days lyvery and provonder	iijs iiijd)

Summa pagine xiijs iiijd

fol 63v

In primis at hattfeld all yat nygth	xvjd)	In die sabati
Item at balduke for our beytyng	vijd)	
Item at Senth Evys all yat nygth	xviijd)	In die do[ca]
Item at Stelton at owr dener	viijd)	In die lune
Item at petroborgth all that nygth	xvd)	
Item in wyn at petroborgth	iiijd)	In die martis
Item for my horse yat day	viijd)	vjs viijd[168]
Item at Staunford commyng to home	iiijd)	
Md yat I payd for leche craffth at london		[169]iijs iiijd

Expens' goyng to petroburgoh at Sanct' botholphe day [17 June 1507]

In primis at brekfast at petroborg	ijd)	
Item for my horse yat day	iiijd)	xd
Item for horse met	ijd)	
Item in ale	ijd)	

Expens' goyng to cambryge

In primis at stelton	viijd)	In die lune
Item at huntyngton	viijd)	ijs vjd
Item mendyng and setting on ij new horse shon	iiijd)	
Item at Cambrig at owr supper	vjd)	
Item in Wyn ye sam nygth	iiijd)	
In primis at the taver' at owr brekfast	vjd)	
Item at dener with my lord dean servands	viijd)	In die martis
Item at Wyn with s' John husey servands	iiijd)	xxijd
Item at owr hosts house at nygth	iiijd)	
In primis at owr brekfast and in wyn	vjd)	
Item at owr dener that day	iiijd)	[In die veneris]
Item in wyn with the clerks off ye cowncell	iiijd)	xxd
Item at owr suppar that day	iiijd)	
Item at owr bedgat in possets	ijd)	

Summa pagine xvjs xd

---

167 Saturday 4 or 11 July

168 this sum refers to all four days

169 this figure is repeated in the margin in the auditor's hand.

fol 64

In primis at owr brekffast	ijd ob)	
Item in wyne to mayster chaunselers servands	iiijd)	In die iuvis
Item at owr deners	iiijd)	iiijs iiijd ob
Item ffor owr horse thoo iij days	xxijd)	
Item at huntyngdon commyng home all ye nygth	xvjd)	
Item ffor beytyng at Stelton uppon ffryday	iiijd)	
Expensys mayd to bugden		
In primis to huggerston	vjd)	
Item at bugden un twysday nygth	xjd)	
Item at (sanct *ins*) Edys at brekffast	ijd)	iijs (v *del*) ixd
Item in wyne ye same morn	ijd)	
Item at owr dener ye same day	iiijd)	
Item ffor owr horse yat wyle	iijd)	
Item at aucunbery all yat nyght	viijd)	
Item at hoggerston beytyngs	vijd)	
Item at stamford	ijd)	

Md yat I hyerd John Redeman to ryde to (m *ins*) breknall	viijd)	
Item to mayster pygot place Rydyng iiij days to ye same	)	
John Redeman	iiijs)	vs viijd
Item to ye same John to Ryde to ye (vycar *del*) abbot	)	
off petroborogth with my ladys letters	xijd)	
Md yat I Rode to petroborogth uppon sanct' Mathew day	)	
[21 September] to haff Ende with ye abbott' ffor	)	
owr lycenc' in expense	xd)	xxs xd
Item ffor ye letter commyssyd ffrom ffrom [sic] my	)	
ladys grace ye kyngys moder	iijs iiijd)	
Item in expensys at crowland	viijd)	
Item ffor master Colston ffor hys fee ij jerneys past	xvjs)	

Summa pagine xxxiijs vijd ob

fol 64v

Expenses

In primis a [writ of] [170]*capias* ffor Maister Cuff off carlby		iijs iiijd
Item expensys goyng to maister Archer place		
In primis ffor my brekffast at Swaffeld	iiijd)	
Item at howham ffor my dener	vjd)	xviijd
Item at Colsterworthe all nygth	viijd)	
Item Ratyd owth maister stonsby dett		iiijs
Item expenses ffor ale to ye bedemen ffor bryngyng in off ye playster	ijd)	
Item expensys in ale to ye bedemen ffor bryngyng in off ye tymbur	ijd)	iiijd

170 writ to an official to seize goods or a person

Expensys a bowth owr wode thys yere

In primis to campyon and to ye plaschers in ale	ijd)
Item to ye plaschers ffor theyr labur	vjs viijd)
Item in bred when ye wode was caryd	xvd)
Item in ale the same tyme	xiiijd)
Item in beffe that tyme	xvjd)
Item in moton	xd)
Item in ffyshe	jd)
Item to ye parsons cart off colsterworthe in ale and bred	jd ob)
Item in spyce yat tyme	jd)
Item to campyon wyffe ffo gyffyng them drynke theyr	xijd)
	[171]xijs viijd ob

Summa pagine xxjs xd ob

fol 65

Expensys abowth owr horse ffro[m] mychelmes the xxij yere off ye Regn' off kyng henry ye vijth [1506] to ye same ffest in ye xxiij yere [1507]

In primis to ye smythe ffor schon and schoyng	xiiijd)	
Item ffor a boschell off peyse	xd)	
Item ffor vj stryke off wootys [oats]	xvd)	
Item to Edward baker for horse bred	xvjd ob)	
Item a new sadull and a brydull with yer pertynyngs	vjs viijd)	
Item allowyd Robert barow ffor ye barn and ye stabull	xxd)	xvjs iiijd ob
Item ffor moyng owr hey	xviijd)	
Item in Ale to ye bedemen ffor yer turnyng and makyng	vijd)	
Item ffor caryyng off ye hey	xvjd)	
Item ffor old hey off Rychard baker presyd	ijs)	
Item ffor schoyng ffrom ye assencion to mychelmes	viijd)	
Item ffor horse bred yat tyme	viijd)	iiijs
Item to ye horse leche	viijd)	
Item ffor bran and grense ffor ye horse all Wyntur	xiiijd)	

Md yat I be lowyd ffor another horse lxviij days *iiijd* a day	xxs
[172]Item payd to Edward baker ffrom sanct' mathew day unto my departyng from the bedhouse	xiiijd
Item in expens' to seve [give] ye person off pauls[173] owr lyfflood and to tell wher all our dett was owyng	ijs

---

[171] this and following sub-totals in right-hand margin

[172] written by Sharpe in his later more hurried hand

[173] the parson of St Paul's church in Stamford was Robert Sheppey, the next warden of the Hospital; see Introduction p13

Summa pagine (xls iiijd ob *del*)
Summa pagine xliijs vjd ob

fol 65v

Reparacions at owr oon place within ye (place *del*) pedehowse [sic] in ye xxij yere of ye regn off kyng henry the vij [1506-7]

In primis an ymage off sanct' blase to ye awtur	xiiijd)	
Item ffor waxe ij li to make ye tapurs off ye awtur in ye chapel	xvjd)	
Item ffor makyng off ye sayd tapurys	ijd)	iijs iiijd
Item ffor waxe j li and ye makyng off ye tapur' in ye chyrche	viijd)	

Reparacion at ye makyng off ye gardyn wall

In primis ffor geduryng off ij lode sand	iijd)	
Item ffor caryyng off ye same sand	vjd)	
Item ffor caryyng ij lode stone ffrom Worthorp	viijd)	viijs xd
Item to ye mason ffor viij days	iiijs)	
Item to hys servand ffor viij days	ijs viijd)	

Reparacion off ye stor howse or off ye scole howse[174] in ye xx yer off k' h' ye vij

In primis to ye (sch *del*) sclaters ffor theyr ernyst	iiijd)	
Item to ye wrytes ffor theyr ernese	iiijd)	
Item to ye parson off senct' mychellys ffor tymbur	vjs viijd)	
Item to andrew stoterd ffor ij cowple sparrys	vjd)	
Item to Roberd martondale ffor iij cowple sparse	xijd)	
Item to carpenters [sic] x days *iijd* a day	iijs iiijd)	
Item ffor ij^c off iiijd nayle	viijd)	liijs vd
Item to ye sclater xj days *vjd* a day	vs vjd)	
Item to hys server xj days *iiijd* a day	iijs viijd)	
Item to bryan stokley off eston ffor m sclate	iiijs vjd)	
Item to loky ffor half m sclate	ijs)	
Item ffor iiij quartur lyme	ijs viijd)	
Item ffor lathe and lathe nayle	xvd)	
Item iij masons and dawbers viij days *vd* a day	xs)	
Item ffor caryng iiij lode off yerth or clay	xijd)	

Summa pagine iij li vs vijd

fol 66

Reparacion at my parler

In primis to Abbott ye wrygth ffor bordyng yeroff iij days *xvd*	xvd)
Item to John benet ffor makyng ye partycion iiij days	ijs)
Item to Wyllam smythe ffor makyng x gret nayllys to ye studs	vd)
Item to Wyllam smythe ffor a (key *del*) key to ye owth [outer?]	)

---

174 This suggests that the storehouse and schoolhouse were the same building, but that is not clear. See Introduction p40

dore and a loke and key to the new dore xd)
Item to Wyllam smythe ffor ij sclottys to ye chamber dore vjd)
Item ffor on sclot to ye parlar dore ijd) xvs ijd
Item to ye same Wyllam ffor makyng ye cowntyng howse key iijd)
Item ffor makyng ye store howse key iijd)
Item ffor a cowple bandys and a par off hookys vjd)
Item iij plaisteres ffor burnyng ye plaister and ffor syfftyng or)
dressyng yeroff iij days *xviijd* a day iiijs vjd)
Item to ye sayd iij plaisteres a bowth ye sayd chambur iiijs vjd)
Item to John paynter ffor payngtyng off sanct' an [Saint Anne] vjs viijd

Reparacion at Robard baroose
In primis to ye sclater ffor ij days xijd)
Item to hys servar ffor ij days viijd) ijs vd
Item ffor a quarter lyme viijd)
Item ffor sclate pynse jd)

Reparacion at Rychard tymyngs
In primis to a sclater j day vjd)
Item to hys server the same day vd)
Item to a mason on day vjd) ijs jd
Item to ye plaisterer ffor mendyng off hys schopp fflorth vjd)
Item ffor rede ijd)

Reparacion at John tomas Wyffe wedow
In primis ffor ffeyng off ye sege vjd)
Item to a sclater ffor on days wagys vjd) xvijd
Item to hys servand ffor ye same day vd)

Summa pagine xxjs jd

fol 66v

[175]Reparacion at thowse wher Wytbred shall dwell
In primis to cary owth the dunge in the yart in ale iijd)
Item a sklater iij days xviijd)
Item to hys server iij days xvd)
Item to iij plaisturers to dryve ye (chambur *ins*) florthe j day xviijd)
Item to the bedmen in ale to ber playster ijd)
Item to a wrigth j day and half to undursett ye chambur viijd ob)
[176]vs xjd ob

[175] there is a marked change of hand at this point; it appears to have been Sharpe writing in a hurry.

[176] this and following sub-totals are in right-hand margin

Reparacion at basal laxton house by the vicarage
In primis to a wrigth ij days to the sewstern and to put)
in sparss into on off the chaumburs xijd)
Item to ij sklaters iij days and half iijs vjd)
Item for pynse to the same house ijd)
iiijs viijd

Reparacion at thangell
In primis to lokkey sklater for coveryng off ij rod off sklat viijs viijd)
Item for iiij quarters lyme ijs viijd)
Item for pynns to the sam warke iiijd)
Item to colyn for iij days poyntyng xviijd)
Item to hys server iij days xvd)
Item to the seid sklaters for poy[n]ttynge off ye barn in (sko *del*))
senth gerg' parysch xjd)
Item for ij pare off dur bands iiijd)
xvs viijd

Reparacion at Skoffgat
Item reparacion to the sklater j day and hys servand xd)
Item for beryng the lym and sklats thydur (in ale *ins*) jd) xjd

Reparacion at Willam clerks
In primis a sklatter on day vjd)
Item to hys server on day vd) ijs vd
Item to the playsterer on day to dryff a chambur florth xviijd)

Reparacion at thomas hondsleys
In primis to benet the wrigth for on day vjd)
Item to lokkey sklater for ij days xijd) ijs iiijd
Item to hys servar for ij days xd)

Summa pagine xxxijs ijd ob

fol 67

Reparacion at John doves in sanct marten parroch
In primis to iij playsterers for ij days warke to dryve the chambur florthe iijs)
Item for rede to the sam chambur ixd)
Item for a horse to cary the plaister thydur ijd)
Item for stuble to the sam place xiiijd)
Item for moyng and geduryng theroff xiiijd)
Item for carege theroff xiijd)
Item for thakkyng *in compoto sequenti*
vjs xjd

Reparacion at Eston
In primis at brian Stokly place to a mason vj days iijs)
Item to hys servand thoose days ijs vjd)
Item for carage off yorthe iiij loods viijd)
Item for caryng off iij lood sand vjd) vijs vijd

Item to a sklater on day	vjd)	
Item to hys servand yat day	vd)	
Item allowed Willam otheram to hys oven makyng	iijs iiijd	
Item reparacion at pylyath		
In primis to To [Thomas] lokkey sklater vij days	iijs vjd)	
Item to hys server vij days	iijs)	ixs
Item for iiij quart' off lyme	iijs)	
Item reparacion at barnek		
In primis to a wrigth for halff a day	iijd)	
Item for a pese to a syd tre	iiijd)	vijd
Item reparacion at wilstropp abowt ye duffcot		
In primis ij quarter off lym	xvjd)	
Item for caryng the lym and sklat	viijd)	iiijs ixd
Item to the sklater iij days	xviijd)	
Item to hys server other iij days	xvd)	

Summa pagine xxxijs ijd

fol 67v

Reparacion at northluffnam

In primis to a wrigth ij days	xijd)	
Item to a mason for iiij days	ijs)	viijs vd
Item to the sklater iij days	xviijd)	
Item to hys server other iij days	xvd)	
Item for iij quarter lyme	ijs)	
Item to carag' off sklat and lyme from Stanford	viijd)	

Reparacion at Carlby

In primis to the gret barn ij spars	iiijd)
Item to ij wrigts for drawyng in off theym	vjd)
Item for bordyng theym the sam day	iijd)
Item a thakker v days uppon the barn	ijs vjd)
Item to hys server v days	xxd)
Item to a thakker xj days uppon ye kyln and other housese	vs vjd)
Item to hys server thoo days	ijs ixd)
Item to hery west to the kyln ix days and other housese	iiijs vjd)
Item to willam markam wrigth ix days	iiijs ~~vjd)~~
Item to robert clerk writh ij days and halff	xvd)
Item to parson off carlby for tymbur and spars	vjs viijd)
Item for rede for the kyln	iiijd)
Item for thak rope	iiijd ob)
Item longland' for stuble and strawe	iiijs vjd)
Item for dawbyng and splentyng ye govell end	viijd)
Item for caryyng iij lood off stuff from stanford	xviijd)
Item for iiij quarter lym	ijs viijd)
Item to the sklater viij days	iiijs)

Item to hys server the sam viij days		iijs iiijd)
Item for pyns to sam house		iijd)
		[177]xlvijs vjd ob

Reparacion at wolstropp by colsterworth

In primis allowed lynsey for a par off posts	ijs)	
Item to the wrigth by gret	js)	iiijs vjd
Item to a mason j day	vjd)	

Summa pagine iij li vd ob

fol 68

Reparacion at northloffnam

In primis at Shyrt hoose to abbott wrigth for iij days	xviijd)	
Item to benet wrigt theyr v days	ijs vjd)	
Item for a C off vjd nayle	vjd)	
Item for a C off iiijd nayle	iiijd)	vjs xd
Item ffor a C off iijd nayle	iijd)	
Item ffor iij par off bands	vjd)	
Item ffor caryyng off old stuff from wytham and for caryng	)	
bords and tymbur from Stanford	xvjd)	

Reparacion off ye cotag' off a roo

In primis for vj lood off stubble or straw	vijs)	
Item for thakyng by grett	vs)	xijs

Reparacion at the myln house [Swafeld]

In primis to Ric' hak for iiij lood stuble	vs)	
Item for watle to the sam house	ijd)	
Item for sevyng wand	jd)	xs iijd
Item to a mason ij days makyng ye wyndose ye gawme	xijd)	
Item for ij lood off mortar	vjd)	
Item to the thakker by gret	ijs vjd)	
Item to ij wrigts for j day to mak wyndose	xijd)	

Reparacion at Stretton

In primis ij quart' lym	xvjd)	
Item to the sklater iij days	xviijd)	iiijs xd
Item to hys server	xvd)	
Item for caryng a lood sand	ijd)	
Item for caryyng the lym and (sand *del*) (sklat *ins*) from stanford	viijd)	

Summa pagine xxxiijs xjd

---

177 in right-hand margin

fol 68v

[178]*Summa totalis stipendiorum custodis confratris et pauper' ac omnium onerum huic domu' elemosinarie pertinent' hoc anno supradicto* lxiiij li xviijs xjd ob

Md yat the warden ys allowed for hys gret laburs and troblese yat he hath had for hys suet off thys almeshouse xxiiijs viijd

Md yat the kyngs counsell hath decred yat the (warden *del*) aldreman off ye gyll off all hallose shall hav or receve off Robert beamonth xv li
The stok now remaynyng ys in letters off rent rolls and other detts an noon in the hands off s' willam sharpp xxxix li viijs jd ob

[The account is signed off with two audit statements; the first written by Sharpe was strongly deleted; the second looks as if it is in the hand of Sheppey. Sharpe's wording of the audit process was not to the liking of Henry Wykes vicar of All Saints in the Market and the patron of the Hospital]

[179](*Probat' est iste compot' xij' dicti Willielmi sharpe custodis dicte dom' elimosinarie per nos henricum Wyks vicarium ecclesie omn' sanctorum in foro et dominum Thomam fforster rectorem ecclesie sti michaelis modo decanum ville Staunford et dominum Willielmum hawkyn confratrem dicte dom' supervisores et auditores cuiuslibet compot' de administrac' bonorum seu officii custodis istius dom' vij° die mensis octobris anno r' r' henrici septimi xx° iij°* del)
ffinis compoti mei Willielmi sharpp dom' elimosinarie

Probat' est iste compot' xij' dicti Willielmi scharpe custodis dicte dom' elimosinarie per me henricum Wyks vicarium ecclesie omnium sanctorum in foro precipium supervisorem et Auditorem pro tempore mee cuiuslibet compot' de administracione omnium bonorum seu officii custodis istius dom' ut patet in statut' dict' dom' vij° die mensis octobris anno dom' m^l et vij° ac anno r' r' henrici septimi xxiij° hiis testibus dom' Thoma ffoster modo decano ville Staunford (dom ins*) Roberto schepey et dom' Willielmo hawkyn confratro dicte dom' et multis aliis.*

---

178 'Total of stipends of warden, confrater and paupers, and all costs this year'

179 The deleted probate statement reads: 'This twelfth account of William Sharpe was approved by us Henry Wykes vicar of All Saints in the Market, Thomas Forster rector of St Michael now dean of Stamford, and William Hawkyn confrater supervisors and auditors of every account of the administration of the goods or offices of warden of this house 7 October 23 Henry VII; the end of the account of me William Sharpp [warden] of the almshouse'.

The second reads 'This twelfth account of William Sharpe was approved by me Henry Wykes vicar of All Saints in the Market the principal (*precipium*) supervisor and auditor for my time of every account of the administration of all the goods of this house as appears by the statutes of the said house 7 October 1507 and 23 Henry VII; this witnessed by Thomas Foster now dean of Stamford, Robert Schepey and William Hawkyn confrater of this said house and many others'

[180]fol 69

[Account of Robert Sheppey for the year 1507-8]

Anno R' R' henrici septimi xxiiij^{o} Compotus xiij

Here folowyth ye xiij acompt' off ye state off yis almesehowse and be me Robert Schepey warden ye fyrst accompth for on hole yere yat ys to sey from ye feste off sanct' michell tharchangell in ye xxiij yere off ye regn' off kyng henry ye vij to ye same feste in ye xxiiij yere off ye regn' off ye same kyng under yis forme

In primis Stoke of ye last acownte xxxix li viijs jd ob
Item thextenthe of owr lyflode yis yeyr lxij li vs vjd ob
Item I sold iiij asches for xijs
Item I resewyd for a kyllyn yat was bornyd xiijs iiijd
Item in batyng of ye bedmen for coreccyons iijs ijd
Item ye stok of ye last acownt and ye extent of owr londs yis yyer with ye asches and ye xiijs iiijd I Resewyd and ye coreccions drawys [amounts to]
v^{xx} li and iij li iiijs ijd
and for stretts of ye cowrt with a eschyp' [sheep?] yat sold
By these parcells foloyng I dyscharge my selfe to xj beydfolk

In primis ye fyrst day off october vs xd)
Item the viij day vs xd)
Item the xv day vs xd) xxixs ijd
Item the xxij day vs xd)
Item the xxix day vs xd)

November

[181]*In ipsa septim' amissus est Johannes* [sic]

In primis the (iiij dey *del*) (v *ins*) day vjs vd)
Item ye xij day vjs vd) xxvs viijd
Item ye xix day vjs vd)
Item ye xxvj day vjs vd)

December

In primis ye iij day vjs vd)
Item ye x day vjs vd)
Item ye xvij day vjs vd) xxxijs jd
Item ye xxiiij day vjs vd)
Item ye xxxj day vjs vd)

fol 69v

Januarius

In primis ye vij dey vjs vd)
Item the xiiij dey vjs vd)
Item the xxj dey vjs vd) xxvs viijd
Item the xxviij dey vjs vd)

---

[180] the hand of Robert Sheppey

[181] admission of John [no other name]

Februarius		
In primis the iiij dey	vjs vd)	
Item the xj dey	vjs vd)	xxvs viijd
Item the xviij dey	vjs vd)	
Item the xxv dey	vjs vd)	
Martius		
In primis ye iij dey (est ma *del*)	vjs vd)	
Item the x dey	vjs vd)	xxxijs jd
Item the xvij dey	vjs vd)	
Item the xxiiij dey	vjs vd)	
Item the xxxj dey	vjs vd)	
April		
In primis ye vij dey	vjs vd)	
Item the xiiij dey	vjs vd)	xxvs viijd
Item the xxj dey	vjs vd)	
Item the xxviij dey	vjs vd)	
Mayus		
Item ye v dey	vjs vd)	
Item the xij dey	vjs vd)	xxvs viijd
Item the xix dey	vjs vd)	
Item the xxvj dey	vjs vd)	
Junus		
In primis ye ij dey	vjs vd)	
Item the ix dey	vjs vd)	
Item the xvj dey	vjs vd)	xxxijs jd
Item the xxiij dey	vjs vd)	
Item the xxx dey	vjs vd)	
Julius		
Item the vij dey	vjs vd)	
Item the xiiij dey	vjs vd)	xxvs viijd
Item the xxj dey	vjs vd)	
Item the xxviij dey	vjs vd)	

fol 70

Augustus		
In primis the iiij dey	vjs vd)	
Item ye xj dey	vjs vd)	xxvs viijd
Item the xviij dey	vjs vd)	
Item the xxv dey	vjs vd)	
September		
In primis ye fyrste dey	vjs vd)	
Item the viij dey	vjs vd)	
Item the xv dey	vjs vd)	xxxijs jd
Item the xxij dey	vjs vd)	
Item the xxix dey	vjs vd)	

Item to my confrater and me for on hole yere xij li
Summa totalis stipendii custodis confratris et pauper' hoc anno est xxviij li xvijs ijd

Annuall charg'
In primis to ye parson off sancte michelys for hys pencion vjs viijd)
Item in expensys for our fownders dyryge vjs viijd)
Item allowyd for gyffyng off our tennants drynke when)
they come vjs viijd) iij li vijs ixd
Item to ye bayly allowyde xls)
Item to master Archer for hys fee vjs viijd)
Item to ye seyd master archer for wythedrawyng ye swyte be)
twen master cufe and us when he was hurte xiijd)

fol 70v

Abatments and dekeys
In primis in all halo paroche ye schopis in ye tenur' off John bacheler abatyde xs
Item abatyd in ye schope by hytt in ye tenur' off John tohmas wyffe ijs
Item abatyd off ye howse next ye tenur' off my lady helmys where ye
pardonar dwellys ijs
Item abatyd in ye place wher richard tymyng dwells be yere iiijs
Item abatyd in ye place wher Whyttbrede dwellys be yere vjs viijd
Item dekeyd holly ye place next ye vicar off all halows xxs (vjs *del*) viijd
Item debatyd in ye clerks howse off all halows vjs viijd
Item dekeyd fully ye place Wher Wyllam baker dwellyd xxvjs viijd
Item dekeyd fully the (C *del*) Crane xxvjs viijd
Item dekeyd fully ye howse Wher Wyllam dwellyd xs
Summa vj li xvjd

Sancte marys paroche
Item debatyd in ye angell xls

Sanct' michell paroche
Item Abatyd in ye howse Where Wyllam pynkkanys dwells vjs viijd

Sanct' martyn paroche
Item debatyd fully ye gardyn place ijs
Item debatyd ye howse Wher ye Wever dwellys iijs iiijd
Item debatyd in bredcrofte with hys perteynyngs iijs iiijd
Item debatyd in our lond yis yere in stanforde felde xvs vd
Item debatyd ye iij acrys off medow att ye small brygs (for owr hors *ins*) viijs
Item debatyd in Skoffgat' in ye hands of ye parson of sent' mychels xijd
[182]Summa iiij li ixd

Debatyd and dekayd in stamforthe
In ye feld and town

Summa lateris x li ijs jd

---

[182] in right-hand margin

fol 71

Dekayd in Worthorpe

In primis ij cottears yis yere	xiijs iiijd
Item j cottear a quart'	xxd
Item dekeyd a slatte pytte for on yere	vjs viijd

Eston

Item dekeyd for a golve[183] longyng to ye gylld howse off owr lady	ijs

Walkote

Item dekeyd in ye same town	xvs viijd

Stretton

Item debatyd in ye cottage	xijs

Northe Wytham

Item dekeyde ye hows wher' george penbery dwellyd	xijs
Item dekeyd holly ye mylln hows	xijs
Item dekeyd ye cottear next scherschaw for holl[184] a yere	(xxd *del*) iijs iiijd
Item dekeyd in Syr willam carters hows	xxd

Twyforthe

Item dekeyd in ye tenur off same town	vijs

Swafeld

Item dekeyd ye mylne hows in ye same town	vjs viijd
Item in falowe brodyng and lyttyllyng	[no sum]

Conthorpe

Item dekeyd in ye seyd town	iijs

Steynby

Item debatyd in ye rent off a syse off John tenman	ijd ob

Summa lateris iiij li vjs ijd ob

fol 71v

Cheffe rents

Item in primis ye tenement in stamford to ye kyng)	
Item the close in bredcrofte to ye kyng)	xxixs
[185]Item j li off pepyr	xviijd
Item ye angell in stamforthe to ye gylde off corpus Xti	xijd
Item ye hows in sent mychel paroche to sent lenards off stamforthe	vjd
Item ye hows att ye malery bryge in all halow parysche to	
m edwarde brown ij yyer	[186]xviijd
Item ye hows in sent' martyn parysche be ye Water syde to gye thorney	iijs

[183] a gable, see *govell* on fol 79

[184] this appears to be a correction from 'half'

[185] this line is inserted at the end of the first line

[186] written over erasure

Item a hows in ye seyd parysche next ye Churche to ye abbey off peterborow	iiijd
Item j hows in ye seyd parysch [*deletion*] on ye same syd next be yond yat to ye seyd abbey	iijd
Item j garden in ye seyd parysch toward ye nonnys off stamforthe to ye seyd abbey	ijd
Item ye fermplace at pyllsyatt to ye seyd abbey	ixs iijd ob
Item j part off a close in pylsyatte felde hyard off gye thorney aforseyd	vjd
Item ye tenement off warmyngton to ye seyde abbey	iiijs
Item ye same place paythe to ye scheryfe (asse *del*) geld off northamtonschyre vjd	
Item ye tenement in barnake payd now to M vincent	ixd
Item ye farme at northlufnam paythe to tomas Bassett	iijs viijd
Item ye seyd place paythe to [thomas *del*] lord sowche	jd ob
Item ye seyd place paythe to ye prior off broke	iijd ob
Item ye hows in eston wher bryan stokley dwellythe paythe to ye kyng	ijs iiijd
Item ye seyd place paythe to ye charter hows in coventre	ijs viijd
Item ye hows in eston where Jon wrytt dwellethe paythe to ye kyng	iijd
Item for ye close foloyng to ye seyd hows be indentur paythe to ye college off tatursale	xvjd
In primis ye manor off Swafelde paythe to lorde grey	ij li xs
Item at Stretto[n] peyd to ye bells	xijd
Item percroft in Swafeld to my lade daleland	xijd
Item in twyford schef to my lade daleland	xijd
Item ye hows nexte ye parsonage in northewitham paythe to s' tomas dalaland	vs vjd
Item ye tenement in barham paythe to ye kyng	jd ob
Item ye land off ye same paythe to ye erle off Westmorelonde	ob
Item ye hows and lande at wylsthorpe to lady eyland	iijd
Summa	vj li xvijs vjd qa

fol 72

Suet' of Cowrt

In primis At Eston at ye kynges Cowrte mercyd	iiijd)	
Item at langdyk for al borow sokn' for ij yer	ijs)	
Item for owr fyne at northluffnam to ye kyngs Cowrt	xijd)	
Item to ye gret Cowrt for swuyng and mercyments	vjd)	vs xd
Item to ye gret leett' for ye prior off broke	vjd)	
Item at Stretton for syuyng and mercyments	vjd)	
Item at Thystylton for syuyng and mercyments	vjd)	
Item at wylstrop at master Elands Cowrt	vjd)	

Stowr of howse

In primis for haf a m of iijd nayl	xiiijd)
Item for ijC of iiijd nayl	viijd)
Item a m of iijd nayl	ijs iiijd)

Item haf a m of iiijd nayl	xviijd)	
Item haf a m of ijd neyl	xd)	xlvijs jd
Item a C of spykyngs	iiijd)	
Item ij dosyn of crests (at ij[d] *ins*)	ijs)	
Item for iij pecys' of tymber yat I bohte of Rob' sted'	iiijs jd)	
Item for cariag' of ye same to thomas taverner	iiijd)	
Item for tymber yat I bohte of Jon fysscher	iiijs viijd)	
Item xlte [40] spars yat I bohte of abbott	viijs)	
Item for iiij seym of lyme in stonnys	vs iiijd)	
Item for a gret band and ij lytyl bands with a hok and a key	vd)	
Item for pauper [paper] al yis yer	iijd)	
Item for fellyng and for kyddyng of owr wode	vijs)	
Item for vj loods of wode caryag	iijs)	
Item for mete and drynk	iijs)	
Item for moyng and makkyng of hey	xiiijd)	
Item for ledyng of ye same hey	xijd)	

fol 72v

In Casuall Expensis and costs

In primis for kepyng of ij Cowrtts ye steward ffees	ijs
Item for owr dynner and swpper at Swafeld	xvjd
Item at Northewyham owr costs yer	xvjd
Item to calys to hys costs goyng to tatersall for byll' yat war nessesary for hws	ijd

Item ye laste yeyr when I went to london to spek with Syr Jon hose for owr stres yat was takken at swafeld for ye xls, my costs [187]ar hyer fol[lowing]

Item my hors hyre to willam skynner	ijs iiijd
Item for hors bred or I went forht	ijd
Item I spent at thomas wyllyams or I went	jd
Item at stelton of my hors	jd
Item at huntyngton my hors and my self	iijd
Item at royston all nyht my hors and my self	vjd ob
Item at wayre my horse and my self	iiijd
Item at London ye fyrst nyght my cost	iijd ob
Item my hors met in London for v deys	xvijd ob
Item on ye morow with archer at brekfast	jd
Item for caryag of us ij be water	ijd
Item at dynner and at sopper and after	vjd ob
Item hyt cost afterword ye tyme I was in London	xixd ob
Item at ware as I com home my hors and my self	iiijd
Item ye nyght at royston my hors and myself	iiijd ob
Item at hwnttyngton my hors and my self	iiijd
also a drynk yat I gaf my hors fer ye bott	vjd
Item at stelton al nyghte my hors and my self	vd ob

[187] in right-hand margin

Item at wamysford my hors jd
Item for Schoyng of my hors iiijd
Item for bornyng of iiij tapyrs (of wax yis yyer *ins*) vijd
[188][Summa] xvs xd ob

fol 73

Item when ye abbot of peterborow had takyn owr stres at pyllysyat Master Ratlyf send thomas tawerner to ye abbott and so for hys sake he delywerd ye stres to a dey and so I went to spek with master pygott and he gaf me cownsell to go up to London to spek with Master breknal and hym togedyr so hyt cost me vjs
Item when I (went *ins*) to my lade[189] to spek with heyr for owr kydds iijs
Item hyt has cost me for goyng to peterboro vij tymes to a gre with ye abbot and I taryed yer sumtyme iij deys iiijs jd ob
Item when owr stres was takon at pyllysyat to thomas tawerner iijd
Item when I went to spek with master breknal on ye mundey in yowl weyk iijd
Item ye abot had of me when I was last with hym xs
Item I we[a *del*]nt to ber ye indentur yat was betweyn ye abot and me to Master pygot yat yt myght be (mad after *ins*) cownsell at london xijd
Item for sawyng of loggs hawf a dey vjd
Item for sawyng of platts a dey xjd
Item peyd to Rob' Barrow for ij crahcs [?] with a mawnger vd
Item yat I spent at dywers tymes when I went to se owr lands iijd
Item for gederyng and caryyng of ij lods of sond viijd
Item I spent of Master clark when he was sent se owr ewydenc' in wyn iiijd

[*Summa lateris*] xxvijs viijd ob

fol 73v

Reparacions in ye bedhows
In primis to hare wryght and to benson of Eston for)
drawyng of ye chamber ower ye closter xiiijd)
Item to chesgat ye Sclater of eston viijd) iijs vd
Item for a loyd ostrey [of straw] and for thakkyng of ye same xviijd)

Item at tymyng' hows for mendyng of a dor band jd
Item yer as jon thomas wyff dwells for makkyng a dor iijd
Item for bands to ye same dor iijd

Item at ye Schop yer as Sche dwellyd for mendyng a peyr of gresyngs iiijd
Item for clensyng a seeg vjd
Item for a loyd of ston and mortar iiijd

---

188 in right-hand margin

189 Elizabeth Elmes who held Wolfhouse manor from whence the kydds came, not Lady Margaret Beaufort

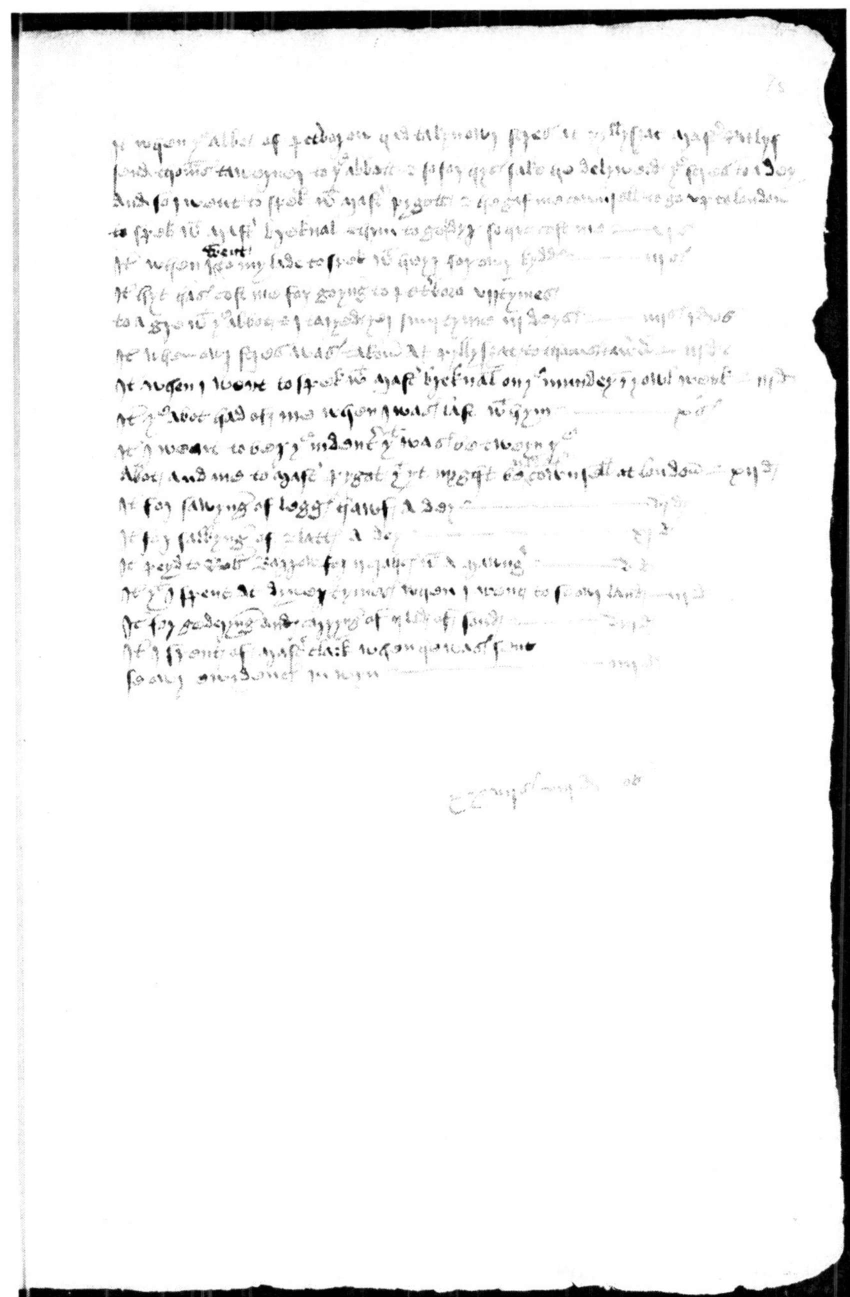

Folio 73 in Sheppey's handwriting: descriptions of his travels in relation to the distraint taken by the abbot of Peterborough are mixed up with building repairs and a payment in wine to the clerk (Bodleian Libraries, University of Oxford).

Item in ye same parysche at Jon toswolds to hare wryght for makkyng a new dor and mendyng a nold dor and for leyyng yn of ij trescholds ixd
Item ij masons ij deys and a haf ijs vjd
Item yer serwer vijd
Item for ij loyds of thornys caryyng and fellyng xviijd
Item for ij bands iiijd
Item a slater a dey and haf ixd
Item for a loyd of strey xiiijd
Item for thakkyng and serwyng [sewing] ye same strey vijd
Item at ye hows neyxt ye vycareg' for clensyng a seyge ixd
Item to a Slater of Worthorpe for hyllyng of ij rood ixs
Item for pwentyng and mendyng besyd yt xijd
Item for iij seym lyme to Jon Jaf ijs
Item for a howk to ye yard dor jd

[190][Summa] xxiijs ijd

Summa lateris xxvjs vijd

fol 74

Reparacions in peter paryche
In primys at ye crane to Chesgat ye Slater of eston for hyllyng a royd and moriiijs
Item for pwentyng iij rod iijs
Item for a seym and a haf of lyme xijd
Item owr tennands at worthorp and perys pwlwer was yer and at wyllam bakkars hows (ij deys *ins*) xxd
Item for strey yat was caryed to ye hows beyownd ye chyrche vjd

[Summa] xs ijd

In sent Andro paryche
Item to ij Sclaters iiij deys mendyng of fawts xxviijd
Item to ye same slaters for hyllyng a Swyncott xvjd
Item ij masons a dey and a haf xviijd
Item yer serwer iiijd ob
Item ijC of lat neyl iiijd
Item for a loyd of erthe iijd

[Summa] vjs jd ob

Item to antony hall ye wryght a dey for makyng ye swyn hows vjd

In sent Mychells parich'
Item to Abbot ye wryght for makkyng of wyndos at pynkkanys hows in ye hal and in ye chamber xd
Item for bands and jemos and for a stabyll ixd

[*Summa lateris*] xvijs xd ob

190 this and following sub-totals are in right-hand margin

fol 74v

In Sent Mare paryche

In primis at ye awngell to antony hall and hys man a dey for settyng up a pentys xjd ob
Item to ij masons vij deys vijs
Item to yer server ijs iiijd
Item for met and drynk to ye bedmen yat dyd help to syf [sieve] iijd
Item for ston vij loyds with ye caryag ijs viijd
Item for vij loyds of mortar caryag xxjd
Item to chesgat ye Slater for leyyng and pwentyng vijs vjd
[Summa] xxijs vd ob

In Sent martyn paryche

Item at Jon dowyff' hows for thakkyng iiij deys xviijd)
Item for a serwer ixd ob) iiijs ixd ob
Item to ij Slaters a dey and a haf xviijd)
Item for a quart' and a haf of lyme xijd)

Eston

In primis at Bryon hows for settyng up a bey in a barn
Item to wyllam skynner for hys carte to cary tymbur yether vd)
Item to a wryght for under settyng and takyng down ijd)
Item for spars sydtreys and balks yat I boyht ijs ijd)
Item to benson ye wryght ij deys xd)
Item to hare wryght and rob wryght and yer man a dey xvd)
Item for wattyllyng and for wattyll xd) viijs viijd
Item for strey yat I boht xiijd)
Item for thakkyng xijd)
Item to ye serwer vd)
Item for thak rop and pak thred iijd)
Item j spent of met and drynk to ye bedmen for helppyng iijd)

[*Summa lateris*] xxxvs xjd

fol 75

Item at ye carwers hows' for ij loyds strey ijs iiijd
Item for thakkyng of ye same strey xijd
Item for hys serwer vjd
Item for mendyng a loke ijd
Item for ij loyds of strey yat ys boht for ye wewers hows and not thakyd ijs iiijd
[191]vjs viijd

Warmyngton

Item for mendyng a chamber florthe xxd)

Worthorpe

Item for mendyng a dowfhos lyme and warkmanchyp xijd)

---

[191] in right-hand margin

Item for mendyng of ij lokks	ijd)	
Northlwfnam		
In primis for iiij bords yat I bohte	xviijd)	
Item xxiiij[ti] legths	xjd)	
Item for vij stolpys	iijd)	
Item for a band and in stabylls	iijd)	xixs xjd
Item to a wryght for makkyng of v dorrs	xxijd)	
Item for ijC neylls	viijd)	
Pyllysyayt		
Item to hare wryght and hys man a dey and haf	xviijd)	
Item for iiij cartful of strey ye pric'	iiijs)	
Item for thakkyng and serwyng of ye same	iijs iiijd)	
Item for makkyng of a peyr of yaytts	xxd)	
Item for mason a dey for mendyng of kyllyn	vjd)	
Item for a loyd of mortar	ijd)	
Item for iiij trasons to ye kyllyn	vjd)	

Summa [*lateris*] xxvjs vijd

fol 75v

Northwitham	
Item for xiiij loyds of strey	xiijs
Item for thakkyng of (and serwyng *ins*) ye same strey	xiiijs viijd
Item for wattyl with ye leying of hyt	viijd
Item at cotteram hows' for makkyng a wall	xvijs vjd
Item for clensyng of ye same wall	xvjd
Item for ledyng of xvij loyds of ston and mortar	iijs viijd
Item for makkyng a gowyl hol and mendyng a nother at Schyrchaw at ye same hows and mendyng a gowyl at coterams hows and makyng ij walls at ye mylyn hows	xvijs viijd
Item for ledyng of ston and mortar	xijd
Item to a Slater at Schyrchaws hows for pwentyng of iiij rode	iijs iiijd
Item to a wryght a dey and a haf	vijd
Item to a nother wryght iij deys	xvd
Item for ij seym lyme	xvjd
Item for viij bands and hoks	xvjd
[Summa]	iij li xvijs iiijd

Swafeld	
Item for makkyng a myllyn ryyn [mill run]	iiijd
Item a wryght iij deys at alyn toppers hows and at Wyllyam yongs	xvd
Item for drawyng a wall at thomas haccs	iijs iiijd
Item for settyng a C asches	xijd

[Summa] iiij li iijs iijd

fol 76

Stretton

In primis for makkyng a Noyffyn and for ston	iijs iiijd
Item for leyyng in of v trasons in a kyllyn	vd
Item for mendyng of a baryn dor and to a wryght	xd
Item for makkyng a perclos' at ye telyors hows	xijd
Item for viij stryks of lyme	viijd
Item to a Slater for workyng yer of	xd
Costs of my hors	
Item for iij stryks of peys and hotts [oats]	xd
Item for all yis yerr for bred	iijs iiijd
Item for schoyng	xvjd
Summa	xijs vijd

The stok now remenyng in my hands os [as] hyt aperys in roll'
of my last acownte and all thyngs alowyd me xxxv li iiijd ob qa

[Audit of Sheppey's account 7 November 1508 by Thomas Morrand vicar of All Saints in the Market]

[192]*Finis compot' mei Roberti Schepey dom' elimosinarie custodis*
Probat' est iste compot' xiij' dict' Roberti Scheppey custod' dict' dom' elimosinarie per me Thomam Morrand vicarem ecclesie omnium sanctorum in foro precipium supervisorem et auditorem pro tempore mee cuiuislibet compot' de administracione' omnium bonorum seu officii custodis istius dom' ut pattet in statutis dict' dom' vij die mensis novembris anno dni m^lo^ v^c^ viij^o^ ac anno r' r' henrici septimi xxiiij^to^ hiis testibus dno Thoma fforster decano ville Staunford dno Willelmo Hawkyn confratre dict' dom' et aliis

[192] 'End of my account Robert Schepey warden of the almshouse.

This thirteenth account of Robert Scheppey warden of the almshouse is approved by me Thomas Morrand vicar of All Saints in the Market church principal supervisor and auditor for my time of every account of the administration of all the goods or offices of the warden of this house as appears in the statutes of the house 7 November 1508 and 24 Henry VII – witnessed by Thomas Forster dean of the town of Stamford, William Hawkyn confrater of the almshouse and others'. Henry Wykes died May 1508.

fol 76v

[Account of Robert Sheppey 1508-9. He did not finish it; John Taylor finalised it]

Anno domini millisimo quingentessimo nono *Compotus xiiij°*
Anno R' R' Henrici octavi j°

Here folowythe the xiiij Accompt off the state off thys almesse howse and be me Robert Schepey Wardeyn the second accompt ffor on holle yer that ys to sey frome the feste off sancte mychaell tharchangell in the xxiiij yere off the Reygn off Kyng Henry the vij to ye same feste In ye fyrste yere off the Regn' off kynge henry the viij[th] undur thys forme

The stok of ye last cownt	xxxv li iiijd ob qa
Thextent of owr lyflod yis yeyre	lxij li (vjs *del*) vs vjd ob
(Item I haf recewyd of olde det of on jon cobler	iiijs *del*)
(Item I haf recewyd of hare west	iijs iiijd *del*)
Item recewyd of ye parson peyk[irk]	ijs iiijd
Item rec' for coreccions yis yyer	iiijs
Item for old tymbur sold to tho westy of seynt merten parysch	xd

(*Summa totalis oneris* lxxxxvij li xixs vijd qa *del*)
(xiijs iijd qa *del*)
(*Inde deductuntur expense' sicut patet in foliis subscriptibus* del).
Summa total oneris lxxxxvij li xiijs jd qa

off thys summa the aforseyd warden dischargyth hym self by thes parcels foloyng

fol 77

A° dni m° v° nono *Compotus xiiij*
A° Regni Regis henr' viij primo

Be theys parcells folowyng I discharge myselfe to x beydfolke

In primis ye v dey october	vjs vd
Item ye xij dey	vjs vd
Item ye xix dey	vjs vd
Item ye xxvj dey	vjs vd
November	
Item ye ij[d] dey	vjs vd
Item ye ix dey	vjs vd
Item ye xvj dey	vjs vd
Item ye xxiij dey	vjs vd
Item ye xxx dey	vjs vd
December	
Item ye vij dey	vjs vd
Item ye xiiij dey	vjs vd
Item ye xxj dey	vjs vd
Item ye xxviij dey	vjs vd

Januarius

Item ye v dey	vjs vd
Item ye xij dey	vjs vd
Item ye xix dey	vjs vd
Item ye xxvj dey	vjs vd
Februarius	
Item ye ij dey	vjs vd
Item ye ix dey	vjs vd
Item ye xvj dey	vjs vd
Item ye xxiij dey	vjs vd

Summa lateris vj li xiiijs ixd

fol 77v

Marcius

Item ye ij dey	vjs vd
Item ye ix dey	vjs vd
Item ye xvj dey	vjs vd
Item ye xxiij dey	vjs vd
Item ye xxx dey	vjs vd
Aprilis	
Item ye vj dey	vjs vd
Item ye xiij dey	vjs vd
Item ye xx dey	vjs vd
Item ye xxvij dey	vjs vd
Mayus	
Item ye iiij dey	vjs vd
Item ye xj dey	vjs vd
Item ye xviij dey	vjs vd
Item ye xxv dey	vjs vd
Junius	
Item ye fyrste dey	vjs vd
Item ye viij dey	vjs vd
Item ye xv dey	vjs vd
Item ye xxij dey	vjs vd
Item ye xxix dey	vjs vd
Julius	
Item ye vj dey	vjs vd
Item ye xiij dey	vjs vd
Item ye xx dey	vjs vd
Item ye xxvij dey	vjs vd

Summa lateris vij li xiiijd

fol 78

Augustus

Item ye iij dey vjs vd

Item ye x dey vjs vd

Item ye xvij dey vjs vd

Item ye xxiiij dey vjs vd

Item ye xxxj dey vjs vd

September

Item ye vij dey vjs vd

Item ye xiiij dey vjs vd

Item ye xxj dey vjs vd

Item ye xxviij dey vjs vd

Summa istius part' liiijs xd

Item to my confrater and to me for on hole yere xij li

Summa totalis stipendii custodis confratris et pauperum hoc anno est xxviij li xs ixd

Annuall charges

In primis to ye parson off sancte mychelys for hys pensyon vjs viijd

Item in expensys for owr fownders dirige vjs viijd

Item allowyde for gyffyng off tenands drynke when thei come vjs viijd

Item allowyde to ye bayly xls

Item to M Archer for hys fee vjs viijd

Item I peyd to master mollysworthe for takyng off a certyn lond in wolstrop and I mwst pey mor [than] I haf peyd vjs viijd

[193]iij li xiijs iiijd

Summa lateris xviij li viijs ijd

fol 78v

Abatiment' and dekeys

In primis in al halo paroche ye schopys in ye tenur' of Jon tomas Wyff abatyd xs

Item ye schope by hyt abatyd and dekeyed j quart' iiijs

Item abatyd of ye hows' wher ye pardoner dwells ijs

Item abatyd of ye tenur wher tymynds dells [sic] iiijs

Item abatyd of ye hows' wher Whyttbred dells [sic] vjs viijd

Item abatyd of ye hows' by ye vycareghe xs

Item dekeyd of ye hows' a[t] yis syd malery bryge xvjs viijd

Item dekeyd wher willam baker dwellyd xxijs viijd

Item abatyd at ye crane vjs viijd

Item dekeyd ye ferryst hows in peter paryche viijs

[194]iiij li xjd

193 in right-hand margin

194 in right-hand margin

Sent' Mare paroche
Item abatyd in ye angell xls

Sent Mychell paroch
Item abatyd of ye hows' wher pynkkany dwells viijs

Sent Martyn paryche
Item abatyd fwlly ye gardyn place ijs
Item abatyd ye howse wher ye wever dwells iijs iiijd
Item debatyed in bredcrofte with hys pertenyngs ijs
Item debatyd in owr lond yis yeyr in stamford feld xs
Item debatyd of owr medowe at smale bryg' xijd
Item debatyd in owr barne in Scoftgat xijd

Summa lateris vij li xviijs

fol 79

Dekeyd and batyd in Worthorpe
Item debatyd in our iiij cotyars by ye yeyr vs
Item dekeyd in on of yem a quart' rent xvjd
Item dekeyd a Sclattpyt in ye same ffeld vjs viijd

Eston
Item dekeyd of a gowell yat longys to our lades gyld ijs

Walcot
Item dekeyd in ye same town xixs

Stretton
Item debatyd of ye cotyars yn ye same town xijd

Norwytham
Item dekeyd ye hows' by ye parsoneghe ijs
Item ye myllyn hows' debatyd viijs
Item dekeyd a lytyl gronde in ye chyrche wardyns hand (for ij yers *ins*) iiijd
Item dekeyd [sic]

Swafeld
Item dekeyd ye hows' yer os ye myllyn stonds vjs viijd
Item dekeyd of haknyng and holyng xijd
Item of jon Tenman of steynbe ijd ob
Item deked [sic] a medow plot calyd brodyng for ij yeyr ijs
Item debatyd of crodon ryggs ijs

Carlbe
Item debatyt in carlbe yis yeyr of hare laxton iijs iiijd

Pyllysyyatt
Item debatyd becaws he was pwt fro ye land yat we had of master torner iijs iiijd

Summa lateris iij li iijs xd ob

fol 79v

Cheff Rents

In primis All ye cheff rents for yis hol yeyr to every lord' drawys	vj li vs xd

Mercyments

Item for mercyments and swuyngs in yis yeyr	vs vjd

Stowr of hows

Item to jon eton of worthorp for ij m and a halff of Slats	viijs iiijd
Item to peyrs pwlwer of ye sam town for a m and a haf of Sclats	vs ijd
Item for caryag of ye same sclats	ijs viijd
Item for tymber yat I boyht of jon toswold	ixs iiijd
Item for tymber yat I boyht of tomas antony	iijs
Item for tymber yat I boyht of Rob' steyd	iiijs jd
Item for tymber yat I boyht of ye parson of sent mychell	ijs viijd
Item for ij dorrs with ij loks yat I boyght cost	xvjd
Item for ij ston ledd and iiij pownds wroght to ley in a goter of jon plwmmer	xvd
Item for iij pownds of soder	vjd
Item for viijC neylls *iiijd* a C	ijs
Item for iij m lat neylls	ijs vjd
Item for a C a half of vj penny nell	ixd
Item for v peyr of bands with hoks	xd
Item for iij (pownds *ins*) wax and for ye makyng	xviijd
Item for mendyng of loks to Jon Smyht	xiiijd

Summa lateris viij li xviijs vd

fol 80

Item for makyng of owr kydds to hare walker	vijs
Item for a stryk whete yat I boyht with ye bakkyng	vjd
Item for iij stryks of malt	xiijd
Item for beyf and moton	xxd
Item for fyllyng of ij bottells and yat ye [they] peyd for ayl os ye cam homwards	vd
Item for caryag of v loyds (kyds *ins*)	ijs vjd
Item for iij lodys of hey yat I boyht for my hors	vs iiijd
Item for hey yat I boyht at ye laterend of yeyr	xijd
Item for bred for my hors at al tymys yis yeyr	iiijs
Item for Schoyng of ye hors al yis yer	ijs iiijd
Item for ij peyr bands cost me	iijd
Item for neylls	[blank]
Item for ston yat I haf had at worthorp pytts	vjd
Item a loyd of plaster	ijs vjd
Item to master tryg for kepyng of owr cowrts	ijs
Item for owr dynner at Swafelld	xvjd
Item at northwitham	xd

Summa lateris xxxiijs iijd

fol 80v

Casuall expenc'

In primis I went to Peturborow be for crystonmes to wyt wedder owr wrytyng wer com home fro london or not hyt was not so hyt cost me ijd

Item I was yerfor feyn to go spek with master pigot and he seyd hys man had lost ye cope so hyt cost me xxd

Item for makkyg a new copy of ye sam indenture iiijd

Item for goyng to London at after crystonmes for to haf had an end with ye abbot and hys atorney was not yer and so I was dyssapwentyd [195]Item to speyk with master torn[er] and with master mollysworthe so yt cost me vjs viijd

Item for calys goyng to tatursall for certeyn ewydenc' hys cost viijd

Item for goyng dywers tymys to owrse [oversee] owr wodds an for mendyng of hegghs xiiijd

Item for rydyng to master pygotts on ye mondey after owr lade dey ye aswmcyon [20 August 1509] to meyt master mollysworthe yer for to bargeyn with hym for yeyrs for sertyn lond in wolstrop and for other thyngs xvjd

Item to ij sawers for sawyng of bords and leggs ewys bord and trasons with other platts iiij deys and a haf iiijs vjd

(Item I spent when I went to spek with *written over erasure*) on godall or ye cheyf rent at cownthorp ijd

Item I spent with archer when he was heyr at mysomer term ijd

Item I gaf hym a grot [groat] to drynk for to be delygent be tweyn my lord [abbot] and me iiijd

Summa lateris xvijs ijd

fol 81

Reparacions in ye bedhous

In primis to hare west and hys fellow for makyng a peyr of new dornys [at ye yard door *in margin*] and a new tresschold and for undersettyng a chamber floryht at ye crane and for makyng a new wyndow at ye hows by jon tomas wife [and for makyng of wyndos *in margin*] at ye hows a yis syd malere bryg iij deys iijs

Item to jon mor ye mason of eston for makyng of a gotter for iij deys xviijd

Item to Thomas aslyn of worthorp for caryyng of vj lods of ston and sand xviijd

In Sent Andro paryche

In primis yer os jerwas coper dwells

Item for ij wryghts for ij deys xxd

Item to jon eton and peyrs pwlwer for iij rods wark in leyng and a haf xvs

Item for iiij rods and a haf pwentyng iiijs vjd

Item for a xj seym of lyme vijs iiijd

Item to tomas tawerner for caryyng of a lod' sond iiijd

[195] This item is run on in the text

Sent mychell paryche
Item yer os pynkany dwellys for pwentyng ij rods ijs
Item for a quart' of lyme and a haf xijd
In Sent peter paryche
Item yer os ye telyor [tailor] dwells for ij rods and a haf to jon eton and perys pwlwer in pwentyng ijs vjd
Item to ye same ij men ij deys and haf pwentyng yer and at ye crane ijs
Item for ij seme lyme yer (and a haf *ins*) xxd
Item for caryage of ij loyds of ston to mak wp ye wall betweyn morrands and hws os hyt was asynyd me of ye qwest at ye gret leet vjd

Summa lateris xliiijs vjd

fol 81v

In Sent mare paryche
Item at ye awngell to antony and hys man for makkyng up ye pentys for hyt was fallyn down and for settyng yn of ij propys to beyr up a chambur at hownsleys hows iij deys iijs
Item to jon etton and perys pwlwer for rewyng [renewing?] a chymney yat was fallyn down and for Sclatyng ye same and ye pentys ye ij iiij deys iiijs
Item for ij seme lyme xvjd
Item for makyng a band of eyrn to bynd a balk with iijd
Item to jon moor of eston for makyng wp ye chymney for ij deys with mendyng a Jame and other places xijd
for hys serwer vjd
Sent martyn parych
In primis at ye hows yer ye weffer dwellys hyt was takon don
Item for takyng down ye hows with a gowyll xxd
Item to hare wryght and hys fellow for settyng up of ij and xxx[te] cowpwlls xjs iiijd
Item to jon etton and perys pwllwer for leyng of ye sclats iiij (rods *ins*) and a quart' xixs
Item for vij seym lyme yat was spent yer iiijs viijd
Item to ij masons for iij deys iijs
Item to yer serwer xijd
Item for caryag' of ston and mortar and sond xxijd
Item for iij M and a haf (of lat neyl *ins*) iijs iiijd
Item for a C of vj penny nel vjd

Item for calys and perkyn and jon holand for ye haf yer iij or iiij deys so ye and I haf spent iiijd

Summa lvjs ixd

fol 82

Item at jon dowf' hows to ij Slaters a dey xijd
Item for a quart' of lym viijd

Eston

Item at Uteram hows for a loyd of strey xvjd
Item to a thaker ij deys and a haf xiiijd
Item to hys serwer vijd
Item to calys and perkyn for helpyng to serwys yer and at ye tother wefers hows iijd
Item for thakrop and for cariag' of ij loyds of mortar erthe vijd
Item to ij Slaters a dey and a haf xviijd
Item for a quarter lyme with ye caryag' ixd

at Bryans hows

Item to tomas antony and hys man ij deys for mendyng of dorrs yatts wyndows ijs
Item for a tre yat was boyht of ye clark of eston vjd
Item for makyng a claspe of eyryn to ye gret yat' ijd
Item to ij masons vij deys for makkyng up of walls and for pargentyng ye dowf' hows vijs
Item for ij loyds of ston iiijd
Item for viij loyds ston and mortar caryyng and a loyd of sond ijs
Item for iij seym lyme yat was spent abowt ye dofcot ijs ijd
Item to calys and perkyn for helpyng to serwys yem yat ye spent ijd
Item to a thakker at ye sam how for mendyng a dey yer ye croys [crows?] had pwllyd owt vjd
Item to hys serwer a dey iijd

Summa lateris xxijs xjd

fol 82v

Worthorp

Item for makkyng a wal betwyn jon eton and peyrys pwlwer a rod wark xxd

Northwytham

In primis to antony hall and to hare[196] and an[o]ther wryght and ye serwands for drayng a hows of vij xx [27] copwll' leyn'hte yat was ron a neynd xxvjs viijd
Item for caryag' of yer stwf yether and hom a geyn ijs iiijd
Item for to geyt stwf to mak scafolds cost me vjd
Item for iij xx brod neyls viijd
Item to a mason for drawyng of (ij cowpwll' *del*) a wall at ye eynd of ye sam barn yat was fallyn down with ye weyht of ye hows iiijs ijd
Item to a wryght ij deys for drawyng yn of ij cowpwlls of ye sam wall and mendyng of dors and wyndos xijd

---

[196] probably hare wright

Carlbe

Item to a wryght iij deys for makyng of dorrs and dornis' and threscholds xviijd
Item to a thakker a dey and a haff ixd
Item hys serwer iiijd

Worthorpe

Item to jon eton and to peyrs pwlwer for makkyng of a wal of a rood wark and mor ijs

Summa lateris xljs xjd

fol 83

Swafeld

In primis At Ryc' hac hows besyd ye kyrk
Item to a mason for makyng up of ij syd walls ye charg' of xix roods cost xxjs
Item for caryag' of mortar and brekyng of ston vijs vjd
Item to a wryght for makkyng up a neynd' of ye sam hows and for mendyng other thyngs iiijs
Item to a thakker and hys serwer ix deys iiijs ixd
Item for thakrop xijd
Item for a C of reeds iijs iiijd
Item for caryag' of ye same reyd' xijd
Item for xij sparrs yat wer boyht xijd
Item for iiij loyds of strey iiijs
Item for ij Sclaters a dey and a haf xviijd
Item for xij stryks of lyme (in stonys *ins*) xviijd

[197]*Summa lateris* ls vijd
Summa total expensorum et allocatorum lxv li xjs jd ob
Summa in superplusag' of the Rents hoc anno nil
Summa *Remanens* xxxij li xxiijd ob qa

[198]off thys Summa Remaynyth in old detts left by master Wyllam Scharp warden afor me as aperyth in a byll -

Item ther Remaynyth in tennands hands of thys last perteynyg to my charge as aperyth by a byll -

[199]finis istius compot' supervisus fuit per me Johannem taylyor deputat' dni thome Morrand vicarii ecclesie omnium sanctorum hac v... a° dni m° vC nono et xxv° die mensis octobris
[200]Per me thomam Morrond probatum est

---

[197] The next section and the page summaries throughout this account are in the handwriting of John Taylor; see his final paragraph.

[198] no totals are included here.

[199] 'The end of this account was supervised by me John Taylor deputy of Thomas Morrand vicar of All Saints 15 October 1509'

[200] written in the hand of Morrand

fol 83v
[*blank*]

fol 84
[Account of Robert Sheppey for year 1509-10]

[201]Ihs
Anno R' R' *henrici octavi ij*° *Compot' xv*m

Heyr folowyth the xv accounte of ye state of yis almysse hows' and be me Syr Rob' Schepey the iiij warden hys theyrd' acounte for on holl yeyr that ys to sey from ye fest of sent mychaell tharchangell in ye fyrst yere of ye Reyne of kyng henry ye viij unto ye sam fest in ye secunde yere of ye Reyng off the same kyng under yis forme foloyng

The stoke of ye laste cownte	xxxij li xxiijd ob qa
The extent of owr lyflod yis yere	iiixxij li (j iij li *del*) vjs
Item ij moorys fools presyd at	iijs iiijd
Item for correccyons yis yere	ijs viijd
Item for ascys yat I sold in bredcroft	xvjd

Summa total onoris hoc anno iiijxxxiiij li xvs iijd (ob *ins*) qa

Be theys parcells foloyng I Dyscharge my selfe to x bedefolke

In primis the v dey of october	vs xd
Item the xij dey	vs xd
Item ye xix dey	vs xd
Item the xxvj dey	vs xd
November	xlijs vjd
Item the ij dey	vs xd
Item ye ix dey	vs xd
Item the xvj dey	vs xd
Item ye xxiij dey	vs xd
Item the xxx dey	vs xd

[202]*Summa lateris* xlijs vjd [sic]

fol 84v
December

Item the vij dey	vs xd)
Item ye xiiij dey	vs xd)
Item the xxj dey	vs xd)
Item ye xxviij dey	vs xd)

[201] in Robert Sheppey's hand

[202] The total should come to 52s 6d. The sub-totals are given by Sheppey in the right-hand or left-hand margin; the page summaries are again in the hand of John Taylor; see end of account.

Januaer'		
Item the iiij dey	vs xd)	
Item ye xj dey	vs xd)	
Item the xviij dey	vs iijd)	
[203]*et ibi mortuus henric' phylyp*		
Item ye xxv dey	vs iijd)	
ffebruarius		
Item the fyrst dey	vs iijd)	
Item ye viij dey	vs iijd)	
Item the xv dey	vs iijd)	
Item ye xxij dey	vs iijd)	vij li
Marcius		
Item the fyrst dey	vs iijd)	
Item ye viij dey	vs iijd)	
Item the xv dey	vs iijd)	
Item ye xxij dey	vs iijd)	
Item the xxix dey	vs iijd)	
Aprilis		
Item the v dey	vs iijd)	
Item ye xij dey	vs iijd)	
Item the xix dey	vs iijd)	
Item ye xxvj dey	vs iijd)	
Mayus		
Item the iij dey	vs iijd)	
Item ye x dey	vs iijd)	
Item the xvij dey	vs iijd)	
Item ye xxiiij dey	vs iijd)	
Item the xxxj dey	vs iijd)	

Summa lateris vij li

fol 85

Junius	
Item the vij dey	vs iijd)
Item ye xiiij dey	vs iijd)
et ibi mortuus est Johannes benlos'	
Item the xxj dey	[204]iiijs viijd)
Item ye xxviij dey	iiijs viijd)
Julius	
Item the v dey	iiijs viijd)
Item ye xij dey	iiijs viijd)

---

[203] death of Henry Phylyp

[204] death of John Benlos; the sum has been amended from 'vs iijd'

Item the xix dey iiijs viijd)
Item ye xxvj dey iiijs viijd)

Augustus
Item the secund dey iiijs viijd)
Item ye ix dey iiijs viijd) iiij li vjd
Item the xvj dey iiijs viijd)
Item ye xxiij dey iiijs viijd)
Item ye xxx dey iiijs viijd)

September
Item the vj dey iiijs viijd)
Item ye xiij dey iiijs viijd)
Item the xx dey iiijs viijd)
Item ye xxvij dey iiijs viijd)

Summa pauperum hoc anno xiij li iijs
Item to my confrater and to me for on hole yeyre xij li
Summa totalis stipendii custodys confratris et pauperi' hoc anno est xxv li iijs

Summa lateris xvj li vjd

fol 85v

Annuall charges
In primis to ye person of sente mychells for hys pensyon vjs viijd
Item in expensys for owr a dirige vjs viijd
Item to M Archer for hys fee vjs viijd
Item a lowyd for ye gederyng of rents xls
Item I peyd to M mollysworthe for takyng a certyn lond' in wylstrope
ye last yere - vjs viijd and yis yeyre xxs
[205] iiij li

Cheyff rentts [206]Item a pond pepper xiiijd
In primis All yis hole yeyre ye cheyf rent drawys vj li xiijd and qa
Item for mercementts and swuyngs drawys vs iijd
besyd yat I was mersyed for a heghe at carlbe at master greysley cowrte
at brasboro iijs
Item to master Tryg for kepyng of ij cowrts ijs
Item for owr dynner at swafeld hyt cost me ijs iiijd
[207]for I had dywerse men of ye contre for to se weder yat colwell deyd
me wrong or not os in fellyng assys [ashes] apon a dyk bank and for
settyng of a kyln wall
Item owr dynner at northwitham xd

---

[205] all sub-totals in this account are in left-hand margin

[206] this line has been inserted to the right of the heading 'Cheyff rents'

[207] marginal total 'vj li xixs qa'

Item I toke a swyt of gorgius pensbere and of hew holme for sertyn mony yat the[y] howte [owed] to yis hows so I tok a wyrte [writ] cost me xxd
And ij alyas capyas [other writs] cost me xxd

Summa lateris x li xixs qa

fol 86

Stoore of hows'
In primis for tymber yat I boyghte of ye parson of sent mychells yt cost me iijs viijd
Item for a rood of bords yat I boyghte of ye same parson vijs
Item for tymber yat I boyght of tomas wytwell xiijs iiijd
Item of ye same tomas for ij leyds ye pryc' viijs
Item for tymber yat I boyghte of Wyllyam skynner iijs iiijd
Item for tymber yat I boyghte yat was ye parsons of stretton ixs
Item for caryage of ye same tymber ijs
Item for tymber yat I boyghte of Roberd sawyge vs
Item for tymber yat I boyghte of Rob' talyer ijs viijd
Item I peyd to jon etton for a M and a hafe of slate vs viijd
Item to perrs pwlwer for haf a M slate xxijd
Item for vj loyds of wal ston to ye same man vjd
Item to jon cordall of eston owr tenand for a rod of boords vijs
Item ye sam jon for ij M latts vijs
Item to ye parson of sent mychells for haf a M latts ijs
Item for a rope to ye bell in ye chappell jd
Item for ij loydys of plaster yat I boyghte cost me iiijs vjd
Item for vij peyre of bands with yer hokks ijs vjd
Item for a trowyll and ij wymbells cost me vd
Item for vj M of latts nells cost me at mydlent feyr iiijs vjd
Item for v C of v penny nells cost me ijs jd
Item for v C of iiij penne nells and a haf xxijd
Item for a booll yat I boyghte ijd
Item to jon holdernes for v deys caryag' of ston and tymber hym self and hys son for mete and drynk xviijd
Item for caryag' of iij loyds sond and a loyd of slate xiijd
Item for iiijC of ij penny neyll xijd
Item for a M of lat nell' cost me xjd

Summa lateris [208]iiij li xviijs vijd

[208] the same figure is in the left-hand margin in Sheppey's hand; the page total is in the hand of Taylor

fol 86v

Item for caryage of owr kyds for a stryk' of qweyt[209]		vd
Item for a haf a seym of Malte [?]		xjd
Item for beyf and motton		xxiijd
Item for iij loyds caryage		xviijd
Item for fyllyng of bottells		ijd
Item for iij lodds of hey yat I boyght		vs
Item for schoyng al yis yere and for prowand [provender]		iiijs
Item for makyng owr kydds		vjs
Item for cryyng ye ij foyll' [foals] at borne and grantam	)	
Item for kepyng yem a hol yeyre	)	xijd
		[210]xxs xjd

A batments and dekeys

In primis in All halo paryche ye schoppe in ye tennur of jon tomas wyff abatyd	xs
Item dekeyd ye schop by hyt for a hol yeyr	xs
Item a battyd of ye hows qweyr tymyng dwells	iiijs
Item dekeyd ye hows qwer ye pardoner dwellyd	xs
Item dekeyd ye hows qwer tosswold dwellt	xxs
Item a batyd of ye hows by ye vyckareg	iijs iiijd
Item a batyd at malare bryge	viijs
Item a batyd at ye crane	vjs viijd
Item a batyd yis yer qwer willam (baker *ins*) dwellyd	viijs
Item dekeyd ye farryst hows in peter paryche	viijs
	iiij li viijs

Summa lateris v li viijs xjd

fol 87

Sent mare paryche

Item dekeyd yis yere in ye angell	v li xs

[211]Sent mychells

Item ye tenur yer os pynkany dwells	viijs

Sent martyns par[yche]

Item dekeyd a gardyn place	ijs
Item a batyd yer as hownsley dwellyd	xvjd
Item a batyd yer of ye wewer dells [sic]	iijs iiijd
Item a batyd in bredcroft with hys perteings	ijs vjd
Item debatyd in owr lond yis yere in ye feylds	vjs
Item batyd of owr myddow at smalbryg	xijd
Item batyd of ye barne in scofgate	xijd

---

209 wheat? see folio 91v

210 this and the next sub-total are in the left-hand margin

211 this heading is in left hand margin

Worthorpe

Item debatyd in owr iiij cottears by ye yere vs

Item dekeyd in on of yem a haf yere rent ijs vjd

Item dekeyd a slatte pytt vjs viijd

Eston

Item a battyd at bryons hows iijs iiijd

Item a battyd a gowyll yat longs to owr lades gyld ijs

Item dekeyd at walcot be yere xixs

Item debatyd at pyllysyat iijs iiijd

Item debattyd of ye ij cottears at stretton xijd

Norwytham

Item a batyd of ye hows be syd ye parsonage ijs

Item a batyd of ye myllyn hows' viijs

Item dekeyd a cottear hows yat ys bornyd by ye water syd ijs

Item dekeyd a lyttyl grond in ye chyrche wardyns honds ijd

Swafelld

Item dekeyd of ye mylyn hows' iijs

Item dekeyd of hakkyng and hollyng xijd

Item of Jon Tenman of steynbe ijd ob

Item dekeyd of a mydow plot calyd brodyng xijd

Item a batyd owt of cradyn ryg' ijs

[212]*Summa lateris* ix li xvijs iiijd ob

fol 87v

Reparacyons in sent andro parych

In primis at Jarwas Coper to Jon Eton and peyrs pwllwer for viij roodys of wark in pwentyng (and mendyng other fawts *ins*) viijs xd

Item for viij seym lyme vs iiijd

In Al halow paryche

Item yer os qwytwyk wyff d[w]ells and ye hows be syd yt to ye god man of ye boro for vj rods pwentyng vjs

Item for iiij seme lyme yat ys not spendyd ijs viijd

Item to a wryght ij days for to mend ower a synke in ye stabyll and for mendyng a mawnger xjd

Item to ij slaters a dey yer os jon tomas wyf dwells and of ye hows by hyt xijd

Item to a mason ij deys for mendyng a wall at ye hows' on ye hyll and a nother wall at tymyngs and a harthston xijd

Sent mychells

Item at pykany hows' for mendyng a synke to colyn and (hys wyf *ins*) ixd

Item for dawbyng a wall yat ye bedmen dyd I gaf yem drynk jd ob

---

[212] this sum is in the right-hand margin wtitten by Sheppey; the page total was written by Taylor

in peter paroch'
Item at ye crane to a wryghte ij deys for undersettyng a chamber
yat was bown to fall xijd

Sent mare parrych'
Item at ye angell to Jo etton for pwentyng and mendyng (oder fawtts *ins*) xviijd
Item for a quarter lyme viijd

Sent martyn paroch'
Item to a wryghte ij deys for makkyng a windo yer os hownsley dells
and to a mason other ij deys for makyng a wal by ye watersyd xxijd
Item for dawbyng up of ij gowyll ends os ye (wewer *ins*) dwells xviijd
Item for a loyd erthe caryag' iijd

[213]*Summa lateris* xxxiijs iiijd ob

fol 88

Reparacyons At northlwfnam
In primis for iiij sem lyme ijs viijd
Item for a loyde sond ye caryag' iijd
Item for vj rodys of pwentyng vjs
Item to a wryght for makyng of dorrs (v deys *ins*) and wyndos and
makyng a lower [louvre] with other thyngs ijs iiijd

Eston
Item for a loyd strey yer os gonbe dwells xiiijd
Item for thakyng ye same strey and serwyng xijd
Item for pwentyng ij roods and mendyng other placs ijs vjd
Item for a quarter and a haf of lyme with ye caryag' ixd iiijd [sic]
for a loyd of sond and slhate to geder iiijd
Item at ye hows' by hyt for a loyd of strey xvjd
Item for serwyng and for thakyng ye same xijd
Item for a loyd strey at utterams' hows' xvjd
Item for thakkyng and serwyng ye same ixd
Item for ij loydys of erthe caryag' vjd

Carlbe
Item for iij loyds of strey iijs vjd
Item for a thakker v deys hys wag' [no total]
Item for hys mett and drynk xvd
Item for of ye sam strey serwyng xvd
Item for ij loyds of mortar vd
Item to a wryght iij deys for makkyng of dorrs wyndos and
dornys with trescholds xviijd

---

[213] this sum was written by Sheppey in the left margin; at the bottom of the page by Taylor

Barhowm

Item for a loyd of strey xiiijd

Item for thakyng and serwyng ye sam xijd

Item for splyntyng and dabyng a gowyl eynd by ye yatt' ixd

[214]*Summa lateris* xxxijs viijd

fol 88v

Warmyngton

In primis for a sydtre and a roftre yat cost ijs ijd

Item to a wryghte ij deys and a haf xiiijd

Pyllysyat

In primys to ij wryghts for settyng up a chamber yat was fled for kepyng up ye hows a loyfft and for leyyng yn of ij walplatts ye ton viiij deys and ye (tother *ins*) iij deys for *vd* a dey drawys iiijs vijd

Item to jon etton for takyng down ye slate and for slatyng hyt a geyn xxd

Item for j seym lyme viijd

Item for neylls yat wer spent at yat tyme cost me xd

Item to ij masons for wyrkyng of a rood and a haff and a quart' after *viijs* ye (quarter *del*) (rod *ins*) xiiijs

Item for caryage of iiij loyds ston xiijd

Item for caryage of xv loyds of erthe ijs vjd

Item to ij Slaters for takyng down a hows' of iij rods wark and a quarter xvs

Item for pwentyng of iiij rods warke ~~xx~~ iiijs

Item for ix seym lyme and a haf vjs iiijd

Item for caryage of ye sam lym vjd

Item for ij loyds of sond caryage vijd

Item for caryag' of iij loyds of wode with ledder fro hom xviijd

Item to ye bedmen for helpyng in wyntter and now in sommer abowte ye wal making I gaf yem to drynk vd

Item for makyng a peyr of gymmoys cost iiijd

Item to a wryght yat dells in wothorpe for vj deys iijs

[215]*Summa lateris* iij li iiijd

fol 89

Swafeld

In primis a wryghte at Ric' hacc hows' and at a nother hows' for leyyng of a roft[r]e and a syddetre dey and a haf viijd

Item at tomas hac' hows' to ij masons for makkyng up a gowyll of a rod wark cost viijs vjd

Item to on of ye same masons for iij deys wark be syd xviijd

---

214 this sum was written by Sheppey in the left margin; at the bottom of the page by Taylor

215 marginal total 'iij li iiijd'

Item for xij loyds of mortar to ye same wark ijs
Item to a wrygh[t]e for makyng up ye gowyll top and for splynttyng ye same and for leyyng in a sydtre in a kyllyn xviijd
Item for dawbyng up ye sam gowyll xvjd
Item for a C neylls and for ij spars vjd
Item at jon holdernes hows' for makyng a wall of a rod wark viijs vjd
Item to ij wryghts for hengyng of ye hows' xijd
Item for a wal platte vjd
Item to a wrygh[t] for leyyng in ye wal plat afor makyng dornys to barn dor ixd
Item for rewyng ye bothom of boyhe [both] ye walls xxd
Item for x loyds of erthe caryag' xxd
Item for caryag' of v bonche of latts fro worthop to pyllysyat ijd

At stretton

Item to a mason viij deys for makkyng a wall iiijs
Item hys serwar met and hyr xijd
Item for v loyds of ston caryag' xvd
Item for iiij loyds erthe car[yag] viijd
Item to a Slater for hyllyng of iiij rod warke xxs
Item for mendyng in other pl[a]ces xijd
Item for iiij seym lym in stonnys with ye car[yag] iiijs iiijd
Item for iij seym lym with latt' yat war c[216] ijs vjd
Item for iij loyds of sond xijd
Item for ij loydys of slate yat I boyhte cost me vs
Item for caryag' of iij loyds of slatte to stretton ijs

Summa lateris iij li xiijs

Summa totalis expensarum hoc anno lxvj li vjs iijd qa
Summa Remanens xxviij li ixs ob

[217]*de hac Summa Remanet in quada' billa antiqua Relicta per dom' Willam Scharp tercium custodem istius dom'* ten pownds fowr schelyngs ijd ob *Et Residuum Remanet in manibus Robarti Schepey dicti custod' computat' Inde alias Responsurus*

fol 89v

[Note added by John Taylor in his distinctive hand on an otherwise blank page. Taylor was deputed by Thomas Morrand vicar of All Saints church and Thomas Forster rector of St Michael's church and dean of Stamford, auditors of the account, to take the audit and make the allowances; he did that on 18 November 1510 before Sheppey, Hawkyn, Morrand and Forster and (for the first time) two of the bedesmen, John Parkyn and John Calays]

---

216 text unfinished

217 'Of this sum, there remain in certain old bills with William Scharp third warden of this house £10 4s 2½d; the rest remains in the hands of Robert Schepey to be accounted for elsewhere.'

Probatus fuit iste compotus Retro scriptus et finitus in nominibus dom thome morrand vicarii omnium sanctorum in foro ville staunford et dom thome forster Rector' ecclesie sancti michael' archangel (ratione factum officii decanatus ins*) hac vice auditorum istius compoti per Johannem taylyor vicarium sancti martini deputatum predictorum thome et thome per eos specialiter electum unanimo consensu utriusque et allocat' per predict' Johannem per eos assignat' hac vice tum coram predicto Robarto Schepey custodo, dno willielmo hawkyn confratro euisdem dom' thoma morrand' predict' thoma forster predict' Johanne taylyor deputat' predict' ac coram duobus pauperibus dict' dom' discretioribus Johanne parkyn Johanne calays decimo (nono* del, *octavo* ins*) die Novembris anno dni millessimo quingentessimo decimo ac A° Regni Regis henr' octavi secundo*[218].

[218] This account written up retrospectively was approved and finished in the name of Thomas Morrand vicar of All Saints in the Market, Stamford, and Thomas Forster rector of St Michael the archangel (by reason of his office of dean *ins*), auditors of this account on this occasion, by John Taylor vicar of St Martin's church, deputy of the said Thomas and Thomas by them specially chosen by the unanimous consent of both of them, and the allowances [were given] by the said John, assigned by them for this occasion before the said Robert Schepey warden, William Hawkyn confrater of this house, Thomas Morrand and Thomas Forster, the said John Taylor deputy and two of the more discrete paupers John Parkyn and John Calays on the 18/19 November 1510, 2 Henry VIII

fol 90

[Account of Robert Sheppey 1510-11; the marginal sub-totals and the page totals are all in the hand of Sheppey]

Ihs est amor meus
Anno RR *henrici octavi iij*° *Compotus xvj*

here folowythe ye xvj acownte of ye state of yis almys hows and be me Syr Rob' Schepey the iiij Wardyn of yis [alms house, the] iiij A counte for a holl yere yat ys to sey from ye fest of sent michaell tharchangell in ye secund yere of ye Reyng of kynge henry ye viij unto ye same fest In ye yeyrd [third] yere of ye Reyne off ye same kyng under yis forme ffoloyng

The stoke of ye last counte	xxviij li ixs ob
The extent of owr lyflod yis yere	iij^{xx}ij li vs
[Space left]	
Summa totalis onoris est In hoc anno	[no total]

Be theys parcell' foloyng I dyscharge my selfe

In primis to my selfe and to my confrater for a holl yere	xij li
Item to viij bedfolke for a hol yeyre	
In primis iiij dey of october	iiijs viijd
Item ye xj dey	iiijs viijd
Item ye xviij dey	iiijs viijd
Item ye xxv dey	iiijs viijd
November	
Item the fyrste dey	iiijs viijd
Item ye viij dey	iiijs viijd
Item ye xv dey	iiijs viijd
Item ye xxij dey	iiijs viijd
Item ye xxix dey	iiijs viijd

Summa pagine (xiiij li xxijs viijd *del*) xxiiij li ijs
[219]*Probatum est per me thomam morrond*

fol 90v

December	
Item the vj dey	iiijs viijd
Item ye xiij dey	iiijs viijd
Item ye xx dey	iiijs viijd
Item ye xxvij dey	iiijs viijd
Januarius	
Item ye therd dey	iiijs viijd
Item ye x dey	iiijs viijd

---

[219] The few audit notes that appear are in the hand of Thomas Forster. Sheppey (as in the last account) wrote his sub-totals in the left-hand margin; the page totals (also written by Sheppey) repeat these.

Item ye xvij dey	iiijs viijd
Item ye xxiiij dey	iiijs viijd
Item ye xxx dey	iiijs viijd
ffebruarius	
Item ye vij dey	iiijs viijd
Item ye xiiij dey	iiijs viijd
Item ye xxj dey	iiijs viijd
Item ye xxviij dey	iiijs viijd
Martius	
Item ye vij dey	iiijs viijd
Item ye xiiij dey	iiijs viijd
Item ye xxj dey	iiijs viijd
Item ye xxviij dey	iiijs viijd
Aprilis	
Item the iiij dey	iiijs viijd
Item ye xj dey	iiijs viijd
Item ye xviij dey	iiijs viijd
Item ye xxv dey	iiijs viijd
Mayus	
Item ye secund dey	iiijs viid
Item ye ix dey	iiijs viijd
Item ye xvj dey	iiijs viijd
Item ye xxiij dey	iiijs viijd
Item ye xxx dey	iiijs viijd

[220]*Summa lateris* vj li xvjd

fol 91

Jun'	
Item the vj dey	iiijs viijd
Item ye xiij dey	iiijs viijd
Item ye xx dey	iiijs viijd
Item ye xxvij dey	iiijs viijd
Julius	
Item ye iiij dey	iiijs viijd
Item ye xj dey	iiijs viijd
Item ye xviij dey	iiijs viijd
Item ye xxv dey	iiijs viijd
Augustus	
Item the fyrst dey	iiijs viijd
Item ye viij dey	iiijs viijd
Item ye xv dey	iiijs viijd

---

[220] This figure also appears in the left-hand margin

Item ye xxij dey iiijs viijd
Item ye xxix dey iiijs viijd

September
Item the v dey iiijs viijd
Item ye xij dey iiijs viijd
Item ye xix dey iiijs viijd
Item ye xxvj dey iiijs viijd
[221] iij li xixs iiijd

Summa pauperum hoc anno (ix li xiijs viijd *del*)
Summa totalis stipendii custodis et confratris et pauperum hoc anno [222]xxiiij li ijs viijd

fol 91v

Annuall charges
In primis to ye parson of sent mychells for hys pencion vjs viijd
Item in expensys at owr founders dirige vjs viijd
Item to master Archer for hys fee vjs viijd
Item peyd to Ric' campion for gederyng rents in swafeld and
Northwitham with ye perteneys yerto xjs
Item A lowy for geyderyng ye rent in stanford and in other plac' and for al other
costs and chargs spent or gyffen with in ye (town *ins*) or withowt os with(in *ins*)
ye cyrcwyt of owr lands or within owr hows' os of owr tenands or other
strangers and for makkyng god' ye rent when (r *del*) ye [they] rwn awey
with ye rent a for owr rekunyng so I to a lowe ye hows ye holl rents xxixs
[223] iij li

Cheyff rents
Item ye cheyff rentts yis yere drays vj li xs qa
Item for merciments and swnygs yis yeyr drawys vijs
Item to hare lace for kepyng a cowrte at nortwitham ye v de of october xxd
Item at owr dynner cost xijd
Item I peyd to master archer for stopyng ye swyt be twyne
jorge penbury and hwe holme yat I had taken a geyn yem vjs ijd
Item for makyng of owr kydds vjs
Item for a stryke of whet with ye bakkyng xiijd
Item for beyf and moton ijs
Item for (to *del*) fyllyng (of ij *ins*) bottells (and *ins*) yat ye dranke at
casterton os yey com homward vjd
Item for a loyd ledyng vjd
[224] vij li vjs iiijd (qa *del*)

Summa lateris x li vjs viijd

---

[221] In left-hand margin only

[222] three attempts have been made to provide a total; two are heavily scored through but appear to read 'xxiij li xixs iiijd' and 'xxiij li xviijs viijd'

[223] in left-hand margin

[224] in left-hand margin

fol 92a[225]

A battments and dekeys

In All halo paryche schop in ye tennur of jon tomas wyf xs
Item ye schop by hyt (abatyd *del*) dekeyd yis yeyr xs
Item ye hows' yer os tymyng dwells abatyd iiijs
Item ye hows' of ye hyll in dekey xs
Item ye hows' be ye wykkareg abatyd iijs iiijd
Item ye hows' by hyt (abatyd *del*) in dekey xxs
Item ye hows' at malery bryg abatyd viijs
Item at the Crane abatyd vjs viijd
Item the howsse ageyns hytt abatyd iij quarters xxijs viijd
Item dekeyd the farrest howse in petyr parysch (xjs *del*) xs
[Summa] [226]v li iiijs viijd

Seynt mary parysch

Item the awngell thys yer dekeyed vj li iiijs
Item in seynt michell parysch abatyd viijs
vj li xijs

Seynt martyn' parysch

Item ther as howndesley dwelled dekeyd a qa and di' iiijs vjd
Item in the same plac' by yer abatyd ijs
Item a Garden plac' dekeyd a yer ijs
Item ther as the wefar dwells abated iijs iiijd
Item abatyd in bredecroft thys yer viijs
Item for iij yer every yer abatyd (be *del*) of ye same rltum [?] behynd in the hole unacownted (xxijs *del*) [227]xvjs vjd
Item abatyd in owr lands yis yer in staunford feeld' xs iijd
Item abatyd at the small brygges xijd
Item abatyd of a barn in skoff gate xijd
[228] [Summa] (iij li xiiijs jd *del*) iij li vijs iijd

Worthorppe

Item the farthest howse in worthorpp in dekey vjs viijd
Item iij cotages besyde abatyd vs iiijd
Item a sklatt pytt dekeyed vjs viijd

Summa lateris (xiiij li *del*) xv li iijs xjd

---

[225] this and the following page are heavily stained

[226] this and all the following sub-totals are in the left-hand margin

[227] this and some of the other corrections to this account were made by John Taylor in his distinctive hand. The page totals are all by Taylor.

[228] both totals in left-hand margin

fol 92av

Eston

Item abatyd in Bryans howsse	iijs iiijd
Item abatyd a govyll yat longs to owr lady gyld'	ijs
Item dekeyd in walcott	xixs
Item abatyd at pyllesgate	iijs iiijd
Item abatyd (t *del*) ij cotears at stretton	xijd
Northwitham	
Item abatyd of the howsse besyde the parsonage	ijs
Item abatyd of the myln howsse	viijs
Item dekeyed a lyttell howsse by ye watur syde	ijs yt was burnd
Item dekeyd a lyttell grownd in the church wardyns handds	ijd
Item a cotear howse dekeyd next ye man[or] plac'	iijs iiijd
Swafeld	
Item dekeyd the myln howse thys yer	iijs iiijd
Item dekeyd of hakyng and hollyng thys yer	ijs
Item abatyd of John denman of rent assis'	ijd ob
Item abatyd at Crowdwn rygges	ijs viijd
	lijs iiijd ob
Stoor off howsse	
Item for a thowsand sklate bowht of ranton son of eston	iijs iiijd
Item for v thowsand latt neyle	iiijs
Item for iiijC and di' of v peny neyle	ijs iiijd
Item for v hundreth of iiij peny neyle	xxd
Item for tymber yat I bowght of Ric karvar	viijs viijd
Item for tymber that I bowght at Northlwffnam	ijs viijd
Item a qweyr of pawper	iijd
Item for vj bwnch off latt	ijs iijd
Item for heggyng abowte owr woode cald swyne how	vs
Item for tymber yat I boyhte of jarwas coper cost me	xijs
	[229] xliijs ijd

Summa lateris iiij li xvs vjd ob

fol 92b

***[At this point, a single sheet written on both sides has been pasted to a stub left in the quire; it has been numbered folio 92b. At one time, it was loose in the book. It is only 9.5 cms wide. It contains a new rental drawn up in 1517-8. Since it belongs properly to folio 125 where it is specifically mentioned, and not to the account for 1510-11, I have printed the text after folio 125; see below pages 292-93*]**

[229] left-hand marginal total

fol 93

[At this point, a different hand appears: it is apparently that of Thomas Williams, as the note on folio 95v reveals]

Store of hows

Item to ye parson of sent michell' for xv copwll spars	vjs)	
Item for a loyde of plaster cost me	xxd)	
Item for ye caryag' of ij loyd' of sond	xjd)	ixs iijd
Item for gaderyng of ye same sond and for doyng mony other	)	
thyngs yat has don gwd to ye hows to calys and perkyn	viijd)	
Item ij peyr of band' with hwks		vd

Casuall charges

In primis for owr stresse yat was taken a[t] swafeld
I went to swafeld to se wat catel war taken yer hyt cost me to content
yem for ye [they] war very wrahte [wroth] vd
Item on ye morow ric' campyon w yonge Ric' hac jon bartylmew and I went
to meyt master hwsse at depyng to desyr hym to se a remyde for hws [us]
bot he come not ther yat dey so they com with me howm yat nyhte and
went ageyn on ye morow and spak with hym so he promyssyd he wold
do ye best he cold and cost me on yem and me theyr and at howm for
her met and mannys mete xxd
Item he sent tomas stok to master browns to haf ye stresse delywerd
bot he wold not in no wysse delywer hyt so ye seyd tomas had of me
with yat I spent with hym xiiijd
Item I was feyn to go to sleford after yat and iij of yes [these] men with
me to se yf any remide wold be ther was iij deys er we cold kno how we
schold do so hyt cost me of yem and meselffe iiijs
Item a sennyt after candelmes I was fen to go to london for ye tennands
had so gret laber with beryng ther catell met and drynk yat [they] cryed owt
of me so yat I was wrke [irked?] of yem hyt cost of my hors and of my self
I was swrhte [surety] ix deys vjs
Item I peyd for wyrt [writ] ijs xjd
[230] xvjs ijd

Summa lateris xxiijs vd

fol 93v

Item when I was come howm and had yis wyrt of replegear[231] then I went to ye
cheryf to haf a warrant to on of hys balys to haf ye catell delywerd he dwells ix
myl be yond spellysbe so I ley at swynsted[232] ye fyrst nyght
a yis syd boston my horse and my selfe cost me vd

---

230 left-hand marginal total

231 writ of replevin or recovery of goods

232 Swinstead manor in south Lincolnshire was given by William Browne to his daughter Elizabeth Elmes; it would have been a sympathetic centre for the warden of Browne's Hospital.

Item on ye moro at boston my hors and myself ijd
Item ye sam nyghte at frysbe[233] wher ye cheryf lyes vjd
Item ye under cheryf was nat hat howm he was at lyncolln so I was feyn to hyr me a gyde hyt cost me fo hys hors and hym selfe xiiijd
Item hyt cost me a[t] horn castell my hors and my self vd
Item at lyncolln ye sam nyghte at sopper ijd
Item for wyn of ye cheryf yat I myghte be sped iiijd
Item at brekfast on ye morow hyt cost me ijd
Item my hors met yat nyght and on ye moro hent nown vjd
Item for waschyng my gown and dyhttyng my hors ijd
Item at ankaster homward my hors and my self iijd
Item at swafeld yat nyght yat I com howm ijd
Item at corbe when ye strese was borrod hyt cost me yer yat dey a pon ye kyngs bayle and of other men yat had down for hws xijd
Item ye[234] loggyd with me a nyght at staunford hys cost vd
Item ye scheryf had of me for serwyng wyrt xijd
Item for iij loyd' of hey for my hors viijd
Item for schoyng yis yer ijs
Item for prowande al yis yeyr ijs
Item for mendyng of haf a dosyn lokks vijd
Item ye smythe in sent mare paryche had ffor oppynynyg of loks ijd

[235]*Summa lateris* xixs vijd

fol 94

Reparacyons

In primis at owr own hows' to a mason dey and a haf ixd
Item to perys pwlwer for iij deys (pwenttyng *ins*) at howm xviijd
Item for mendyng a pentys (on ye hyl *ins*) and a swynkot (at malerybryg *ins*) a dey vjd
Item for iij sem lym with yat was spent at ye wal ijs
Item for pwentty yer as pytt' dwell' iiij rods iiijs
Item for ij seym lyme (and a haf and a stryke *ins*) xxjd
Item to jarwas coper for a ryng to a leyd ijs
Item to plwmmer for settyng on ye sam and for soderryng of ij ledds xijd
Item for a C neylls to ye same leds ijd
Item for iij lods of erthe and a loyd at howm ixd
Item to ij masons and yer serwar for settyng ye ij leds (a dey *ins*) xijd
Item to yer serwar a dey yer iiijd
Item a loyd of erthe yat was spent at ye malery bryg iijd
Item to ye sam masons for makkyng of ij wall' there os wytwyk wyf dwell' an theyr sarwar a dey xvjd

---

[233] The sheriff of Lincolnshire was Sir Robert Dymoke of Scivelsby by Horncastle.

[234] the name of the official is missing – it may be the king's bailiff

[235] this sum is both in left-hand margin and page total

Item to habbot wryght for makk a new dor and mendyng other thyngs ixd

[236]xviijs jd

Sent martyn parych

Item to Rob' wrygh and hys fello for drawyng ye hows yer os hownsley dwelt and for leyyng in of iij balks with a wal plate iiijs vjd

Item to peyr' pwlwer for hyllyng of a rod and iij quarters vjs ixd

Item for pwentyng ij rods and a quart' ijs iijd

Item for iiij deys of deytall wark ijs

Item for iiij sem lym and a haf iijs

Item for to help to tak down ye sclats to a knafe nykkol iijd

Item for caryage of tymber thydder and howm viijd

Item for caryyng of haf a M sclat iiijd

Item for caryyng of a loyd erthe iijd

Item for caryyng of a loyd of ston iiijd

Item for settyng of vij bonche of latt' at eston vd

Item to ij masons and hyr serwar a dey xvjd

xxijs jd

Summa lateris xls ijd

fol 94v

Reparacyons

Item at ye whytwyks and at ye hows' by hyt for mendyng at ye stabyll wyndo and for makyng a dor at wytwyks ij deys xijd

Item to ye slater yat dwell' in peter paryche for pwentyng of ij rods wark and haf a deys wark at wytwyks and ye hows' by hyt ijs iijd

Item at tymyng' for fewyng a gwtter and mendyng a plot and settyng on a crest and for mendyng a pentys and other fawtts at ye h[ows] by hyt xvd

Item to habott wryghte for haf a dey at ye sam hows' iijd

Item a[t] tymyngs for makkyng a wyndow and mending a peyr of gresyngs vjd

vs iijd

Sent mare paryche

Item at ye angell to a wryght of tynwell for makkyng of ij bwlkes for viij deys warke iiijs

Item to abbot ye wryth iij deys for makkyng gwtter with a pentts and for settyng yn a frank post with a stod xviijd

Item to ye slater in peter paryche for hyllyng of ye same gwtter and mendyng in other places iij deys and a haf iijs

Item for ij seym lym and a loyd sond xixd

Item for a C of led nell yat was spent ther ijd

Item to abbot a dey for mendyng of dorrs and wyndos in sent mychel paryche vjd

Item at jon dows' in sent martyn paryche for ij loyds of thornys and for heggyng ye same ijs

[236] this and following sub-totals in left-hand margin

Item for a loyd of thornys caryyng fro wolfhows to a gardyn
in sent martyn paryche viijd
xiijs vd

Summa lateris xviijs viijd

fol 95

Reparacyons at northlwfnam
Item for makkyng a barne of iij beys with ij peyr of brod dorrs I cownand [covenanted] with ye tennand be gret for ye takyng down and settyng up os in wryght craft mason wark for strey and for thakyng for xxxs
Item for haf a C red and for caryage ijs viijd
Item for a C neylls of vj penny nell vjd

Eston on ye hyll
Item for a loyd strey yat was thakkyd of ye ij cottears at jak wryght cros' xvjd
Item to a thakker ij deys and to hys serwar of ye sam xvjd
Item for a loyd of erthe with ye caryage ijd
Item to coper of tynwell for makyng a frame to ye well at carwar' hows and for makkyng of standers and trescholds and mendyng of dors at deys hows and at cordall vj deys and a haf iijs iijd
Item for a loyd strey yat was thakkyd at deys hows' xvjd
Item for ij deys thakkyng and serwyng ye sam xvjd
Item to a wryght a dey at gwnbeys hows' for helpyng of a yat vjd
xlijs vd

Warmyngton
Item I cownand with ye tennand for tymber and for wa[r]kmans hyr for mendyn of a kylyn hows and in al other places for vs

At Barnak
Item to jon eton for pwentyng of viij rods of wark viijs
Item for vj sem lyne with ye caryage iiijs vjd
Item for a loyd of sond iijd

Pyllysyate
Item to a mason ij deys xijd
Item to hys serwar vjd
Item for ij loyds erthe vjd
xixs ixd

Summa lateris iij li ijs ijd

fol 95v

At wylstrope Reparacyons
Item (a *ins*) wryght for makyng ye hal dor and mendyng of other dorrs and thresscholls (ij deys *ins*) xijd
Item for ye makkyng of a new kyllyng ye whych ys not os yet endyd has cost me xxs

Stretton

Item to Rob slater yat dwellyd at ye boyr for hyllyng a quart' xvd
Item for ij deys a wark in pwentyng and hys serwar xvjd
Item a mason ij deys with hys serwar xvjd
xxiiijs xjd

Summa lateris xxiiijs xjd
Summa totalis expensarum hoc anno lxiij li xviijs viijd ob
[237]*Probatum est per me thomam Morrond*
Summa remanens in tenement' xvj li xjs ijd
et quod billa Relicta per dom Willam scharpe x li iiijs ijd ob

[238]*ffinis istius compot' supervisus fuit per Tomam Willyams deputat' dni Thome Morrand vicarrii ecclie omn' sanctorum in foro hac vice A° dni m° d° xj° ac anno r' r' henrici viij' iij° hiis testibus dno willielmo hakyn confratro (Johanne* del) *Johanne calis cum aliis*

fol 96
[*Blank*]

[237] in the hand of Thomas Morrand

[238] 'the end of this account supervised by Thomas Williams deputy of Thomas Morrand vicar of All Saints in the Market for this occasion 1511 and 3 Henry VIII, witnessed by William Ha[w]kyn and John Calis'

fol 96v

[Account of Robert Sheppey for the year 1511-12; it is in Sheppey's hand. There is no audit statement at the end of the year]

ihs

Anno R' R' *henrici octavi iiij*° *Compotus xvij*°

Heyr folowythe the xvij acownte of ye state of yis almys hows and be me Syr Rob' Schepey ye iiij wardyn of yis [house] hys v acownt' for a hole yer yat ys to sey from ye fest of sent michaell tharchangell in ye iij yere of ye Reyng of kyng henry ye viij of yat name unto ye sam' fest in ye iiij yere of ye Reyng of ye same kyng affter yis form foloyng

The stok of ye last Acownt drawys xxvj li xvs iiijd ob

The extent of owr lyflod' yis yere iij^{xx} ij li vs

Summa totalis on[er]orum est in hoc anno [no total]

I dyscharge my self be thes' parcells foloyng

In primis to viij bedfolk at yis dey yat ys to sey
The iij dey of October iiijs viijd
Item ye x dey iiijs viijd
Item ye xvij dey iiijs viijd
Item the xxiiij dey iiijs viijd
Item the xxxj dey (iiijs viijd *del*) vs iijd
yat dey enteryd lankton

November
Item ye vij dey of november vs iijd
Item The xiiij dey vs iijd
Item ye xxj dey vs iijd
Item The xxviij dey vs iijd

Summa [lateris] xliiijs iijd

fol 97

December
Item The v dey vs iijd
Item ye xij dey vs iijd
Then departyd hare mylner
Item ye xix dey iiijs viijd
Item ye xxvj dey iiijs viijd

Januarius
Item ye secund dey vs iijd
yat dey enteryd henre mosundew
Item The ix dey vs iijd
Item ye xvj dey vs iijd
Item The xxiij dey vs iijd
Item ye xxx dey vs iijd

Februarius
Item The vj dey vs iijd
Item ye xiij dey vs iijd
Item ye xx dey vs iijd
Item The xxvij dey vs iijd

Marcius
Item The v dey vs iijd
Item ye xij dey iiijs viijd
That dey margaret departtyd from yis hows' to heyr son
Item ye xix dey iiijs viijd
Item The xxvj dey iiijs viijd

Aprilis
Item The secund dey iiijs viijd
Item ye ix dey iiijs viijd
Item The xvj dey vs iijd
yat dey enteryd kateryn golsmythe
Item ye xxiij dey vs iijd
Item The xxx dey vs iijd
yat dey departyd hare mosundew
Item I peyd for waschyng of clothys and for dyhttyng of met and serwyyng yem v wykk' xviijd

Summa lateris v li xijs xjd

fol 97v

Mayus
Item The vij dey iiijs jd
That dey was Renold[239] expwlsyd
Item ye xiiij dey iiijs jd
Item ye xxj dey iiijs jd
Item The xxviij dey iiijs jd

Junius
Item The iiij dey iiijs jd
Item ye xj dey iiijs jd
Item ye xviij dey iiijs jd
Item The xxv dey iiijs jd

Julius
Item The secund dey iiijs jd
Item ye xix [sic] dey iiijs jd
Item ye xvj dey iiijs jd
Item ye xxiij dey iiijs jd
Item The xxx dey iiijs jd

---

239 perhaps Thomas Reynolds, admitted 1497.

Augustus
Item The vj dey. iiijs jd
Item ye xiij dey iiijs jd
Item ye xx dey iiijs jd
Item The xxvij dey iiijs jd

September
Item The iij dey iiijs jd
Item ye x dey iiijs jd
Item ye xvij dey iiijs jd
Item ye xxiiij dey iiijs jd

Summa pauperum hoc anno xij li iijs vijd
Item to my confratr' and to me self for on holl yere xij li
Summa totalis stipendij custodis confratris et pauperum hoc anno est xxiiij li iijs vijd

fol 98

Annuall charges
In primis to ye person of sent michels for hys pensyon vjs viijd
Item in expensys at owr fownder' dirige vjs viijd
Item peyd to archer for half hys fee iijs iiijd
Item peyd to hare lace for kepyng of ij cowrts at northwitham and ye other haf fee vs
Item peyd for dynner at boythe cowrtts xvjd
Item a lowyd for gederyng of owr rents in swafeld and northwitham with ye pertener' yert [240](xijd *del*)
Item a lowyd for gederyng ye rent in stawnford and in other placs and owerseyng of reparacions and for geyl [?] spenc' and rewards[241] os in gyffyng ageyn sumtym *jd* sumtym *ijd qa* grote and for makkyng gwd ye rent' of yem yat nohte ar xls
Summa iij li xijs iiijd
Item for makkyng owr kydds vjs
Item for caryage of yem hom iijs iiijd

Cheyf rentts
Item the cheyf rents yis yere drawys vj li vs
Item a pownd pepper xiijd
Item mercymentt' swuyngs drawys yis yere vijs
Item for iij loyds of hey for my hors viijs
Item for prowand and for schoyng ijs
Item I peyd to ye taxe at swafeld vs

Summa lateris xj li vd

---

240 marginal note 'nota'

241 a sub-total is inserted at this point 'xls'

fol 98v

Stor of hows

Item primis for ij M Sclate and a haf	xjs vjd
Item for tymber yat I boyhte of Masterys tryg	iijs
Item for a tre yat I boyghte of ye plwmmer	xxd
Item for xiij copwl sparrs yat I boyghte cost	vjs vijd
Item for ij M latts with ye caryage fro eston	vijs viijd
Item for v M of v penny neyll' a[t] symon and jwde dey[242]	viijs
Item for iiij M lat nell'	iijs ijd
Item for iijC of iiij penny neyl	xijd
Item a C of iij penny neyll	iijd
Item for vij stok lokk	ijs iiijd
Item for iij dossyn of baston rope	xxjd
Item tymber yat I boyght of ye peynter be yond ye watter	vs
Item for ij peyr of bands with hokks	vijd
(Item for a tre yat I boyghte of ye plommer	ijs *del*)

Summa lateris lijs vjd

fol 99

A batments and dekeys

Item in sent mare paryche at ye angell dekeyd and battyd	vj li iijs iiijd
Item in sent michaell paryche (deke *del*) abatyd	viijs
Item in alhalo paryche a batyd ye schop in ye tenur of jon tomas wyf	xs
Item the schop by hyt a batyd	iiijs
Item the hows' yer of tymyng dwell' a batyd	iiijs
Item the hows' of ye hyll' a batyd	iijs iiijd
Item the hows by ye wyccareghe a batyd	iiijs viijd
Item ye hows by hyt a batyd	iijs iiijd
Item ye hows at malery bryge	viijs
Item ye crane yis yer dekeyd and a baty a haff yer	xvjs viijd
Item ye hows os jon thomas dwell' dekeyd and battyd	xvjs viijd
Item ye farryst hows in peter paryche dekey	xs
Item in sent martyn paryche os hownsley dwelt dekeyd	ijs
Item a gardyn plac' in ye sam paryche	ijs
Item theyr os ye wefar dwell' a batyd	iijs iiijd
Item in bredcroft yis yere	viijs
Item a battyd and dekeyd in owr lands yis yer in staunford feeld'	viijs vjd
Item a battyd at smal bryg	xijd
Item a battyd of owr barn in schofgat	xijd
Item in worthorpe iij cottears in dekey yis yeyr	xxjs iiijd

Summa (lateris ins) xij li xixs ijd

242 i.e. at the fair in Stamford held at St Simon and St Jude tide under the charter of 1481

fol 99v

Eston

Item at Bryans hows a batyd	iijs iiijd
Item a batyd a gowyll yat longs to owr ladys gyld	ijs
Item dekeyd in walkot	xixs
Item a battyd ij cottears at stretton	xijd

Northwitham

Item a batyd ye hows be syd ye parsonaghe	ijs
Item a batyd of ye myln hows	viijs
Item dekeyd a lytyl hows be ye water syd yat was bornyd	ijs
Item dekeyd a lytyl grond in ye chyrchwardyn hands	iijd
Item dekeyd ij cottears yis yere	vjs viijd
Item dekeyd at wylstrope	xijd

Swafeld

Item a battyd of ye myln hows	ijs iiijd
Item a battyd in hollyng and hakkwnyng	xijd
Item a batyd of jon tenman	ijd ob
Item a batyd of crodon ryggs	iijs iiijd

Reparacyons at eston

Item to perys pwlwer for pwentyng xix rood' wark	xixs
Item for a xj sem lyme with ye caryag' fro clyff	vijs xjd
Item for ij loyds of sond with ye caryag'	vd
Item to a mason ij deys for makkyng of wall' at gondobe hows and at deys hows with hys serwar	xxd
Item for a loyd strey and a loyd erthe at utterams hows	xxd
Item for thakkyng of ye sam strey and serwyng	xiiijd
	xxxjs xd

Summa lateris iiij li iiijs

fol 100

Reparacions

In primis in staunford theyr os jon tomas has taken ageyn ye crane	
Item to ij masons macyall and moor for takkyng down a wall of of [sic] a rood' wark and a quart' and making hyt up	xs
Item a dey wark of ric' uffyngton and hys serwar	xjd
Item for caryag of ij loyd' ston fro worthrpe	viijd
Item for caryag' of v loyd' of erthe and ij lod' sond	xxjd
Item for caryag' of iiij loyd' of slatt' to ye sam hows'	xijd
Item for caryag' of ij loyd' of tymber and bryngyng ij home	ixd
Item for car[yag] of ij loyd' of tymber to hows	vjd
Item to marcyall of poll parrych for settyng up of xix copwll' of sparr' *vd* a copwl be syd iiij pryncypal copull'	ixs
Item to ye wryght for makyng a peyr of dorns	vjd
Item to Rob' sayg' for settyng on of telfett dey and a half	ixd

Item to on James a slater for iiij rood' wark and a half in leyng new xixs iiijd
Item for v sem lyme yat was spent yer and in other places iijs iiijd
Item for takkyng down ye old hows xijd
Item to ye same slater for hyllyng and pwentyng at ye farryst hows in peter paryche and at ye cran[e] and ye hows by hyt and at ye angell for hys warkmanschyp xxs
Item for x sem lyme vjs viijd
Item at whytwyk' wyf' hows to ij masons for makkyng at ye chymney and a threschold and at malere breyg and at hom' xvd
Item for cariag' of ij loyd' of ston and ij loyd' of marter xiiijd
Item to marcyal of eston for settyng a led and mendyng a greys ixd
Item a loyd of erthe iijd
Item to jarwas coper for a reyng to ye leyd ijs
Item for settyng hyt on iijd
Item for [deletion] ijC neyll iiijd
Item for a peys of leyd yat was wrohte to ley in ye gotter os ye telyer dwell' vijd
Item to ye plommer in sent Andro parych for leyng hyt in iiijd

Summa lateris (iiij li *ins*) iijs jd

fol 100v

Reparacyons
Item for a mason iiij deys in schofgat for makyng a wal ijs
Item hys serwar xviijd
Item for makkyng game [sic] wal a deys wark ixd
Item for careag' of a loyd ston and a loyd mortar vd
Item at pytts hows for haf a loyd sterey ixd
Item to a thakkar a dey with hys serwar ixd
Item at jarwas copers to a wryghte ij deys xijd
Item to Ryc' uffyngton a dey and a haf with hys serwar xiiijd
Item peyd jon marciall of poll paryche for makkyng a dor and ye grond of a well and wyndos and settyng yn a theschold with other thyngs iij deys and a half xxd
[243]at ye crane

in sent mychell par[yche]
Item for fewyng a synk to on scherwod xiiijd
Item to calys and perkyn for helpyng ther xijd
Item for caryyng of ij loyd' of mortar theder vjd
for caryyng awey v loyd' of ston and iiij loyd' of myrre xxd
Item to Rob' tomson for bornyng of ij loyd' of plaster and for workyng hyt part at ye angell and part in sent micaell and tymyng' iiijs iiijd
Item for a haf a loyd strey at ye farryst hows in peter paryche ixd
Item a loyd strey at jon dooffys be yond ye water xviijd
Item a thakkar a dey and a half with hys serwar xiiijd

[243] in right-hand margin

Reparacyons at Worthope

Item for ij loyd' of strey with ye caryage fro eston	iijs
Item for ij loyd' of mortar	iijd
Item to a thakker iiij deys	ijs
Item hys serwar mett and hyre	xiiijd

Summa lateris xxviijs vjd

fol 101

Reparacyons at Swafeld

Item Ric hacc' hows' for hewyng a rowftre and leyyng in ye same in ye hey hows ij deys	xijd
Item for a loyd of wattyll yat was spent yer and thomas hac' hows' and for wattyllyng ye sam	xd
Item for ij loyd' of strey	ijs
Item for a thakker iiij deys	ijs
Item to hys serwar	xd
Item for drawyng a barn yer os ca[m]pyon dwell'	iiij(d *del*)s
Item to a mason for makkyng a wall yer os alyn topper dwell' of vj rood' wark iij foote to a rood	vjs viijd
Item to ye same mason for ij deys wark in ye sam yard besyd with hys serwar	xviijd
Item for caryag' of ston and mort [sic]	ijs

Northwitham

Item for ij loyd' of strey yat was spent at ye myllyn hows and at ye hows be ye watersyd	ijs iiijd
Item to a thakker iiij deys with hys serwar mett and hyer	iijs vjd
Item for caryag of ye sam strey with loyd' of mortar	xijd
Item to mason for makkyng deys wark and a halff of a wall and undersettyng a chamber at ye hows be ye watersyd and makyng a mwdwall with hys s[erver]	xij [sic]
Item at ye manner plac' theyr dyd slyf down ye on syd al ye thak yat for I boyghte iiij loyd' of strey	vs iiijd
Item yer was a thakker ix deys with hys serwar	vjs viijd
Item a loyd of wattyl with with [sic] ye caryag' cost	xijd
Item for ij loyd' of mortar	iiijd
Item a wryght ij deys for mendyng of barndors	xd

Summa lateris xlijs xd

Summa totalis expensarum hoc anno iij^{xx} ij li xiiijs jd

Summa remanens in tenementts xvj li ijs ijd

[244]*Et quoad billa (antiqua* ins*) relicta per dom William Scharpe* x li iiijs ijd ob

[245]*Probatum est per me thomam morrond*

---

244 'some old bills remain with William Scharpe'

245 this and all such notes are in the hand of Morrand

fol 101v

[246]Heyr ys ye end' of Acownt except certyn wod yat was soold in a wode callyd swynhaw to ye walor of iij or iiij ackers os yyt [as yet] unacowntyd so remeyng' at yis (tyme *ins*) in ye wardyns hands an so he to be cowntabyll yerpon

[246] in Sheppey's hand

fol 102

[Account of Robert Sheppey for the year 1512-13. The last pages of this account are missing]

ihs

[247]*Anno Regni Regis henrici octavi quinto* *Compotus* xviij

Her foloweth the xviijth acowntt of the state of thys Almys hows and by me Syr Robt Schapay the iiijth warden of thys [house] hys vjth acowntt' for a hole yer that is to sey from the feste of seynt michaell the archawngell in the iiijth yer of the Reign' of kyng henry the viijth of that name un too the same feste in the vth yer in the Reign' of the same kyng affter thys foorm folowyng

The stok' of the last acowntt (old and new *ins*) drawys xxvj li vjs iiijd ob
The extentt of owr lyfelod' thys yer lxij li vs

Item ther remayneth ij acres of wode at the end' of the last acowntt and a roode and a halff hys was sold affter *xxxs* an acre theroff the hole swm drawys iij li xjs
Item of that the parson of collysworth had for the tyth vijs viijd
Item the Sales man for fellyng and for [blank space] ye wode vjs
Summa totorum onerum est in hoc anno iiij^{xx} li [248]xij li[249] iiijd ob

Wheroff I dyscharge my selff by theys parcells folowyng with yis ij roys (roys a boun *ins*[250])

(Septembe *del*)

October
In primis payd to ye beydmen the fyrst dey of october iiijs jd
Item the viijth dey iiijs jd
Item the xvth dey iiijs jd
Item the xxij dey iiijs jd
Item the xxix dey iiijs jd

November
Summa lateris xxxiiijs jd

fol 102v

Item the vth dey iiijs jd
Item the xijth dey iiijs jd
Item the xixth dey iiijs jd
Item the xxvj dey iiijs jd

December
Item the thyrd dey of december iiijs jd

---

247 in Sheppey's hand

248 heavy deletion illegible

249 in other words, the total is iiij^{xx}xij li [£92]

250 reading uncertain

Item the xth dey	iiijs jd
Item the xvijth dey	iiijs jd
Item the xxiiij dey	iiijs jd
Item the xxxj dey	iiijs jd
Januarye	
Item the vij^th dey	iiijs jd
Item the xiiij^th dey	iiijs jd
Item the xxj dey	iiijs jd
Item the xxviij^th dey	iiijs jd
ffebruarye	
Item the iiij^th dey of february	iiij^s jd
Item the xj dey	iiijs jd
Item the xviij^th dey	iiijs jd
Item the xxv dey	iiijs jd
March	
Item the iiij^th dey of march	iiij^s jd
Item the xj dey of march	iiijs jd
Item the xviij^th dey	iiijs jd
Item the xxv dey	iiijs jd

Summa lateris iiij li vs ixd

fol 103

Apryll	
Item the fyrst dey of aprll	iiijs jd
Item the viij^th dey	iiijs jd
Item the xv^th dey	iiijs jd
Item the xxij dey	iiijs jd
Item the xxix dey	iiijs jd
Maye	
Item the vj^th dey of maij	iiij^s jd
Item the xiij^th dey	iiijs jd
Item the xx' dey	iiijs jd
Item the xxvij dey	iiijs jd
June	
Item the thyrde dey of june	iiijs jd
Item the xth dey	iiijs jd
Item the xvij^th dey	iiijs jd
Item the xxiiij dey	iiijs jd
Julye	
Item the fyrst dey of julye	iiijs jd
Item the viij^th dey	iiijs jd
Item the xv dey	iiijs jd
Item the xxij dey	iiijs jd
Item the xxix^ne dey	iiijs jd

August
Item the vth dey of August [251]iijs vjd
Item the xij^th dey iijs vjd
Item the xix^th dey iijs vjd
Item the (xxj *del*) xxvj dey iijs vjd

Summa lateris iiij li (iiijs vijs vjd *del*) ixs xd

fol 103v

September
Item peyd the secund dey of September iijs vjd
Item the ix^th dey iijs vjd
Item the xvj dey iijs vjd
Item the xxiij dey[252] iijs vjd
Summa xiiijs

Summa pauperum hoc anno xj li (xvjd *del*) iijs viijd
Item to my confrater and to my selff xij li
Summa totalis stipendij custodis confratris and pauperum hoc anno
xxiij li (xvjd *del*) iijs vjd

Annuall charges
In primis payd to the parson of seynt michall for his pension vjs viijd
Item in expens' at our fowndars dirige vjs viijd
Item payd to henr' lacy for his fee vjs viijd
Item payd for the stwards dynnar at North withom and at swafeld xvjd
Item payd for gaderyng of the rentt at swafeld and north withom to Ric' campion xjs
Item alowyd for gaderyng the rent in stanford and in odder places and for necessary expens' and rewards as in gevyng ageyn sum tyme jd [unfinished]

Summa lateris xxiiij li xvjs (viijd *del*)

fol 104

[This account jumps from annual charges into reparations without any heading. The next account does the same]

Seynt Clement parysch
Item to a mason for makyng a wall in owr barn yard in skoff gate hyred by grett ijs viijd
Item for iij lood' of erth ixd
Item for ij lood' of ston viijd
[253]iiijs jd

---

[251] there is no record of any departure from the almshouse at this time

[252] there is no sign of any payment on 30 September, presumably in the next account part of which is missing; see folios 104-5.

At Eston of the hyll
Item to a wryght ij deys at a gwtter xijd
(Item for a lode straw with the karyage *del*)
Item at john cordale hows to perys pulver for layyng a gwtter
and ij rood' warke besyde in poyntyng iijs iiijd
Item for tymber that was spent in the same gwttar xvjd
Item for ij seem off lyme that was spentt ther and att gwnby howsse xvjd
Item at gunby hows for poyntyng of the dwffcote a dey and a halff ixd
vijs ixd

Summa lateris xjs xd

fol 104v

Pyllsyate
In primis to jamys skclater his man and his servand for (poyntyng *del*)
(hyllyng *ins*) of iij roode warke and a quart' xiiijs vijd
Item for karyage of iij lood' of sklatte xviijd
Item for a lode of sand iijd
Item for iiij seem off lyme ijs viijd
[254]xixs

Swafeld
In primis ther as holdernes dwell' (for *del*) to a mason for makyng of
a wall of a rood' wark save halff a quarter vijs
Item ther att the same howse to a wryght for undersettyng
the howsse a dey vjd
[255]Item ther as willyam gelyn dwell' (fo *del*) to a mason for making wpp
a wall of a roode warke and a qwarter ixs
Item for kariage of vij lood' of mortar xiiijd
Item for plaschyng the hegge in northow iijs
xxs viijd

Summa lateris xxxixs viijd

[Some folios have been lost between fols 104v and 105; the end of the account for 1512-3 and the start of the account for 1513-4 are missing.

---

253 this and the next sub-total are in the right-hand margin

254 this and the following sub-totals are in the left-hand margin

255 in left-hand margin

fol 105

[Part of the account of Robert Sheppey for the year 1513-14. In this account, the sub-totals in the margins are in the accountant's hand; the 'summa' at the bottom of the page when they appear are in a different hand, that of John Taylor, again the auditor.]

December	
Item the (vij *del*) (ij *ins*) dey	iiijs jd
Item the (xiiij *del*) (ix *ins*) dey	iiijs jd
Item ye xxj dey	iiijs jd
Item ye (xxvij *del*) xxiij dey	iijs vjd
that dey dyed langton	
Item ye xxx dey	iijs vjd
Januarye	
Item ye vj dey	iijs vjd
Item the xiij dey	iijs vjd
Item the xx dey	iijs vjd
Item ye xxvij dey	iijs vjd
ffebruarius	
Item the iij dey	iijs vjd
Item the x dey	iijs vjd
Item the xvij dey	iijs vjd
Item the xxiiij dey	iijs vjd
Marcius	
Item the thyrd dey	iijs vjd
Item the x dey	iijs vjd
Item the xvij dey	iiijs jd
that dey enterd nicholas burreene [?]	
Item ye xxiiij dey	iiijs jd
Item the xxxj dey	iiijs jd
Apryll'	
Item the vij dey	iiijs jd
Item the xiiij dey	iiijs jd
Item the xxj dey	iiijs jd
Item the xxviij dey	iiijs jd
	[256]iiij li ijs xd

fol 105v

Mayus	
Item ye v dey	iiijs jd
Item the xij dey	iiijs jd
Item the xix dey	iiijs jd
Item the xxvj dey	iiijs jd

---

[256] this and all sub-totals in this account are in the left-hand margin

June	
Item the secund dey	iiijs jd
Item the ix dey	iijs vjd
that dey departyd parkyn	
Item the xvj dey	iijs vjd
Item the xxiij dey	iijs vjd
Item the xxx dey	iijs vjd
July	
Item the vij dey	iijs vjd
Item the xiiij dey	iijs vjd
Item the xxj dey	iijs vjd
Item ye xxviij dey	iijs vjd
August	
Item the iiij dey	iijs vjd
Item ye xj dey	iijs vjd
Item the xviij dey	iijs vjd
Item the xxv (dey *ins*)	iijs vjd
September	
Item the fyrst dey	iijs vjd
Item the viij dey	iijs vjd
Item the xv dey	iijs vjd
Item the xxij dey	iijs vjd
Item the xxix dey	iijs vjd
	iij li xixs xjd

Summa pauperum hoc anno ix li xviijs iijd *probatum est*[257]

fol 106

Item to my confrater and to my self	xij li
Summa totalis stipendii custodis confratris et pauperum hoc anno	xxj li xixs xjd

Annuall charges off thys yer

In primis payd to the parson of seynt michael ffor his pension	vjs viijd
Item in expens' at owr fowndars dirige	vjs viijd
Item payd to henry lacy for kepyng of cowrtt' and for hys fee	vjs viijd
Item payd for gaderyng of the Rentt of swafeld and north wythom to Richard Campion	xjs
[258]Item for gaderyng of the rentt in staunford and in oder places and for all oder necessary expens' and rewardds yis yer	xxxs

[257] total corrected and approved by auditor

[258] two sub-totals in left-hand margin, one deleted and the other not deleted; the first figure for each is lost in the binding but the remainder are as follows: (... li xixs xd ob qa *del*) and [x] li vjs vjd. This second sub-total in turn has been corrected by the auditor at the foot of this section.

Item for makyng of kydd' thys yer vjs
Item for karyag' of the same kydd' ixs
Item for chefe rentts thys yer iij li (xijs *del*) vjs iiijd qa
of thys seyd chefe rentts is abated thys yer in swafeld that hath been payd in tymes past with certeyn lands purchesed of s' John huse and Xristofer brown to the valor by the yer iij li xvjd Thys seyd swm to be abated of the old acowntt
Item for cheef rentt bought of John Thorney owt of the hows by ye water syd beyond the brygg in seynt martyn parysch iijs
Item payd to hym for the purchasse of the seyd iijs v mark
and for the makyng of the indenturs and makyng (oder wrytyngs *ins*) of the same ijs
Item for a pond of pepper xiiijd

Summa x li (vjs vjd *del*) xvijs jd qa

fol 106v

Item for amercimentt' and essoygnes vijs viijd
Item for casuall charges and (stor of howse *del*) (Item *ins*) to the eyd of the kyngs dwtey xxs
Item at swafeld to the xv^th^ xs
Item at Northwithom to the xv^th^ vijs iiijd
Item for karyyng of ij lood' sand' home to our howse vjd
Item for karyyng off leyd' from ye grey frers and to the grey frears xijd

Stoor off howse

Item for x m^l^ latt neyle vijs xjd
Item for v hundreth of ij penny neyle xd
Item for v hundreth of iij penny Neyle xvd
Item vC off iiij penny neyle xxd
Item for a roode of boord' viijs
Item for (a *del*) ij thowsand sklate viijs
Item for karyag of the same sklate and for ij Thowsand moo sklates ijs viijd
Item for kariage of a lood sklate to northwithom viijd
Item to abbot the wryght for hewyng of tymber vd
Item for reparacions of owr chappell and for the castyng of a foder of leyd and leyyng of ye same also for ij webbs of leyd that I bowght of the plummar that cost me in money xxs vacat[259]
and besyd yat I gave hym to boote [also] x ston off leyd
Item for leyd that I bowght of a glasear (v *del*) iij ston xiiijd
Item for vj ston off leyd that I bowght of a Tynkar besyde ijs iijd
Item payd to the plummar for leyyng of ij foodyr and for kastyng of on' foodyr and for takyng wp the gwttars and leyyng down ageyn for his labur and hys servaundd' xxs

[259] 'vac' in left margin; 'vacat' in right margin - the item has been cancelled/disallowed

of theyse charges payd john bendlowse (alias john myddilton *ins*) at the owr of hys deth to me beeyng warden [260]xxs

[261]Summa iiij li viijs

fol 107

Item the same john bendlowse payd of his goods remaynyng afftyr hys deth vjs viijd

Item john parkyn payd to the same charges of hys goods afftyr hys deth vjs viijd

(I *del*) And so of theys reparacions made uppon owr chappell remayneth no mor charges bot xs jd (to owr howse costs *ins*) besydes the gyffts off theym that be goon whose names ar' a for rehersed

Item payd to Robt beymond for (the redemption of [hys special writ *del*] *ins*) hys patentt that he had gevyn owt of owr howse by owr seale vj li xvjs viijd beside the dett that he awght to the hows

Abatementts And dekeyse

In all halow parysch a schopp in the tenur of m henr' ward xs
Item the schopp by hytt abatyd' iiijs
Item ther as tymyng dwell' abatyd' iiijs
Item the howse of the hyll in dekey a quart' rentt xxd
Item abatyd' of the same howse iijs iiijd
Item the howse by ye vicarag' abatyd' iiijs
Item the howse by hytt abatyd' ijs
Item the howse at malary bryg' abatyd' xs
Item the crane is abatyd' thys yer vjs viijd
Item the howse ageyn hytt abatyd' xs
Item the howse ageyn bynwark[262] is in dekey xs
Item the awngell in seynt mary parysch vij li
Item in seynt michaell parysch abatyd' xs
[263]xvij li xijs iiijd

Summa xviij li vs viijd

fol 107v

Sent martyn parysch
In the howse by ye water syde a halff yer in dekey vjs (viijd *del*)
Item abatyd of the same howse ijs
Item a gardyn place abated' and dekeyd' ijs
Item ther as the weyfar dwell' abatyd' iijs iiijd
Item abatyd' in bredcrofft viijs

[260] this sum of 20s is to be deducted from the total

[261] this figure, which is repeated from the left-hand margin, appears to be the page total

[262] This is the house referred to as 'the furthest house in St Peter's parish'

[263] this figure in the right-hand margin appears to be a different page total

Item abatyd' of our land' thys yer ijs viijd
Item abatyd' off a barn in skoff gate xijd

Worthorp
Item abated' in ye cotear ther as the dwff cott is iijs
Also in iij cotears besyde hytt abatyd' vs
Item of theym halff a yer in dekeye ijs vjd[264]

Eston
Item abatyd' ther as bryan dwell' iijs iiijd
Item a govyll yat longg' to our lady gyld' ijs

Walkott
Dek(e *ins*)yde owr land' in that town' xixs

pyllegate
Item abatyd at pyllesyate iijs iiijd

Stretton
Item ffor ij cotears at stretton xijd

Barham
Item a howse in barham abatyd' ijs

Cowntesthorpp
Item a [*deletion*] close in dekey in Cownthorp iijs
[265]iij li ixs ijd

Swafeld
Summa iij li ixs ijd

fol 108

Item abatyd of the myln howsse ijs iiijd
Item abatyd in hollyng and hakennyng xijd
Item abated' in Croydon Rygges iijs iiijd

North wythom
Item abatyd' of the howse besyde the parsonage ijs
Item abatyd' of the myln howse viijs
Item abatyd' of the heyd plac' thys yer vjs viijd
Item iiij cotears in dekeye xiijs iiijd
Item a cotear by ye water syde yat was brentt ijs
Item a lyttyll grownd (dekeyd *ins*) in the church wardens hands iijd
Item dekeyd' at wolsthorpp xijd
Item john Tenman of steynby for rentt assis ijd ob

Reparacions
In primis at the Crane (v *del*) in seynt petyr' parysch to a wryghyt a dey and a halff for makyng off a frame to the well xijd
Item to perys pulwer for poyntyng of iij roods of wark at the awngell iijs

---

[264] a different sum has been erased and the sum of 'ijs vjd' inserted

[265] in left-hand margin; the page total has been inserted below the next sub-heading

Item to the same perys for hyllyng a swyn skott ij deys warke xijd
Item for a mason ij deys ther as fostar' dwell' in seynt andrew parysch for amendyng of a gresyng and oder warkes xijd
Item payd to a wryght for skyrtyng of a door and amendyng of ooder dwrs and thresholdes a dey and di' ixd

[266]Summa xlvjs xd ob

fol 108v

Item for a seme lyme and a halff that was spentt att the awngell xijd
Item for halff a seem yat was spentt att Tymyngs howsse iiijd
Item a lode of sand to the awngell iiijd
Item peyd to abbott for a dey wark yer os hanforth dwell' vjd
Item for caryag' of a loyd eyrth hom to owre oyn hows' iijd

North Wythom

Item viij lood' off Straw bowght for thak xijs
Item (to *ins*) the thakkar and hys servar viijs

Wolsthorpp

Item for amendyng the barn at wolsthorpp iijs vd

Reparacions at Swafeeld

Item for a roode wark of wallyng at alyn toppar hows xxjd
Item at margarett Jamys howse for a dey and a halff wark xiijd
[267]Item at strowsons for wod and warkmanschypp of hys kyln howsse xxijd
Item for iiij lood' of mortar viijd
Item for iij lood' of ston iijd
Item gyffyne to ye bedmen at sertyn tymys when the haf doyne for well of ye hows vjd

[268]xljs xjd

fol 109

Warmyngton

Item for makyng iij bayyes of a barn that was faln Down to a wryghyt hyred by greete to make hyt ageyn xs

[269]Summa xljs xjd
Summa totalem expensarum hoc anno iij^{xx} li iij li viijs vijd ob qa

The sume remaynyng yn the stoke or yn the wardens hands and yn a byll left be s' William Scharp yn old dett xxvij li xvs vd qa

---

266 this sub-total is in the left-hand margin and at the foot of the page

267 in left-hand margin; the final figure has been corrected

268 in left-hand margin; there is no page total but a total has been inserted by Taylor on the following page.

269 this and the next few lines are in Taylor's hand; Sheppey resumes with the heading 'Compot' xx'

[Unnamed account but in the hand of Robert Sheppey for the year 1514-15. The page totals were again made by Taylor as auditor, not by Sheppey]

Compot' xx' ihs

Anno regni regis henrici octavi vij^o compot' xx' her foloweth the xx acownt of ye state of ye almys hows' for a hol yere that is to sey from ye fest of sent michaell the arcangel in the vj yeyr of ye reyn of kyng henri the viij of yat name un to ye the [sic] same fest in ye vij yere of ye ren of ye same kyng after yis forme foloyng

The stok of ye last acowntte old and new drawys xxvij li xvs vijd qa
The extent of owr lyflod' thys yere lxij li vs
Summa totorum [sic] *onerorum est in hoc anno* iiij^{xx} li and x li vijd qa

Wherof I dyscharg' my selff by theys parcell' foloyng

[270](In primis peyd to ye bedmene ye xxix dey of september iijs vjd *del*)
Item the vj dey of october iijs vjd
Item ye xiij dey iijs vjd
Item ye xxj dey iijs vjd
that dey enterd barkar
Item ye xxviij dey iiijs jd
[271]xvs ijd

Summa xvs ijd

fol 109v **ihs**
November
Item the thyrd dey of november iiijs jd
Item the xth dey iiijs jd
Item the xvij dey iiijs jd
Item the xxiiij dey iiijs jd

Item [sic] December
Item the fyrst dey iiijs jd
Item the viijth dey iiijs jd
Item the xv dey iiijs jd
Item the xxij dey iiijs jd
Item the xxix dey iiijs jd

January
Item the vth dey iiijs jd
Item the xijth dey iiijs jd
Item the xixth dey iiijs jd
Item the xxvj dey iiijs (jd *del*) viijd
that dey enterd Tomlyns of hys wags

---

[270] see fol 105v

[271] in left-hand margin

ffebruary

Item the secund dey	iiijs (jd *del*) viijd
Item the ixth dey	iiijs (jd *del*) viijd
Item the xvj dey	iiijs (jd *del*) viijd
Item the xxiij dey	iiijs (jd *del*) viijd

March

Item (the *ins*) secund dey	iiijs (jd *del*) viijd
Item the ixth dey	iiijs jd
Thys dey departyd jankyn worthyngton	
Item the xvj dey	iiijs jd
Item the xxiij dey	iiijs jd
Item the xxx dey	iiijs jd

Summa iiij li xiijs iiijd

fol 110

Aprill

Item the vij dey	iiijs jd
Item the xiiij dey	iiijs jd
Item the xxj dey	iiijs jd
Item the xxviij dey	iiijs jd

Maij

Item the iiijth dey	iiijs jd
Item the xj dey	iiijs jd
Item the xviijth dey	iiijs jd
Item the xxv dey	(iiijs jd *del*) iijs vjd
That dey departyd barkar	

June

Item the ffyrst dey	iijs vjd
Item the viijth dey	iijs vjd
Item the xvth dey	iijs vjd
Item the xxij dey	iijs vjd
Item the xxix dey	iijs vjd

Julius

Item the vj dey	iiijs jd
That dey enterd willam geff	
Item the xiij dey	iiijs jd
Item the xx dey	iiijs jd
Item the xxvij dey	iiijs jd

August

Item the thyrd dey	iijs vjd
that dey departyd Tomlyns	
Item the xth dey	iijs vjd
Item the xvijth dey	iijs vjd
Item the xxiiij dey	iiijs jd

That dey enterd tho Walsch[272]

Item the xxxj dey	iiijs jd
Summa iiij li iiijs vijd	

fol 110v

September

Item the vijth dey	iiijs jd	
Item the xiiij dey	iiijs jd	
Item the xxiiij dey	iiijs jd	
Item the xxviij dey	iiijs jd	
Summa	xvjs iiijd	
Item to my selff and to my confrater		xij li
Summa totalis stipendii custodis confratr' et pauperum hoc anno		xxij li ixs vd

Annuall Charges Off thys yer

In primis ffor cheffe rentt' thys yer	iij li xjs iiijd ob qa
Item for amerciamentt'	vjs ixd
Irem payd to the parson of seynt mychell for hys pension	vjs viijd
Item in expens' at owr fowndar dirige	vjs viijd
Item peyd to henry lacy for hys fee and for kepyng of Cowrtts	vjs viijd
Item payd for gaderyng of the rentt' of swaffeeld and Northwithom and oder places to Ric' champion	xjs
Item for gaderyng of rentt' of staunford and oder places and for reward' thys yer	xxxs
Item for makyng of owr kyddes	vjs
Item for karyage of the same kydd'	viijs
Item for a pownd off peyper	xvjd
Item for ij lood' plastwr	vs
Item for vj dosen of Crest'	vs iiijd
Item for boord' bowghyt of the tenande's of northwythom	iijs
Item for vj boord' bowght of Johan stoderd	xvjd
Summa	viij li ixs iiijd ob qa

fol 111

Stoore of howsse

In primis for viij thowsand of latt nayles pric of a thowsand *xd* the hole swm	vjs viijd
Item for iiijC off ij penny neyle	viijd
Item for three hundreth of spykyngg'	xvd
Item for iijC off thre penny neyle	ixd
Item for iij thowsand latt bowght of a man of harryngworth	xijs

[272] written underneath this entry is 'manl' - it is not clear what this means

Item for thre thowsand sklate batterd and booryd	xijs
Item for ij m sklate	viijs
Item for a thowsand and a halff of sklate	vjs
Item for halff a thowsand of sklate	ijs ijd
Item for karyage of the same sklate from the pytt' to staunford to dyvers places	ijs iiijd
Item for halff a roode boord bowght of john cordall	iijs viijd
Item for tymbre bowghyt of john ward	iiijs iiijd
Item I ask alowanc' for rydyng to london at wytsundey was a twelffmoneth to make the end' betwyx s' john huse and me that cost me for my horse mete my servand and my selff	xiiijs
Item I payd to my master and tyll an oder sergeaunt for drawyng indenturs and oder wrytyngs	vjs viijd
Item to master clerk for a reward	iijs iiijd
Item for wrytyng of the instrumentt'	vjs viijd
Abaatementts And dekeyse	
Item a schopp in all halow parysch in the tenur off master henry warde abated	xs
Item a schopp by hytt in dekey a halff yer	vs iijd
and theroff abatyd thys (yis haf yere *ins*)	ijs
Item a howse in the tenur' of Richard Tymyngs abated	iiijs
Item a cotyard howsse uppon Cleymowntt abated	iijs iiijd
Summa	v li xiiijs xd

fol 111v

Item a howse by the vicarag' abatyd	iiijs
Item a howse by hytt abatyd (yis yer *ins*)	ijs
Item the same howsse in dekey a halff yer'	viijs
Item the howse at malarey brygg abatyd	xs
Item the Crane abatyd	vjs viijd
Item the howse owr ageyns hytt abatyd	ixs viijd
Item the howse in bynwark in dekey	xs
Item the Awngell in seynt mary parysch abatyd	vj li xiijs ijd
Item in seyt myschell parysch abated	xs
Item Seynt martyn parysch [sic]	
Item the hows by ye water syde in dekey	xvjs
Item a gardyn place dekeyd	ijs
Item ther as the weyfar dwell' abatyd	iijs iiijd
Item abatyd in skoff gate	xijd
Item abated in Bradcrofft	viijs
Item abatyd in owr land' thys yer	iijs
Worthorppe	
Item abatyd ther as the dwff howse is	iijs
Item abatyd of the oder three Cotyars	viijs
Item on' of theym in dekey a halff yer	ijs

Eston
Item abatyd ther as bryan dwell' iijs iiijd
Item (aba *del*) dekeyd in owr lad' gylde ijs

walcott
Item dekeyd in owr land' in that town' xvjs iiijd

Summa xiij li xxd

fol 112

Pyllesgate
Item abatyd at Pyllesgate iijs iiijd

Stretton
Item ij Cotyars abated xijd

Item Barham [sic]
Item abatyd in barham ijs

Cownthorpp
Item abatyd in Cownthorpp iijs

Swafeeld
Item abatyd of the myln howsse ijs iiijd
Item abatyd in hollyng xijd
Item abatyd in Crowdon rygg' iijs iiijd

Northwythom
The ferm place in dekey a hole yer' iiij mark'
Item at the (pars *del*) howsse beyond the parsonage abaated ijs
Item a Cotege dekeyd ijs
Item three cotag' in dekey xs
Item a lyttell grownd dekeyd in the church warden' handd' iijd

Wolsthorpp
Item abatyd at wolsthorpp xijd
Item dekeyd at john Tenman ijd ob

Summa iiij li iiijs ixd

fol 112v

Reparacions off Staunford
In primis at owr own' howsse to a sklattar for poyntyng viij roode warke viijs
Item to a mason for amendyng of s' wyllyams [Hawkyn] chymney vjd
Item for ij stoonys bowghyt of m' ley xijd
Item for halff a seym lyme iiijd
Item for iiij lood' of sand xijd
of thys money I debate ijs that I had of Jenkyns
Item to a sklatar at whytwyk' wyffe howse for a rode and a
quarter hyllyng vs vijd
Item for iij roodes and a halff poyntyng at that hows and
at pytts howsse iijs vjd

[273]Item for a jagge of strey xijd
Item for amendyng of a glasse wyndoo at whytwykk' xijd
Item to john feyrchyld of Tynwell for makyng a door at whytwyk' hows and for mendyng of swyn cote dwrs and mendyng durs and threshold' as pytt' dwell' and for a dur yat was made to the broode yaat' at barnak iiij deys and a halff ijs
Item ther as Tymyng dwell' for mendyng of ij lokk' with a band tyll a dwr vd

In petir parysch

Item at the Crane to a sklaatar for ij rood' and a quarter hyllyng xjs iijd
Item for three rood' poyntyng iijs
Item for iiij deys warke theyr and for ij deys wark at John Thomas howse poyntyng and amendyng off fawtes iijs
Item for a loode of sand iijd

Summa xxxixs xd

fol 113

Item for the farthest hows in petir parysch to willam Ives mason for makyng a chymney by greyte vijs
Item for takyng down of the same viijd
Item for Cariage of v lood' off ston xxd
Item for karyage of vj lood' of mortar xxd
Item for a seyme and a halff of lyme that was spentt at the chymney xijd
Item for a loode strey that was spent ther' xvjd
Item to a thakkar and hys servar viijd
Item for makyng Cleyn of the yard' iijd

Ar laryfax

Item for ij roode hyllyng and ij rood' poyntyng and ij deys wark of a man xiijs
Item for a loode of sande iijd
Item for iiij yard' of evys boord' iiijd

Seynt martyn parysch

In primis for makyng of a new kechyn to ij masons iiij deys and a halff iiijs vjd
Item to ij servars xxd
Item for viij lood' of ston ijs viijd
Item for ij lood' of mortar vjd
Item (s *del*) for vj Cwppull spars ijs vjd
Item to a wryghyt for settyng it up ij deys and a halff xvd
Item for makyng of a dwr and threschold' vjd
Item for a loode of sand iijd
Item for halff a thowsand sklate and the carayge ijs vjd

Summa (l xlijs *del*) xliiijs ijd

[273] line inserted

fol 113v

Worthorpp

Item for ij lood' straw	iijs viijd

Eston

Item for a stulp and mendyng of gunby yaats (and *ins*) a lode of strey spent at (T *ins*) dey hows	iijs
Item at eston' for a loode strey to utteram hows	xviijd
Item gundby howse to ij sklatars (vj deys *ins*)	vjs
Item for eys borde and for a bonch of latt	vjd
Item for evys boord' at the same howse	ijd
Item for ij spars	vjd
Item for settyng wp of the same	ijd
Item for a loode of sand'	ijd

Swafeeld

Item at Campion howsse to a wryghyt for settyng in of iiij post' and ij balk'	js iiijd
Item to a mason for iij roode warke	iijs
Item for wattlyng wand' and for wattlyng	ijs
Item to a wryght a dey for mendyng of margarett Jamys Rooffe of hyr howsse	vjd
[274]Item for wattyll heggyng and kepyng the wood'	ijs vjd

North Wythom

Item to a wryght for settyng in of ij balk' and for makyng of a chawmbyr rooffe	iijs iiijd
and for mendyng off dwrs	ixd
Item for ij balk'	js iiijd
Item to a sklatar iij deys poyntyng and amendyng off fawtes	xviijd
Item for a seym and a halff off lyme	xijd
Item for (s *del*) a loode of sand'	iijd
Item for karyage of halff a thowsand sklate	xd
Item for xij lood' of streye	xvijs

Summa lijs

fol 114

Stretton

In primis to ij wryghyt' ix deys (and di' *ins*)	ixs vjd
Item to a mason (vj *del*) thre deys and a halff	iijs vjd
Item to theyr servar	xiiijd
Item for a joyst tree in the hall pric'	iijs iiijd
Item for sawyng of trasons to ij sawers for three deys	iijs
Item for ij lood' of plaster with the karyage	vs viijd
Item for halff a seyme lyme	iiijd

[274] line inserted

Item for free ston to the geawmbb'	vd
Item for karyage of ij lood' wod with fellyng from swynow	xijd
Item for ij vertvales to a yate	ijd
Item for neylys hook' and a band' to ye wyndosse	ijd
Item for xxiiij seym lyme besyd certen lyme afor wrytten that was spent in dyvers places	xvjs
Wolsthorpp besyde Colsterworth	
Item for straw and wattyll	xvjd
Item to thomas Cok' for makyng of a ston wall at Eston at gunby howsse	iiijs
Item for karyage of ij lood' ston (to ye same wall *ins*)	iiijd
Summa	xlixs xjd

fol 114v

Warmyngton	
Item for vij lood' of strey	viijs ijd
Item for drawyng and thakkyng of the same	vs viijd
Item for thak rope	iijd
Item for Reed'	ijs vjd
Item for vj lood' erth	xijd
Item to a mason a dey wark' and hys servar	viijd
Item for makyng wp of wall' to ye same barn	vijs
Pyllesyate	
Item for a mason ij deys and hys servar	xviijd
Item to a sklatar for takyng wp a guttar iij deys	xviijd
Item for a seym' of lyme	viijd
Item for a peyr of gymmos	vd
Item for thak rop	iijd
Summa	xxixs vijd

[275]*Summa totalem exspensarum solucionem et decani'* [sic] *hoc anno* lxiiij li xvs vjd ob qa
Et ad huc remanet in manu computant' predict' hoc anno xxv li vs jd

---

[275] total of expenses, payments and decays[?] this year £64 15s 6 ¾d and thus remains in the hands of the said accountant £25 5s 1d

fol 115

[Unnamed account for 1515-16; Thomas Williams may have written it; Thomas Forster (TF) dean of Stamford audits – see probate signature at bottom of every page to folio 119v.]

Ihs est amor meus

anno r' r' henrici octavi compotus xx' primus her folowehte the xxj acownt of the state of thys allmys hows for a holl yere that ys to sey from ye fest of sent mychaell the arcangell in the vij yere of ye reyn of kyng henr' ye viij of yat name unto ye same fest in the viij yere of the reyn of the same kynge

The stoke of ye last acounte old and new	xxv li vs jd
The extent of owr lyfloyd thys yere	lxij li vs

wher of I dyscharg' me by theys parcell' foloyng

October	
I payd the v dey to viij bedmen	iiijs viijd
Item the xij dey	iiijs viijd
Item the xix dey	iiijs viijd
Item the xxvj dey	iiijs viijd
November	
That dey enteryd wyllam drywer	
Item the iij dey	vs iijd
Item ye x dey	vs iijd
Item the xvij dey	vs iijd
Item the xxiiij dey	vs iijd
Item ye last dey	vs iijd

Summa xliiijs xjd *per me* T F *decanum*

fol 115v

December	
Item the vij dey	vs iijd
Item the xiiij dey	vs iijd
Item ye xxj dey	vs iijd
Item the xxviij dey	vs iijd
Januarii	[276]Summa xxjs
Item the iiij dey	vs iijd
Item ye xj dey	vs iijd
Item the xviij dey	vs iijd
Item the xxv dey	vs iijd
ffebruarius	Summa xxjs
Item the fyrst dey	vs iijd
Item ye viij dey	vs iijd

[276] these sub-totals were written by Thomas Forster

Item the xv dey	vs iijd
Item the xxij dey	vs iijd
Item the laste dey	vs iijd
Marcius	Summa xxvjs iijd
Item the vij dey	vs iijd
Item ye xiiij dey	vs iijd
Item ye xxj dey	vs iijd
Item the xxviij dey	vs iijd
Aprilis	Summa xxjs
Item the iiij dey	vs iijd
Item ye xj dey	vs iijd
Item the xviij dey	vs iijd
Item the xxv dey	vs iijd
Maius	Summa xxjs
Item the ij dey	vs iijd
Item ye ix dey	[277]iiijs viijd
Item ye xvj dey	iiijs viijd
Item the xxiij dey	iiijs viijd
Item the xxx dey	iiijs viijd
	Summa xxiijs xjd

Summa total' vj li xiiijs ijd *per me T.F. decanum*

fol 116

Junius	
Item the seyxte dey	iiijs viijd
Item ye xiij dey	iiijs viijd
Item ye xx dey	iiijs viijd
Item the xxvij dey	iiijs viijd
Julius	Summa xviiijs viijd
Item ye iiij dey	iiijs viijd
Item the xj dey	iiijs viijd
Item ye xviij dey	iiijs viijd
Item the xxv dey	vs xd
yat dey enteryd rob holand and hary [sic]	
August	Summa xixs xd
Item the fyrst dey	vs xd
Item ye viij dey	vs xd
Item ye xv dey	vs xd
Item the xxij dey	vs xd
Item the xxix dey	vs xd

[277] there is no indication of the departure which took place at this date

September	Summa xxixs ijd
Item the v dey	vs xd
Item ye xij dey	vs xd
Item the xix dey	vs xd
Item the xxvj dey	vs xd
	Summa xxiijs iiijd

Item to my selff and to my confrat' xij li

Summa totalys stipendii custodis confratr' et pauper' hoc anno xxv li xs jd

Summa total' xxv li xs jd *per me T.F. decanum*

fol 116v

Cheyf rent'

Item in primis ye tenement' in staunford to ye kyng	xxixs
Item a pounde pepper ye pryce	xvjd
Item the angell to corp' Xti gylde	xijd
Item ye hows in sent mychell parych (to sen lenard' *ins*)	vjd
Item ye hows at malery bryg to thomas wyllyams	ixd
Item in sent martyn paryche ij howsys with a gardyn towarde the nunys	ixd
Item the feyrm place at pyllys yatte to ye abbot of borro	ixs iijd ob qa
Item for a closse in ye sam felde to master thorney	vjd
Item for owr ferme at warmyngton to ye sam abbot	vjs iijd
Item to ye cheryf of northhamton schyre	vijd
Item for ye ferm in barnak to master fynsed [Vincent]	ixd
Item for a naker land yat we haf of the parson of sent mychell to master wynsed	ijd
Item owr londe in eston on ye hyll pey[t]he to ye kyng	ijs (jd *del*) iiijd
Item to ye prior of coventre	ijs viijd
Item to ye wardyn of tatersall	xvjd
Item owr land at carlbe to master coffe	xijd
Item the tenement at barhome payth to ye kyng	jd ob
Item to ye eyrle of westmorland	ob
Item a tenement in wylstrope paythe to master eyland	iijd
Item a tenement in northluffnam paythe to master basset	iijs viijd
Item ye same place peyhe [sic] to ye lord sowche	jd ob
Item the seyd place peyth to ye prior of broke	iijd ob
Item a tenement at stretton peyth to ye bells	xijd
Item at swafeld to (s' *del*) master bagott	xijd
Item a tenement besyd ye parsonaghe at northwithham to m baggot	vs
Item a tenement in twyford peyh to ye sam man	xijd

[278]*Summa lateris* iij li xs vd ob qa *per me T F decanum*

[278] the whole line in the hand of Forster

fol 117

merciment' and swuyng'

Item a mercyment with a swuyngs at ye kyngs corte	vd
Item at ye prior of cowentre cowrte	iiijd
Item for warmyngton owndyll and pokbrok	xvijd
Item at langdyk hwndyrthe	xijd
Item at barhame at ye kyngs cowrte	vd
Item at wylstrope at master eland cowrt	vd
Item at northlwfnam for owr fyn at ye kyng' corte	xijd
Item mercyd at ye kyng' leytt'	vijd
Item at ye prior' cowrtt'	vijd
Item at stretton m	vd
Item at tyssyllton cowrt	vd

[279]Summa vijs *per me T.F. decanum*

Abatment'

Item abatyd in owr landys in al placyss thys yere in part of other cowntts	xj li (xvjs *del*) vjs iijd ob

Dekeys

Item dekeyd in stawnford' and in other partt' of owr lande thys yere	iij li xvijs iiijd

Annuall charg'

Item at owr fownder' yere dey	vjs viijd
Item to ye parson of sent mychell'	vjs viijd
Item to hare lace for kepyng cowrt' and for hys torney fee	vjs viijd
Item to master colson for gedering ye rent at swafeld and in other placesse	xiijs iiijd
Item for gederyng rent in staunford' and in other placesse a(nd *ins*) for hors kepyng and for (e *del*) other expenc'	xxvjs viijd
Item for makkyng owr kydys	vjs
Item for cariage of ye same kyd'	ixs
Item to ye eyd at martylmas to ye kyng	xxs

[280]*Summa expens' istius lateris* iiij li xvs *per me T F decanum*

fol 117v

Store of hows

Item for half a rod of borde yat was spent at stretton northwitham and in other placesse	iiijs
Item for tymber yat I bohte of jon warde	xiijs vjd
Item for a peys of tymber yat I boyht of my ost [host?]	xvjd
Item for ij spar' and iiij barrys' yat weyr sawne to a yatte	xijd
Item Item [sic] for neyll' at symon dey and jude	iiijs
Item for neyll' yat I boyhte at mydlent	vjs

---

[279] line inserted - hand of Forster

[280] the whole line in the hand of Forster

Item for tymber yat I boyht iij pecys of fylyps owr tenand xxd
Item for ij m sclat yat cost me viijs
Item for ij m and a halfe yat I boyht of jon wynter xs
Item for vj sem lym yat I had at ye austyn frerys iiijs
Item for vj sem yat com fro clyff iiijs vjd
Item for a xj seym lyme yat I had at trinyte kylyne vijs iiijd
Item to ij sawer' for sawyng stander' legg' eywys bord' ijs vjd
Item for banddys and hokkys yat I boyht of masterys Dyat cost me xviijd
Item for band' and hok' yat I boyht of jon elred xiiijd
Item for a loke of ye sam mane vd
Item for caryag' of iij loyd' of sond' to owr oyn hows xd
Item to ij sawer' iij deys for sa[w]yng of a bord kebbyll ijs viijd
Item for viij dosyn crest' vjs iijd
Item for goyng to london (ys *ins*) thym twelmond to speyk with master hosse master breknall and with master pygot to mak a neynd off owr land' betweyn master hwsse and hws - they myghte not tend' hyt yen bot they promysyd me they wold make a neynd heyr at a sysse xvijs
Item docter royston had of me for the copy off my brother syr wyllyams wyll vs
Item for caryage of ye slat yat I boyhte of wynter to owr oyn hows and for takkyng theym down xiiijd

Summa lateris v li iijs xd *per me T F decanum*

fol 118

Reparacyons In stawnford
In primis In sent tandrowe paryche theyr of os hwe mason dellyth for iiij rodys and a half of hyllyng xixs (ixd *del*)
Item for takyng up a gotter and leyyng hyt agayne xd
Item to hym seylf for makkyng a wall betwyn masterys tryg and hus ixd
Item a loyd of ston and loyd of mortar vijd
Item for ij loyd' off sand viijd

In alhalo paryche
Item at george glower' hows iij rod' and a half (pwentyng *ins*) iijs vjd
Item to a mason a dey and a half with hys serwar xiijd
Item for a loyd off ston and ij loyd' off mortar xd
Item a loyd sond iijd
Item at ye god wyf qwytwyk' in pwentyng iij persons viijd
Item to a wryghte for makkyng of dorr' stander' and for mendyng a dor at gorges iiij deys xxd
Item for a loyd of thorns with ye caryage xijd
Item a[t] phylyp hows ij schater' [sic] ij deys with theyr serwar xiiijd
Item to a wryght for mendyng of a [281](pl *del*) palle ij deys (ijd *del*) xd
Item at emson hows to a mason with hys serwar ij deys xxd

281 this word has been amended and cannot now be deciphered with confidence

Item ij loyd' est [eft?] ston ij loyd' of mortar xiiijd
Item ij sclater' with ther serwar half a dey viijd
Item to abbot for tornyng a partycyon and mendyn of a dor and wyndos a dey and (a *ins*) half viijd
Item theyyr afor caryag' a loyd of sond iijd
Item as wynter dwell' for mendyng a heche and a loyd eyrth vd

in peter paryche

Item at jon tomas iij deys and a half (pwentyng *ins*) iiijs viijd
Item at bottons ij sclater' a dey and a half (with yer serwar *ins*) in pwentyng (xviijd *del*) ijs
Item a a loyd sond iijd
Item theyr os tymyng dwellyd to on slater haf a dey and for mendyng a loke vd

Summa lateris xlvs *per me T F decanum*

fol 118v

Item At ye Awngell to ij slater iiij deys for mendyng of ij gotter' with other fawtt' vs iiijd
Item a loyd of sond iiijd

in sent martyn parych

Item at jon dowff' hows' for iij loyd' of strey iiijs vjd
Item thakkyng and serwyng of the sam strey iijs iiijd
Item be the watersyde for hyllyng off iij quart' warke iijs iiijd
Item for mendyng fawtt' besyd ij deys xxd

at pyllysyatte

Item to ij slater' and ther serwar for iiij rod' warke and a half iiijs vjd
Item for mendyng off fawtt' ij deys ijs viijd
Item for a loyd of basterd ston with ye caryag' vijd
Item for a loyd of mortar ijd
Item a mason ij deys xijd
Item for caryage a loyd of sclat form [sic] eston pytt' vd
Item for caryage of lyme and crest' from stanford viijd
Item for a loyd sond iijd
Item for makkyng a heche at ye gat dor iiijd

Barnak

Item ij sclater' a dey and theyr s[erver] for (f *del*) mendyng fawt' xvjd

warmyngton

Item for reparacyons down at warmyngton ye last yere and the other yere afor that besyd yat was set in xjs ixd

Worthorpe

Item for iij loyd' of strey iiijs ijd
Item for thakkyng and serwyng the sam vijs ixd
Item for ij loyd' of mortar iiijd

Summa lateris ls vd *per me T F decanum*

fol 119 [*A new hand starts here*]

ihc

Eston

In primis for makyng off a yate att Gonneby howse to a wryte iij days	xviijd
Item for makyng of aney [a new] yate att the kervers to a wryght ij days	xijd
Item for makyng of barr' to the same yate	ijd
Item for the tree yat the barr' wer' made of	iijd
Item att uttrames howse for ij lood' stoble	iijs
Item for thakkyng iij day and servyng with ij lood' mortar	ijs iiijd

Northluffenham

In primis to ij Slater' for iiij roode (and a half *ins*) warke poyntyng att Skarborows howse	iiijs vjd
Item for carriag' of iiij quarter of lyme theyr	viijd
Item to the said slaters (and ther server' *ins*) for leyng and mendyng of defaut yer	xiiijd
Item for takyng downe of slate and tymber from the dowfcote toppe	viijd
Item for cariag' of the tymber to Staunford	vjd
Item for a loode of Sande	iijd
Item to a wryght for v days worke about the makyng of ij greet wyndows and mendyng of doores	ijs vjd

Stretton

In primis to a mason for v days werke	ijs vjd
Item to server of the mason for v days	xxd
Item for v lood' of ston and for the cariag' of ye same	xxd
Item for mete and drynke to a plasterer for x days	xxd
Item to ij Slater' and ther server for ij days	ijs iiijd
Item for cariag' off lyme and a lode Sande	vijd

Summa lateris xxviijs xjd *per me T.F.decanum*

fol 119v

Swafeld

In primis (ta *del*) to a wryght for mendyng fawt' in dywer' places	xvjd
Item to a mason and hys s[erver] ij deys at campyons hows	xviijd
Item a loyd of ston and ij loyd' of mortar	vjd

Carlby to ij slater' and ther serwar a dey and a half	ijs ijd
Item for caryag' of ston and lyme and for sand	vjd
Item to a wryght for settyng up of ij copwll' a dey	vjd
Item for ij spar'	vijd

Wylstrope

Item to ij slater' for hyllyng a rode warke and pwentyng half a rod	vs
Item for caryag' of a loyd ston eys [eves] bord' and latt' fro staunford	viijd
Item for seyttyng a seym of lym (and a half *ins*) at swafeld and for ye lym and for sand	xxd

[282]Item to the sam slater' for mendyng of fawt' besyd xijd
Item to a wryght for iij deys and for tymber to a rwftre xxd

(So *del*) Northwitham
Item for thakkyng of xij loyd' of strey and for serwyng of ye sam the last yere os yyt not cownttyd xiijs iiijd
Item for reparacyons down by master colston yis yere
Item for strey yat he boyhte ixs
Item for caryag' of ye sam strey xviijd
Item to a thakker for thakkyng of ye sam strey vijs ijd
Item for serwyng of the thakkar xvj deys vs iiijd
Item peyd for thakrope and for iiij bord' and for nell' xxjd
Item for a mason ij deys at ye gret place viijd
Item for serwyng and bordyng of ye sam mason vjd
Item for a loyd ston and for vij loyd' of erthe xxd
Item for a loyd of strey and thakkyng of ye sam ijs

Summa lateris iij li *per me T F decanum*

fol 120
Summa totalem expensarum et solucionum hoc anno iij^{xx} li iij li xiiijs ijd qa
Et ad huc remanet in manu computant' hoc anno xxv li vs jd

[282] these two lines inserted after account had been written up

fol 120v

[Account for the year 1516-17. This account appears to be in the hand of Thomas Williams. The page totals are in the hand of the auditor, probably Morrand]

Anno R' R' *henrici octavi ix° compotus vicessim' ij*

Her foloes the xxij[ti] a cownte of ye state of yis almes hows for a holle yere that ys to sey forme [sic] the feste of sent mychaell ye arcangell In the viij yere off ye reyn of the same kyng henri the viij off yat name unto ye same fest in the ix yere of the reyn off ye same kyng

The stok of the last acownte olde and new [no totals]

The extent of owr lyfloyd thys yere

Wher of I dyscharge my self by theys' parcell' foloyng

October

Item I peyd to ye x bedmen (ye iij dey *ins*) as hyt remenyd in the laterynd off ye last payment' to ye sam bedmen	vs xd
Item the x dey	vs xd
Item ye xvij dey	vs xd
Item the xxiiij dey	vs xd
Item the xxxj dey	vs xd
November	
Item the vij dey	vs xd
Item the xiiij dey	vs xd
Item the xxj dey	vs xd
Item the xxviij dey	vs xd
December	
Summa	lijs vjd[283]

fol 121

Item the v dey	vs xd
Item ye xij dey	vs xd
Item the xix dey	vs xd
Item ye xxvj dey	vs xd
Januarius	
Item the ij dey	vs xd
Item ye ix dey	vs xd
Item the xvj dey	vs xd
Item ye xxiij dey	vs xd
Item the xxx dey	vs xd

283 sum corrected from 'xlvjs viijd'; this and the other page totals are in the hand of Morrand but there is no signature

ffebruarius

Item the vj dey	vs iijd
[284]*ac die mortuus est respyn*	
Item ye xiij dey	vs iijd
Item the xx dey	vs iijd
Item ye xxvij dey	vs iijd

Marcius

Item ye vj dey	vs iijd
Item the xiij dey	vs iijd
Item ye xx dey	vs iijd
Item the xxvij dey	vs iijd

Aprilis

Item the thyrde dey	vs iijd
Item ye x dey	vs iijd
Item the xvij dey	vs iijd
Item ye xxiiij dey	vs iijd

Summa lateris v li xvs vjd

fol 121v

Maius

Item the j dey	vs iijd
Item ye viij dey	vs iijd
Item the xv dey	vs iijd
Item the xxij dey	vs iijd
Item the xxix dey	vs iijd

Junii

Item the v dey	vs iijd
Item ye xij dey	iiijs viijd
yat dey dyed henry [sic]	
Item the xix dey	iiijs viijd
Item the xxvj dey	iiijs viijd

Julii

Item the iij dey	iiijs viijd
Item ye x dey	iiijs viijd
Item ye xvij dey	iiijs viijd
Item the xxiiij day	(iiijs viijd *del*) vs iijd
yat dey enteryd Rob' Hall	
Item the xxxj dey	vs iijd

[284] death of Respyn [pauper]

August'
Item the vij dey vs iijd
Item ye xiiij dey vs iijd
Item the xxj dey vs iijd
Item ye xxviij dey vs iijd

September
Item the iiij dey vs iijd
Item ye xj dey vs iijd
Item ye xviij dey vs iijd
Item the xxv dey vs iijd

Summa lateris v li xijs

fol 122

Item to my self and to my confratrer [285] xij li
Item the some of ye hole stypend' of ye wardyn and hys brother and ye bedmen for a hole yere xxv li xiiijs ijd

[286]*Summa totalis pro presbitaris et pauperibus* xxv li xiiijs ijd

Cheyf rentt'
Item the cheyfe rentt' yis yere os the[y] apeyr in last cownte drays iij li xs vd ob qa

Mercymentt' and swuyng' yis yere vijs

A batment'
Item a batyd in owr landys thys yere

Dekeys
Item dekeyd in ye feldys and in towne of stawnford and in other part' of owr land yis yere [287]xiiij li viijs iiijd ob

Annuall charg'
Item at owr fownder' yere dey vjs viijd
Item to ye parson of sent mychell' vjs viijd
Item to hare lace for kepyng owr cowrtt' and to be of consell with hws vjs viijd
Item to master colson fo gederyng ye rent in swafeld northwiththam and other places xiijs iiijd
Item for gaderyng of rentt' in staunford and other places and for doyng cost of owr tennand' when ye com and for gyffyng yem now a jd and now a nother and for hors hyr and meyte xxvjs viijd

Summa xxj li xs xd qa

[285] marginal note 'vacat'

[286] in Morrand's hand

[287] This total covers both abatements and decays

fol 122v

Item for makyng owr kyddys yis yere	vijs
Item for caryag' of ye same kydd'	ixs
Item to the kyng' eyde at martylmes	xxs
Item to master baggot for dyschargyng hws of al manner repracyons at northwithham wylstrope and twyford be a covande mayd be Indentturs yat I haf peyd hym (for ye teyrm of xl yere[288])	viij li

Store of hows

[289]Summa ix li xvjs

[290]Item for tymber yat I boyghte of a pentter be yonde ye water	ijs
Item for v m lat neyll' yat was boyhte at symon and jude	iiijs ijd
Item for half a m of ij penny neyll'	xd
Item for iiijC iij penny nyell'	xijd
Item ix m lat neyll' yat was boyght at mydsomer feyr	vijs vjd
Item for half a m iijd neyl	xvd
Item for iijCof iiij penny neyl	xijd
Item for iiijC of v penny neyl	xvjd
Item for iijC of v penny (di *del*) neyl (with ye [291]alowans *ins*)	xiiijd
Item for iiij vertwall with iiij hok' for to heyng [hang] yatts at eston on peyr at swafelde a nother peyr	xijd
Item for half a m slate yat caryed to estton with ye caryag'	ijs vjd
Item half a m yat was carryd hom to owr oyn hows' with ye caryag'	ijs vijd
Item for a m and a half (of slat *ins*) yat was caryd beyond ye water to the weffares hows'	vjs vjd
Item for caryag' of ye sam slat (to wyllyam knot *ins*)	xijd
Item for ix sem lyme yat I had at ye trynytes yat was spent at hoyme and beyond ye water	vjs
Summa	xxxixs xd

fol 123 [*A quite different hand wrote the following section*]

ihs

Stamford Reparacions

In primis at owr awn howsse for a Coveryng to the Canopye with a sylk frynge with skowryng and dyghtyng of the same to agnes Claypole	ijs
Item to a glasear for amendyng the chappell wyndose and in oder plac'	xijd
Item for new cloth to the amendyng of iij vestmentt' *xijd* that was reysed of the dede mense good'	

---

[288] in left-hand margin

[289] this sub-total for the 'annual charges' has been inserted below the heading for the following item

[290] left-hand margin 'Nota xijd'

[291] a discount of jd for bulk purchase

Item payd to three sklatars for takyng down and settyng wp of ij roods wark and a quarter xs
Item for halff a Thowsand sklate (with the karyag' *ins*) ijs vijd
Item for karyage of ij lood' of sand vijd
Summa xvjs ijd

petyr' parysch
Item at John Thomas to ye same sklatars a dey and a halff ijs
Item (for *del*) alowed to ye same john Thomas for amendyng of a stable xijd
Item to john feyrchyld wryghyt for studdyng of a Chawmbyr syde at ye same howse a dey vjd
Item at willam britton' howsse for mendyng of a wyndoo a dey vjd
Item to ij sklaters and theyr servar' halff a deye at the howsse wher tymyng' dweld viijd
Item for ij bandd' and a hooke to the wyndoo iiijd
Summa vs

fol 123v

Saynt martyn parysch
Item for vj cwppull spars j wall plate and halff a plate ij Catt' iijs vjd
Item to john feyrchyld for wyrkyng ther x deys in settyng wp of a Chawmbur rooffe ther as the weyvar dwell' vs
Item ij sklatars and theyr servand' for takyng down the same chawmbyr and settyng it wp ageyn iiij roode warke and mor' xviijs
Item ffor a thowsand sklate and a halff with the karyage viijs
Item for ij lood' of sand with gaderyng and karyage viijd
Item at the howse by the watersyde a wryghyt ij deys for studdyng of a howsse syde and amendyng oder fawtes xijd
Item to empson and oder ij felowes for dawbyng and splyntyng of the same vijd
Item a lode of erth iijd
Item a lode of ston for ye growndsole iijd
Summa xxxvijs iiijd

Eston at whytwell' howsse
Item to john feyrchyld for settyng wp a yate and ij stulpes and ij spurnes three deys xviijd
Item I bowghyt the stulpes and the spurnes of whytwell' wyffe for xd
Item at gunby howsse to the same wryght for makyng ij swynkott dwrs and leyyng in vj spars in the swynkott and skyrtyng of the greyte yaat' iiij deys[292]

Summa lateris xljs viijd

[292] figure lost in binding

fol 124

Item to ij sklatars and theyr servar halff a dey viijd
Item at john Cordall' to the same wryghyt for makyng ij peyr of Dwrnes a threschold and a boord to mend a Dwr and a leyge for the town yate hys labur *ijs*, the Dwrnes the threschold the boord and the legge I boughyt of John Cordale that cost me xd
Item the same John Cordale asks alowanc of me for xiiij trasons that he cawsed to be leyd of hys kyln for theym and the warkmanschyp' of the same (iiijs *del*) iijs
Item to thomas Daye for a lode of straye with the karyage ijs
Item for a Thakkar a dey and a halff ixd
Item hys servar the seyd dey and halff vd
Item to ij sklatars and theyr servars ij deys at John cordall' ijs viijd
Item for halff a thowsand sklate (with ye karyage *ins*) ijs vjd
Item for ij seym (lym that cam from Clyff *ins*) xvjd

Pyllesgatte
Item for iij peecys of tymber xijd
Item to the wryghyt' for wyrkyng the seyd peec' xvjd
Item to a thakkar iiij deys xxd
Item to (a *del*) (hys *ins*) servars to the sam thakkar xxd
Item for Reed' to wattell xiiijd
theys reparacions wer doon to a barn syde that fell down with parte off the wall

Summa lateris xxiijs

fol 124v

ad huc Pyllesyate
Item for a thakkar amendyng of an oder barn viijd
Item for ij bunch of thakrope ijd
Item for mendyng of a gresyng to a wryghyt with a step to ye same iiijd
Summa xiiijd

Stretton
Item to iij sklattars iij deys iiijs
Item to a wryghyt a dey for makyng a stabull door' vjd
Item for a mason a dey vjd
Item for ij seym lyme xvjd
Item for a lode of sand iijd
Summa vjs vijd

Swafeld
Item at tomas stroson hows for drawyng in a barne wall iiijs
Item to a wryght for hewyng of iij bord' logg' viijd
Item to same wryght for sawyng a rod of bord iijs iiijd
Item to same wryght and hys man iij deys at Rob' nyccolson hows' for makkyng of new yatt' and dorr' ijs

Item to ye seyd wyght [sic] for settyng up a new royffe ower a chamber at rob' nyccoll' hows	iiijs
Item for xv sparr' yat I boyght of wyllyam yong	xxijd ob
Item for vj spar' boyght of hare lawtton	ixd
	Summa xvjs vijd ob

Summa lateris xxiiijs iiijd ob

fol 125

Item of nyccoll topper iiij sparr'	[MS torn]
Item jon tyd on spar	jd ob
Item to tomson for iiij sparr'	vd
Item for heggyng of xxiiij polle at owr wode	xviijd
Item at stroson hows' for ixC nell'	ixd
Item for thakrope to ye same hows'	iijd
Item to sceywyn mason at campyons hows' a dey	iiijd
	Summa iijs ixd ob

[A different hand is responsible for the following entries, probably that of Richard Dykelun, the new warden]

Dns' Robt' Schepey custos huius dom' elemosinarii decessit penultimo die (mens' ins) *Januarii A° dni 1517*[293] *et A° r' r' henrici octo ix°*

[294]*Ricardus Dykelun in decretis bacularius electus est in custod' supradict' dom' xj° die mens' ffebruarii A° dni et A° r' r'* (*h'* ins) *octavi supradict' a quo die et A° sepedict' dictus Ricardus computat sumpt' et emolumenta (ad dict' dom' pertinent'* ins) *usque ad festum sci Michael archangeli in A° dni 1518 et A° r' r' henrici octavi 10°. Et iste est compotus vicessimus iij dom'*

---

[293] this figure and the following figures in this paragraph are in Arabic form; this records the death of Sheppey on 30 January 1517/8

[294] 'Richard Dykelun bachelor in decrees was elected as warden of the above house on 11 February 1517/8 and 9 Henry VIII, from which date Richard accounted for the costs and emoluments belonging to the said house to Michaelmas 1518, 10 Henry VIII; and this is the twenty third account of the house'.

[The start of the account of Richard Dykelun for the year 1517-18]

Anno r' r' henrici octavi x° Compotus istius dom' xxiij'
[295]*In primis M[em]o[ra]nd' est quod dom Willielmus Tylle confrat' dom' elemosinar' rec' per manus Thome Wyllams ex legato dni Willelmi Hawkyns iij° die ffebruarii A° supradict'* xls *de quibus retinuit sibi* xiijs iiijd *pro salario suo a retro existent pro termino Nativitati dom preteriter et insuper soluit ix pauperibus pro stipendiis suis a penultimo die Januarii usque ad vj^{ta} die marcii hoc est per quinque septimanas* xxvjs iijd
et insuper dedit in supradict' Ricardo nunc custodi vd et sic eq' (*de* ins) *dict'* xls
Item recepi de dict' domino Willielmo confratro pro lecto predecessor' viijs

[296]*Item de dimidio bonorum duorum pauperum s[cilicet] Will'* (*vjd* ins) *et Roberti Hall* (ijs viijd *ins*) *summa* iijs ijd
Onus computat' terrarum et tenementorum hoc anno ut per j billam[297] *annex' hinc compoti extendit cum aliis fructis recept' ad summam* xliiij li (xvjs *del*) xjs iiijd

[298]*Computas' exonerat' se a supradict' summa per sequenc'*
In primis pro stipendiis pauperum a sexto die marcii usque secundem diem octobris videlicet ix pauperibus (xxjs *ins*) *per mensem et octo pauperibus per spacium xxvj septimanarum* (vj li xvjd ins) - Summa vij li ijs iiijd
Item pro stipendio custodis et confratris sui per tres terminos anni ix li
Summa totalis stipendii custodis confratris et pauperum xvj li ijs iiijd

fol 125v
[page badly worn and torn; text is faded; part is illegible]

[Illegible line ending in] xs vd ob
Summa [chief rents], amercyments, fines and swuytt' iij li xvijs vd ob qa
Item j li pric' pepyr xviijd

---

295 'Memo that William Tylle confrater received from Thomas Williams from the legacy of William Hawkyns on 3 February 40s from which he retained 13s 4d for his arrears of salary for the Nativity term and he paid to the bedesmen for their stipends from 30 January to 6 March, that is five weeks, 26s 3d; and therefore he gave to the said Richard now warden 5d and this amounts to the said 40s. And he [Richard] received from William confrater for his predecessor's bed 8s'.

296 'Half the goods of two paupers, i.e. William (6d) and Robert Hall (2s 8d) – total 3s 2d. The charge on the account of the lands and tenements this year as by a bill annexed to this account extends with other profits received to £44 11s 4d'

297 this is the 'new rental' now bound between folios 92 and 93; it is printed below on pages 292-93.

298 'From which sum the accountant discharges himself as follows: In primis the stipends of the paupers from 6 March to 2 October, namely nine paupers for one month (21s) and eight paupers for 26 weeks (£6 16d) total £7 2s 4d. And the stipend of the warden and confrater for three terms £9'

Annuall chargs thys yer

In primis to (ye *ins*) parson of Sent mychell vjs viijd
Item to henry lacy for kepyng of our cowrt' vjs viijd
Item to master colson for gederyng Rent at swafeld Northwithham and oyer plac' xiijs iiijd
Item for gaderyng Rent at Stamford and oyer plac' and for reward' thys yer xxs
Item for makyng of a M kydd' and halfe a C vjs
Item for cariag' of the same xxj loode xs vjd
Item for fellyng makyng and caryage of our medow ijs

Store of howse

ffor vij pec' of tymbyr bowte by the warden decessd xijd
Item for mendyng of a Nett[299] cownand [covenant?] by ye same warden viijd
Item for iij pownde waxe (ijs *ins*) and makyng of vj li (*iijd* ins) ijs iijd
Item for nayle bowte at mydlenty fayr halfe a thowson Splynte (*viijd* ins) nayle iij peny nayle (*xijd* ins) iiij peny nayle (*xvjd* ins) iijs
Item for mendyng ij lokks and makyng of a key vd
Item payde to the parsun of powlys [St Paul's] for a Spone vjs viijd
Item expens' made for apperans at lugborgh[300] aforne my lorde of lincoln officers at ye swte off Bawchon ixs jd
Item to knotte to schew our londs in Stamford felds ijd
Item at ye ffayr of Simond and Jude halfe a M v peny nayle xixd)
Item halfe a M iiij peny nayle (*xv*[*d*] ins) j M iij peny nayle(*xxijd* ins) iijs jd)
Item ij M Splynte nayle ijs iiijd)

[301]Summa vijs

Item to m' dene for goyng to m' pygoote for horse (*xijd* ins) and expense (*ijs viijd* ins) iijs viijd
Item to ledy nettun to m' Schawncelar [Chancellor] for our costs xvjd
[302]*Item pro vino ad celebrandum a fest' annunciacionis v^s m' usque festum Michael'* xxd
Item for sendyng to london to m' pygot for divers cawsys of our howse xiijs iiijd

Stamford Reparacyons

ffor iiij lode thorne to wytwykk' and Dowsys howse for fellyng and caryeg' of the same iijs viijd
Item to a hecter [?] of the same iiij days (*xvjd* ins) and a servar iij days (*ixd* ins) ijs jd
Item for makyng of a henkyll and a hoke and mendyng of a lokke at ye Angell iiijd
Item for iiij loode of thakk to Dowsys howse and carters and ye Stabyll in ye beede howse viijs

---

299 or 'Mett'

300 I have been unable to identify this location where the bishop of Lincoln's officers held court

301 right-hand margin

302 Wine for celebrating from the feast of the Annunciation of BVM to Michaelmas

Item for strawyng and drawyng of the same thakke	xijd
Item to a thakkar and servar by the space of iij days	iiijs xjd
Item to a masun and hys servant at divers placs by [illeg]	vjs viijd
Item for v loyde of mortar and stone to ye same [illeg]	xvd

Summa pagine xj li ijs ijd [?] Prob' est

NEW RENTAL 1517-8

fol 92b

[The following text is a new rental drawn up in early 1518, probably by Dykelun or one of the auditors. It is written on a slip of paper now pasted between folios 92 and 93; it is the 'bill' mentioned on folio 125].

Tenannds in Stamford	
...[illeg] in ye pultre market	nil
In paroch' omnium sanctorum	
William Styanabye for half-year	iijs
Mariota *soror* Rankyll	vs
Alicia Baly	xvjs
M Carter *pro di' ann' in festo ad vincula sti Petri*	vijs
Wytwyk *vidua*	xvjs
Philipp' at malery bryge	xijs
In paroch' Sti Pet'	
Willielmus Botun in ye Crane	iij li
John Thomas	xviijs viijd
A nodyr howse	nil
In paroch Sce Mare	
Laurencius Vawse *in signo An'li* [Angeli]	xxxiijs iiijd
In paroch' Sci Mi'l	
Rector *pro horreo* [barn] in skyfegate	vs
Thomas hanforde	xs
In paroch' sci Andree	
Hugo Masun	xvs
In paroch' Sci Martini	
Johnes Dowse	xiijs iiijd
Johnes Stevenson	xs
Johnes Jhonsun	vjs vjd
Eston	
Robertus Gunby	xlvjs iiijd
Thomas Dey	viijs
William Hutterham	vijs
Johnes Carver	vijs
Johnes Cordall	xvjs

Worthorppe

Thomas Smyth	vs iiijd
Robertus Harte	vs
Willielmus Rydall	ijs vjd
Petrus pulver	vs

Pyllsyate

Cuthbertus Bownde	xlvjs viijd
Berneck – Walkotte	nil
Wermyngton	xxs
Wylstroppe	xxs
Barham	xiiijs
Carlby	xxs
Sowth Wytham	xijs

Nortwitham Twyforde Wolstroppe Colysworth Sewsterne Gunby Steneby
Thomas Bagotte iij li vd

fol 92b *verso* [303]

Swafeld
[304]*ut patet Rotul' curie ibidem* xij li xviijs vjd

Stretton	xxxviijs viijd
North lufnaham	iij li

[305]*De terris et pratis in campis Stanford*

ffor Bredcrofte of (ye *del*) the parson of Sent Clements

Item of Robert Carby for iiij akyers	ijs
Item o[f] John Grene for iij akyrs	xviijd
Item of John Warde for iiij akyrs	ijs
Item of Gervis cooper for iiij akyrs	ijs

[306]*Summa tot' istius bylle* xliiij li xiijs xjd

[307]*Summa totalis* xliiij li xiijs ixd

303 the reverse side is written from bottom of the sheet upwards

304 'as appears by the court rolls'

305 'lands and meadows in Stamford fields'

306 this is written in a different hand - the reading is uncertain.

307 written in a different hand; this figure is not completely clear.

APPENDICES

I: Tables of accounts

- **a) annual balances**
- **b) disposable income**
- **c) disbursements**

II: List of bedesmen and bedeswomen 1495-1517

III: Documents from Browne's Hospital archives

- **a) statutes of the Hospital**
- **b) Delalaund deeds**
- **c) donation board**

IV: Documents from the National Archives relating to suit between the gild of All Saints and the Hospital:

- **a) Court of Chancery**
- **b) Court of Requests**

V: Itinerary of London visits 1506-7

VI: The date of the book

APPENDIX I: TABLES OF ACCOUNTS

Table 1: the annual balances

	Stock and new additions	estates (the charge)	total charge	expenditure
1495-6 Coton	20 0 0	61 13 7½	81 13 7½	44 8 4¼
1496-7 Coton/ Taylor	31 10 5¼	62 6 2¼	93 17 7¾[308]	85 0 9¾
1497-8 Taylor	8 7 6 [sic]	62 2 5	71 5 11[309]	64 16 3¾
1498-9 Taylor	6 12 11¼	62 2 5	68 15 4¼	49 8 1 ¾
1499-1500 Taylor	33 13 10½	62 15 1	96 8 10½	56 16 4
1500-1 Taylor	39 12 7½	62 7 5	102 0 0½	56 10 2¼
1501-2 Taylor	45 9 10¼	62 15 10½	108 5 8 ¾	62 15 10½
1502-3 Taylor	45 9 10¼	62 17 0½	128 6 10¾	83 8 9¼
1503-4 part Sharp				
1503-4 part II: Sharp missing				
1504-5 Sharp missing				
1505-6 Sharp missing				
1506-7 Sharp	68 11 8	62 5 6½	131 7 2½	63 18 11½ 1 4 8
1507-8 Sharp	40 16 7½	62 5 6½	103 4 2	no total
1508-9 probably Sheppey	35 7 6¾	62 5 6½	97 13 1¼	65 11 1 ½
1509-10 Sheppey	32 9 3	62 6 0	94 15 3¾	66 6 3¼
1510-11 Sheppey	28 9 0	62 5 0	90 14 0	63 18 8½
1511-12 Sheppey	26 15 4½	62 5 0	89 0 4½	62 14 1
1512-13 Sheppey; account incomplete	26 6 4½	62 5 0	88 11 4½	not complete
1513-14 income missing				63 8 7 ¾
1514-15	27 15 7¼	62 5 0	90 0 7¼	64 15 6 ¾
1515-16	15 5 1	62 5 0	77 10 1	63 14 2 ¼

308 the total of 93 1 9¾ is deleted and the correct total inserted

309 correct total should be £70 9 11

Table 2: Disposable income (calculated)

	estates	decays/abatements	chief rents /amercements	total (calculated)
1495	61 13 7½	3 6 0	6 3 3¼/ 7 11	54 16 5¼
1496	62 6 2½	3 18 10	6 9 1¼/ 4 6	51 13 9¼
1497	62 2 5 RB	5 4 2	5 0 1¼/ 4 0	51 13 7¾
1498	62 2 5 RB	3 12 6	5 19 10¼/ 4 0	52 6 1¾
1499	62 3 5 RB	8 1 10 DA	5 19 10¼/ 4 3	47 17 5¾
1500	62 3 5 RB	7 1 11½ DA	5 19 8¼/ 3 8	48 18 2¼
1501	62 15 10½[310] RB	8 2 0 D 1 6 3 A	6 0 1½/ 2 4	47 5 2
1502	62 15 2½ RB	5 8 1½ D 2 5 8 A	6 0 9¾/ 5 0	48 15 7¼
1503[311]	recd from tenants[312] 5 8 3½			
1506	62 5 6½	14 1 4 DA	missing/ 5 0	
1507	62 5 6½	14 16 6½ DA	5 17 6½/ 5 10	42 4 7½
1508	62 5 6½	11 1 10½ DA	6 5 10/ 5 6	44 12 4
1509	62 6 0	14 7 5	6 1 1¼/ 5 3	41 13 2¾
1510	62 5 0	17 16 3½	6 10 0¼/ 7 0	37 11 8¼
1511	62 5 0	15 12 1½	6 6 1/ 7 0	39 19 9½
1512	62 5 0	not listed	not listed	
1513[313]		18 19 11½	3 15 4¼/[314] 7 8	39 2 0¼
1514	62 5 0	18 11 0	3 11 4¾ / 6 9	40 0 10¼

---

310 includes additional items not listed

311 Taylor's account for the first few months of this year

312 Robert Beomond's name is deleted from this account, these sums had been paid to the warden directly

313 The start of this annual account has been lost but the account is also badly kept

314 note to say £3 0 0 chief rent in Swayfield to Corby has been abated in perpetuity.

1515	62 5 0	3 17 4 D 11 14 3½ A	3 10 5¾ / 7 0	42 15 10¾
1516		14 8 4½ DA	3 10 5¾ / 7 0	

Table 3: Disbursements

	Bedes-men	Annual charges	Holding courts/ suits and amerce-ments	Casual	Stoor	Repar-acions	Miscellan eous
1495-6	15 10 8	8s 8d	18 4½ / 7 11	19 9	10 3	13 10 5	7 5½
1496-7	19 3 4[315]	in casual costs	18 9 / 4 1	17 10 11 13 6	4 0 2	7 4 7 5 15 0	3 11 1½
1497-8	17 17 0	22s 6d	1 1 0 / 4 0	14 7½	17 10	17 15 9	2 5 0
1498-9	17 1 3	22s 6d	1 0 0½ / 4 0	7 10	-	5 9 2	2 0 0
1499-1500	17 14 8	22s 6d	1 0 9 / 4 3	1 8	9 10	8 0 10	2 0 0
1500-1	12 7 11	22s 6d	nil / 3 8	5 11	3 0	12 7 0	4 19 2½
1501-2	16 1 5[316]	22s 6d	nil / 2 4	2 13 3½	3 17 11	11 10 10	no sum
1502-3	16 9 2	22s 6d	10 11 / 5 0	10 11	5 4 2½	30 17 7	1 0 0
1503-4 part			4 7 (part year)	6 7	4 4	no sum	
1506-7	14 11 1	3 11 8	no mention / 5 0	3 15 8	3 8 9	10 13 7	2 4 8
1507-8	16 17 2	3 7 9	3 0 (in casual) / 5 10	1 7 8½	2 7 1	14 4 11	12 7
1508-9	16 10 9		no mention / 5 6	17 2	3 0 4	10 15 8	
1509-10	13 3 0	4 0 0	8 6 (in chief rents) / 8 3	-	5 19 1	24 9 9	

[315] for the first year and part of the second year, the bedesmen and women were paid at 8d per week; thereafter at 7d per week

[316] From January 1503, the total establishment was reduced from 12 to 11.

1510-11	12 2 8	3 0 0	12 7 [?] / 7 0	16 2	4 12 5	7 5 11	
1511-12	12 3 6	3 12 4	no mention / 7 0	-	2 12 6	7 14 5	
1512-13	11 13 0	1 2 5	no mention / 7 8	-	4 8 0	2 11 6[317]	
1513-14	9 19 11		no mention / 7 8	1 17 10	6 16 8 5 8 2	2 8 8	
1514-15	10 9 5		no mention / 6 9	-	4 10 10	10 15 6	
1515-16	13 10 1	4 15 0	no mention / 7 0	-	5 3 10	9 4 4	
1516-17	13 13 2	3 0 0	no mention / 7 0	-	1 19 10	5 7 10	
1517-18		3 13 2	no mention / no mention	-	2 11 2	no total	

317 some of reparations are listed under 'Stoor'

APPENDIX II: LIST OF BEDESMEN AND WOMEN 1495-1517

Bedesmen

Name	admitted	death or departure
Thomas Brugge[318]*	1494 or earlier	died Jan 1499
Thomas Andrew*	1494 or earlier	
Thomas Normanton*	1494 or earlier	
John Burgoyne*	1494 or earlier	died 2 August 1503
William Blackbourn	1494 or earlier	died Sep 1497
Richard Sutton	1494 or earlier	died March 1497
Robert Johnson	1494 or earlier	died June 1496
Henry Walch	1494 or earlier	died April 1497
dom George Keele (clerk)*	1494 or earlier	
[319]John Cantyng*	1494 or earlier	died 3 Sep 1500
William Hesull[320]*	adm July 1496	dep Sep 1500
Thomas Reynolds*	adm April 1497	exp May 1512
Richard Bulkeley*	adm Aug 1497	expelled July 1498
Thomas Bentley*	adm Oct 1497	licence for absence for two weeks July 1500 but did not return
William Bacon[321]	adm Oct 1498	died 29 Sep 1500
William Umfrey	adm Oct 1499	died 14 July 1500
John Stretton	adm 31 Jan 1501	
John Lynley	adm 20 June 1501	
Edmund Grenham	adm 27 June 1501	
John Midylton *alias* Bendeslow	adm 7 May 1502	died June 1510
There are no records from Jan 1504 (when there were nine residents) to Oct 1506 (when there were ten residents).		
Thomas Sleng[322]		died Jan 1507
Henry Phylyp		died Jan 1510
Harry Mylner		dep Dec 1510
John Perkyn	adm Aug 1507	dep June 1514
John [Calays?]	adm Nov 1507	
... Langton	adm 31 Oct 1510	died Dec 1513
Harry Mosundew	adm Jan 1512	dep 30 April 1512
unnamed		departure Aug 1513

318 those with * are named (with the two bedeswomen) as witnesses in a deed of December 1498 by Sir Thomas Delalaund to the Hospital, see Appendix III.2; those without dates of departure probably died or left during the gap years of 1504-6.

319 Wright gives J Cantasy

320 Wright gives 'Resul'

321 one entry reads 'Baker' in confusion with a tenant of that name; the 1498 list gives Bakon

322 those without a date of admission were presumably admitted between 1504 and 1506.

incomplete Oct-Nov 1513; in Sep 1513, there were six residents, in December seven residents		
unnamed	adm Oct-Nov 1513	
Jankyn Worthington		dep March 1515
Nicholas Bureene?	adm March 1514	
… Barker	adm Sep 1514	Barker dep May 1515
… Tomlyn	adm Jan 1515	Tomkyns dep Aug 1515
William Geff	adm July 1515	
Thomas Walsch	adm Aug 1515	
William Driver	adm Nov 1515	
unnamed	adm Sep 1515	
unnamed		departure May 1516
Robert Holand	adm July 1516	
Harry …	adm July 1516	Henry … died June 1517
Respyn		died Feb 1517
Robert Hall	adm July 1517	

Bedeswomen

Elizabeth Huntley	1494 or earlyer	died 8 Jan 1503; her place appears not to have been filled
Mathilda Huntley	1494 or earlyer	departure unknown, probably 1504-6; her place was probably filled by Margaret
Margaret	adm sometime between 1504 and 1506	departed "to heyr son" 12 March 1512
Katerine Golsmythe	adm 16 April 1512	

APPENDIX III: DOCUMENTS FROM HOSPITAL ARCHIVES

1. THE STATUTES OF BROWNE'S HOSPITAL, STAMFORD

Wright (Domus Dei *pp 28-53, 459-474) used two different sources for his Latin and English texts of the statutes of the Hospital. The English translation now appears to have disappeared but it contained material which was not included in the Latin text. The Latin text was taken from a late seventeenth century copy still in BH archives now in Lincolnshire Archives Office (LAO, BHS1/2) but now damaged. This includes some important material which Wright did not use, so this material is given below. A more detailed note about these statutes will be posted on the website of the Stamford and District Local History Society, www.stamfordhistory.org.uk.*

The following translation from the Latin of the statutes of Thomas Stokes (1495) is taken from that of Wright. I have made a number of changes to modernise some of the English, but it retains something of its nineteenth century flavour.

From LAO, BHS 1/2

Statuta domus Eleemosinarie Willi Browne de Stamford
compilavit Tho Stokk habens Regiam authoritat' sub lettris patentibus [*Statutes of the almshouse of WB of Stamford compiled by TS having authority of royal letters patent*]

Willus Browne Mercator de Stapulis fundavit Anno dni 1495[323] decimoduo decembris Anno Regis henr' septimi decimo [12 December 10 Henry VII, i.e. 1494]
Jophannes Cotton primus Custos, Willus Hawkins primus confrater. Thesaurus in Cista Anno dni centum et novemdecim libri undecim solid' et undecim denar'

[*WB merchant of Calais Staple founded [the Hospital] in 1495 22 December 10 Henry VII [1494]. John Cotton first warden, William Hawkins first confrater. Cash in chest this year £119 11s 11d]*

Then appointment of John Rippingdon as warden 1557 and Richard Snowden as confrater 1564.

From English translation of statutes formerly in BH archives and used by Wright:

To all Christian people to whom this writing shall come, I Thomas Stokk clerk, canon of the cathedral church of York, by virtue and authority of letters patent of our Lord, now King Henry VII, by a certain writing of mine[324] sealed with my seal and also signed with my own name by my own hand, dated at Stamford the twenty-second day of December in the year of our Lord 1494 and in the year of

---

[323] Browne founded the first Hospital in 1475 but died in 1489; Stokes founded the second Hospital on 22 December 1494 and promulgated the statutes on 9 October 1495 before he died later in October 1495. Hence the date here of 1495 (quite clear).

[324] This document of 22 December 1494 is not now extant; the same date appears on the donation board, see below.

the lord king the 10th, have in reality made, ordained, founded and established for ever an almshouse at Stamford consisting of one warden, a secular chaplain, and one confrater, also a secular chaplain, to celebrate according to my ordinance or the ordinance of my executors or of any of them Divine service for ever and to pray for the good estate of our lord king and of Elizabeth his consort Queen of England, and of Reginald Bray knight and Catherine his wife, and of me Thomas Stokk and of Elizabeth Elmes and William Elmes, while we live and of our souls when we shall have departed this life, and especially for[325] the souls of all the faithful departed. And I have assigned, ordained and appointed my well-beloved in Christ John Cotton, a secular priest, to be first warden of the almshouse, and also William Hawkins, a secular priest, to be the first confrater of the almshouse, and have instituted and put them the warden and confrater in real possession of the almshouse; and furthermore by virtue and authority of the said letters patent, by the same writing of mine, I have decreed, made and ordained certain ordinances concerning the almshouse, as appears more fully in the said writing of mine concerning the foundation of the almshouse, reserving to myself during my life power and absolute authority over the almshouse, the warden and confrater and their successors, and also over the profits, revenues or possessions or whatever things are bestowed or will hereafter be bestowed upon the same warden, confrater or their successors, [and the power] of further ordering, publishing, interpreting and declaring and also of making, establishing and ordaining any other ordinances whatsoever, and also of subtracting and altering ordinances made at the pleasure of myself Thomas Stokk; over which I, Thomas Stokk, desirous to bring to its due end that which was so well begun, have ordained certain honest and reasonable statutes and ordinances, to be observed hereafter by the warden and confrater and their successors, and also by the twelve poor of each sex, mentioned in my said writing as to the foundation. The which statutes and ordinances are known to be necessary and profitable, not only for the governing of the warden, confrater and their successors and of the twelve poor of each sex, but also for the possessions and goods of the almshouse, now had or hereafter to be had, and also profitable for the increase of God's worship, the prosperity of the living, and the salvation of souls departed; the name of Christ being first called upon for a sure and perpetual mercy, and therefore I proceed as follows:

I Statutes to be strictly observed

I will, determine and ordain that all statutes and ordinances contained in the said writing concerning the foundation of the almshouse by me in the same writing of mine published, made and ordained, be never hereafter infringed but steadfastly held and inviolably observed for ever. Also I will, appoint and ordain that in a certain capital messuage with a chapel and other buildings in Stamford upon Clay Mount, there be established for ever a certain almshouse commonly called 'William Browne's almshouse', for the invocation of the Most Glorious Virgin Mary and of All Saints to the praise and honour of the Name crucified; in

[325] this prologue does not mention William Browne and Margaret

which almshouse, I will, appoint and ordain by these presents that hereafter for ever there shall be there one warden and confrater, and also twelve poor of each kind or sex, namely, ten men and two women, under the reasonable rule and governance of the warden and confrater and their successors, that they may pray for the good estate and the souls of the said intercessories; the which poor men and poor women I will that they be single and not married.

II The oath of the warden

Furthermore I will, appoint and ordain that he who shall be admitted to be warden or confrater of the almshouse shall on his first admission publicly in the chapel of the almshouse before me Thomas Stokk whilst I live, and after my death before my nephew William Elmes, and after the death of us both before the dean of Stanford for the time being or at least before the vicar of All Saints in the Market for the time being, and before the poor of the same house for the time being, laying his hand upon the holy Gospels of God, swear personally under this form:

> I, [JC] to be admitted warden (or confrater) of the almshouse of William Browne of Stamford, do swear that I will to the utmost of my power in all things maintain the interests and profit of the house, and will not reveal the secrets of the said house to the damage and prejudice of the same. Also, that I will hold and inviolably observe, as far as concerns me, all the statutes and ordinances concerning the said house according to the plain, literal and grammatical understanding of them; and to the utmost of my power I will cause them to be kept and observed by others; and that I will not admit any other statutes and ordinances, interpretations, counterfeits, injunctions, declarations or other expositions impugning or repugnant to, derogating from or contrary to, these present ordinances and statutes or the true meaning of any of them made by any other than by the consent and will of the founder; nor will I accept or consent to them or any way allow them; nor will I at any time obey them, nor in any manner use them or any of them within the said almshouse or out of it, tacitly or expressly. Also that I will not be a detractor, secret whisperer or criticiser or a provoker of hatred, anger, discord, envy, contumely, brawling or any manner of quarrelling whatsoever. Nor will I unlawfully carry on conspiracies, confederations or illicit pacts against the ordinances and statutes of the said house or to the prejudice or trouble of anyone dwelling in the same house; nor will I myself (so far as in me lies) in future procure or permit these things to be done by others in any way whatever, nor will I lend or give counsel, help or favour to any such things or to any one of them; and that, so far as I am able and so much as belongs to me, I will by all ways and means possible keep and cause others to keep and maintain the tranquillity, peace, profit, interests and honour of the almshouse and the unity of all dwelling therein. And that I will faithfully observe all and each of the ordinances and statutes of the house so far as they concern me; otherwise, without any kind of resistance, I will undergo willingly and submit myself to the penalties to be inflicted and ordained for the offender in the premises or in any of the ordinances and statutes of the house; and I will faithfully observe them according to the true force, form

> and effect of the ordinances and statutes of the almshouse. All these things I will in my own person faithfully observe, so help me God and these Holy Gospels of God.

III The oath of the paupers

[326] .. that all and each of the poor persons of either sex admitted or hereafter to be admitted to the almshouse, on their first admission publicly in the chapel before me, Thomas Stokk while I live and after my death before my nephew William Elmes during his life, and after the death of us both before the dean of Stamford for the time being and before the warden, the confrater and the rest of the poor of the almshouse, each of them laying his or her hand upon the Holy Gospels, shall personally swear after this form [*English*]:

> I, A B, depose and actually sware by these Holy Evangelics which I bodily touch, that from henceforth I will not show nor outwardly disclose the secrets and councils of this almshouse to the hurt and prejudice of the same, and I shall well and truly keep and observe, to my power, all the laudable ordinances and statutes of the almshouse as much as to me appertaineth. So help me God and all the Holy Saints by this Holy Book.

IV General election.

..that when and as often after my death and after the death of my nephew, any warden or confrater or any of the twelve poor of the almshouse shall depart or be removed from the house for any cause for which he ought to be removed according to the ordinances, statutes and constitutions made or to be made by me, Thomas Stoke, for the rule, government and direction of the almshouse, or by any other manner shall be removed from the house, or shall wholly by free will depart from thence, that then the dean of Stamford for the time being and the vicar of the parish church of All Saints in the Market for the time being, within fourteen days following after the death, departure or removal, shall nominate, appoint, admit and put into real possession another fit person in the room of the warden, confrater, man or woman so departing, removed or leaving. And if it shall happen that the dean or vicar or their successors, within fourteen days after any warden, confrater or poor person of the almshouse shall depart or be removed or expelled from the house or shall voluntarily depart thence as agreed, shall not have named, appointed, admitted and placed in actual possession another sufficient person in the place of him or her so departing, removed or removing, that then and so often the heirs of William Browne and their heirs, within another fourteen days then immediately following, shall name, appoint, admit and put into actual possession for that time only a fit person in the place of the last warden, confrater or poor person so departing, removed or willingly retiring and of the same sex. If not, then the Alderman [of Stamford] and the abbot of Croyland; if not, then the bishop of Lincoln; and if not, *ad infinitum* etc.

---

[326] I have omitted the phrase 'Furthermore I will, appoint and ordain …' from each of the remaining statutes

V Form of admission

.. that every nomination, institution, admission and appointment of warden and confrater of the almshouse be made and granted to each of them, the warden and confrater, by a writing formally made and sealed, to have and to hold unto himself for the term of his life according to the ordinances, statutes and constitutions hereafter specified. Also that every nomination, institution, admission and appointment of each of the ten poor men and two poor women of the almshouse hereafter to be made shall be made by word of mouth only, to have and to hold unto themselves for the term of the life of every one of them, according to the ordinances, statutes and constitutions made and hereafter specified in this behalf.

VI General correction

That if any of the warden, confrater and twelve poor or their successors be or shall be a waster, destroyer or consumer of the goods of the almshouse, or be notoriously perjured in not observing any of the previous statutes or those coming afterwards, or if he be or shall be an open fornicator or adulterer, or incorrigible or unduly and habitually a frequenter of a tavern or taverns or a keeper or breeder of hawks and hounds, or be intolerably offensive to the harm of the almshouse or a provoker of hatred, anger, discord, envy, insults, strife, brawling or quarrels of any kind, or be notoriously known as guilty of any notable crime which may bring discredit upon the almshouse, and being thus notoriously known and having not lawfully cleared himself of what is so known or cannot clear himself of the same, or otherwise shall be convicted thereof or any one of them before his ordinary, let him immediately *ipso facto* be removed and expelled from the almshouse and from that time forward let him lose all his benefits in the same.

VII Against manual work

.. that none of the poor men or women of the almshouse, after his or her admission, shall occupy himself or herself in any servile manual or labouring work or in any manner carry on the same publicly or privately, save when they are so engaged in repairing and mending their own necessaries, and even that let it be done secretly in their own rooms at especially fitting times to be allotted and assigned by the warden and confrater.

VIII The poor to be elected and their condition

.. that those who after my death by my present ordinance shall have the right to prefer any poor man or woman to the almshouse when the place of any one shall be vacant, shall admit only a fit person (putting aside all excessive affection and corruption of entreaty and bribe), one who is lowly, devout and poor and not having any other way of getting a living, and who knows thoroughly the *Lord's Prayer*, the *Angelic Salutation*[327] and the *Apostles' Creed.*

---

[327] the Magnificat

IX Concerning the infected

.. that no leprous man or woman shall be admitted or placed in the almshouse. And if any one of the almshouse, after admission thereto, shall become leprous or infected by any other infirmity repulsively noisome to his or her fellows, he or she ought to be removed by me, Thomas Stokk, during my life and after my death by my nephew William Elmes during his life, and after the death of both, by the dean of Stamford and the vicar of the parish church of All Saints in the Market of Stamford for the time being, lest he infect or be horribly loathsome to his healthy fellows. And let him betake himself to some other place where he may be admitted, and during his or her life, let him or her receive their daily allowance by this present ordinance granted and assigned to them for their relief, and I will that he or she be reputed as one of the number of the house for his or her life.

X Of absence

That neither the warden, nor any of his successors, wardens of the almshouse, nor the confrater, nor any of his successors, shall in any manner absent himself hereafter from the house for one whole month in the year, continuously or by broken periods, without my leave whilst I live, and after my death, without the leave of my nephew William Elmes, and after the death of us both, without the leave of the vicar of the parish church of All Saints in the Market of Stamford, and then only for honest and fitting causes; provided always that either the warden or the confrater and their successors for the time being, be personally resident in the almshouse for the keeping and preserving of good government in the house, so that both are not absent at the same time. And that none of the twelve poor of the almshouse in any manner absent themselves hereafter from the same for one whole day without the leave of the warden of the house, if he shall be present, or in his absence without the leave of the confrater; the which confrater I will that he always be, in the absence of the warden, sub-warden or deputy of the warden. And that his leave be not granted unless pressing necessity require or some reasonable cause, approved of by the warden or confrater, urge it.

XI Mutual help

.. that the sick, weak and helpless poor of the house shall be very diligently looked after and helped with all daily necessaries by their fellows who are healthy and strong, and especially by the women of the said house for the time being.

XII General exercises

.. that on every weekday either the warden or confrater shall, all excuses laid aside, say Mass in the chapel of the almshouse at seven o'clock in the morning or near thereto; which Mass, all the poor of the house are bound to attend; and that the other shall celebrate his Mass every weekday in the parish church of All Saints in the Market in the chapel of the Blessed Virgin Mary[328]. And that on

[328] the burial chapel of William Browne

every Lord's Day or feast day, both the warden and confrater shall celebrate Mass in the church of All Saints in the Market where I will and ordain that they then attend and assist in the choir of the church at High Mass in the morning and at both Vespers and Compline, unless a reasonable cause hinder; provided always that if any of the twelve poor be so cast down by infirmity or weakness that he or she shall not be able to come to the church upon feast days, I will that then one, either the warden or confrater, celebrate and say his Mass in the chapel of the almshouse upon such feast days to the spiritual refreshment of the afflicted one.

XIII The exercises of warden and confrater

.. that daily throughout the year at two o'clock in the afternoon, the warden and confrater say by turns in the Chapel of the almshouse for the souls of William Browne and Dame Margaret his wife, also for the souls of me Thomas Stokk and of William Elmes when we shall have been taken away from this life, and for the souls of our parents and benefactors, and all the faithful departed, holy services for the dead, namely the *placebo* and the *dirige* with the customary psalms and collects; and when they are finished and said, let the warden and confrater say by turns the psalm *de profundis* with this prayer following: 'Incline, O Lord, thine ear to our prayers, whereby we as suppliants earnestly pray for Thy compassion that Thou wouldest absolve the souls of Thy servant William Browne and of Margaret his wife, the souls of Thy servants, me Thomas Stokk and William Elmes, when we shall have departed this life, and the souls of all the faithful departed, from every bond of their sins, that in the glory of the Resurrection among the Saints and Thine Elect, they may peacefully be refreshed through Christ our Lord. Amen. May they rest in peace. Amen.' And that then every one of the twelve poor say, for the souls of the said intercessories, the *Lord's Prayer* once with the *Angelic Salutation* and the *Apostles Creed*. And also that the warden and confrater and the wardens and confraters their successors shall every Wednesday and Thursday say the *Requiem Mass* for the souls of the aforenamed, in place and manner above said, if a reasonable cause do not hinder.

XIV Exercises of the poor

.. that each of the twelve poor and their successors, so long as they live, every day in the morning when they have risen from their beds and again in the evening when they retire to rest, shall kneeling on their knees in the chapel, say the *Lord's Prayer* five times, the *Angelic Salutation* five times and the *Apostles' Creed* once, with special and mindful commendation of the said souls in the words prescribed, unless, it may be that any one of them, through infirmity or weakness of body, shall not be able to come into the chapel. Such a one, nevertheless, is bound to say the same prayers in his or her chamber while he or she cannot get to the chapel. And that each of the poor men, at other empty and more convenient hours every day, if not hindered by weakness or by any other lawful or reasonable cause, is to say for the welfare of the souls of the above-named three psalms of the glorious Virgin Mary, and both the poor women, on account of their constant occupation in serving the rest of their fellows, shall be bound to say two psalms of the Blessed Mary every day at least. Also, I will that daily, morning and evening, the *Lord's Prayer, Angelic Salutation* and *Apostles Creed,* having been said and completed in the chapel, one of the poor men, a senior of them, shall say openly in English: '*God have mercy on the souls of William Browne of Stamford and Dame Margaret his wife, and* (after my death) *on the soul of Mr Thomas Stokk, founder of this almshouse, and their fathers and mothers and all Christian souls*'. And that all the rest of the poor shall respond, '*Amen.*'

XV Residence

.. that the warden, confrater and twelve poor and their successors, all and every of them, shall be required to inhabit and continually to reside within the said almshouse and its precincts, as do other poor commonly reside or are obliged to reside in like almshouses and hospitals. And that each of the ten poor men shall have in the almshouse, at the decision of the warden or in his absence of the confrater, one room separate to himself, there only to remain and to lodge; and the two women shall have a room common to them, there to remain and lodge together.

XVI The seal and common chest

.. that the warden, confrater and their successors have a common seal and a common chest for themselves and for the twelve poor; in the which chest the common seal and papers, letters, charters, writings and treasure of the almshouse shall be placed and kept safe; which chest, let it be placed and guarded in a secret and secure place within the precincts of the said house. And for the same chest let there be three keys always, each key having its own special lock, of which keys one shall be in the keeping of me, Thomas Stokk, while I live, and at my death in the custody of the vicar of the Church of All Saints for the time being; and another of the same keys in the charge of the warden of the house for the time being; and one of the ten poor men for the time being, well known for his discretion and morals, shall have charge of the third key. So that no one of them presume to hold all three of the keys, or two of them together, nor shall anything be sealed with the common seal without the consent of all the keepers of the keys for the time being.

XV The inventory

.. that the warden of the house for the time being shall have for ever the government and rule of the house, and of the confrater and of the poor for the time being, also the administration of all rents and goods of the house. And immediately after the admission or preferment of any future warden into the house, the same warden, before he meddle with or have any administration of the house, let him make a full and faithful inventory of all the goods of the house found there at the time of his promotion or admission, in my presence while I live or of my deputy in this behalf, and after my death in the presence of my nephew William Elmes or his deputy herein, and after the death of both of us in the presence of the vicar of All Saints in the Market for the time being or of his deputy herein as required by the warden, and of two of the more discreet of the poor men.

XVIII The account

.. that every warden of the house for the time being, every year within one month after the feast of St Michael the Archangel, shall be bound to render a faithful account of all his administration of and in the revenues and goods of the almshouse before me, Thomas Stokk, while I live or my appointed deputy, and after my decease before William Elmes, my nephew or his appointed deputy; and always before the vicar of All Saints in the Market for the time being or his appointed deputy; and also before the confrater of the house; also before two of the more discreet poor men of the same house; the which vicar I ordain and appoint chief supervisor of every audit. And I appoint, ordain and assign by these presents the same vicar for the time being, for his labour in this task, to receive and have yearly five marks[329] of lawful English money out of the surplusage of the revenues of the house after the necessary charges of the same house, if the surplusage of the rents of the house will extend so far (but if they be too little, then as far as the surplusage shall happen to extend at the keeping of every such audit) by the hands of the warden for the time being, if he, the vicar, shall be diligent for the augmentation of their yearly maintenance, having duly commended to God the souls of William Browne and Dame Margaret his wife and also the souls of me, Thomas Stokk, and of my nephew William Elmes, when we shall have departed this life, and of the souls of our parents and of our benefactors and of all the faithful departed. But if the vicar shall be (which God forbid) negligent in the premises and shall not show himself diligent in performing the premises, then I will that his pension of five marks be altogether kept from him by the warden for the time being, and for that turn, let one half of his pension be given to the dean of Stamford for the time being, that he may undertake the labour and faithfully execute effectively the business of the vicar in these premises, but the other half of the pension shall be reserved for the necessary uses of the almshouse, and so yearly, so often as the vicar shall be remiss. And this said [i.e. the account rendered], and it having been done and completed every year [i.e. audited], I will then that the same warden for the time being, in the presence of the keepers of the keys for the time being, be bound to place and lock up in the common chest the book of his audit for that year and all the money remaining over (*superfluentes*) of the revenues of the house, over and above the charges of the same and over and above the pension assigned as said, for the full satisfaction of those who are then present and for the memory of those coming after them, to be kept in safe custody, so that out of such money remaining over the necessary repairs of the house whenever they shall happen and other ordinary charges falling upon and occurring to the same may be better paid and the expenses thereof better met.

XIX Not holding any other benefice

.. that it shall not be lawful for the warden for the time being, nor for the confrater there for the time being, to combine his office or service in the house with any benefice, dignity or ecclesiastical office, or to obtain or hold any other

---

[329] £3 6s 8d

benefice or ecclesiastical office or farm or other promotion whatever (on which he shall be able to live comfortably) with the same office or place in the almshouse; but that immediately after the warden or the confrater shall have obtained any other benefice or ecclesiastical office, with cure or without cure, or farm or any other promotion whatever on which he may be able to live comfortably, that then he shall be bound, in deed, name and word (*re, nomine et verbo*), to resign the office of warden and service of confrater in the almshouse and from thence be utterly removed without any hindrance or contradiction whatever. And that immediately another new warden or another confrater in the almshouse shall be elected and preferred into the place of him so removed or resigning, according to the form formerly laid down by me, and so shall it be so often as a suchlike case shall happen.

XX What may be received beyond stipend of the house

.. that if and as often as any one of the twelve poor of the almshouse comes into a living of four marks a year *de claro*[330] by inheritance, or in any other way shall be increased to such a yearly revenue over and above his or her former allowance, that then and so often, *ipso facto,* such poor person so advanced or increased shall be entirely removed from the almshouse and that another poor person in his or her place shall forthwith be provided for the same almshouse and placed in the same after the prescribed form. Also if any one of the poor, after admission to the house, be increased above the sum of twenty shillings *de claro* and under the sum of four marks in revenues and advancements, spiritual or temporal, or in any other way, that then one half of the true value of such living to which he or she is so increased shall, without guile or fraud, be placed every year in the common chest of the almshouse, to remain there so that it may be converted to the use of the almshouse when so required; and that the poor person so augmented may obtain or have the other half thereof, together with the portion of a poor person of the same house to be assigned later[331]. Otherwise he or she who shall not have observed the present ordinance, let him or her forthwith be removed from that almshouse and from all profits of the same, and let another poor person in his or her place be provided for the same almshouse in the form prescribed.

XXI Concerning the duty of the women

.. that the women of the almshouse for the time being be and carry themselves as the 'mother figures' (*matres-familiae*) of the house, and so bear themselves in washing and other things befitting honest women, and (so far as is decent) be completely attentive and useful to the poor men in their necessities.

XXII Who shall correct misdoings

.. that the defects of the warden and of the confrater of the almshouse for the time being shall be reformed and corrected or punished by me, Thomas Stokk

[330] i.e. 'net'; four marks was £2 13s 4d

[331] in statute 24

whilst I live, and after my death by my nephew William Elmes during his life, and, after the death of both of us, by the dean of Stamford and the vicar of the church of All Saints in the Market for the time being, either by taking away the stipend of them, the warden or confrater, for a week, more or less, according to the quantity and quality of their offences at the discretion of the correctors, or by depriving and removing them, the warden or confrater or either of them, from their office and service, stipend, interest and place which he had in the same house, if the fault (*pertinacia*) of one or other of them require it.

XXIII Of any infirmity of the warden or confrater

.. that when the warden or confrater of the almshouse for the time being, through their own negligence or ill government, happen to fall or come into any long-term sickness so that the masses or other divine services cannot, at least in time of their infirmity, be celebrated by the warden or confrater, that then another fit and honest chaplain be provided during their sickness, at the cost of the warden or the confrater thus disabled by sickness, out of the stipend belonging to him, for saying in the almshouse masses and other divine services which do and ought to belong to the warden or the confrater, as long as such infirmity endure or be found in him. And if and so soon as the warden or the confrater shall recover from his sickness, that then he shall cease from his exhibition[332] to the chaplain, and he who was before sick and is now restored to health, let himself celebrate the masses and other divine services and undertake and perform, as becomes him, the cure and duty imposed on him.

XXIV The several salaries

.. that the warden of the almshouse shall have and receive from the revenues of the almshouse for his salary, stipend or pension, ten marks of lawful English money to be paid by his own hands; and the confrater for the time being is to be paid and receive for his labour or pension yearly by the hands of the warden for the time being eight marks of lawful English money at the four usual periods of the year, namely, at the feast of St Michael the Archangel, Christmas, Easter, and the Nativity of St. John the Baptist, in equal portions[333]. Also I will that every man and woman of the twelve poor shall have and receive by these present statutes out of the revenues of the almshouse, by the hands of the warden for the time being, seven pence of lawful English money for their maintenance, to be paid at the end of every week without any delay.

XXV Chest for vestments

.. that the warden, confrater and poor shall have in the almshouse another chest for the chalices, vestments, ornaments and other goods of the almshouse, guarded by two keys and two locks; of which keys I appoint that one of them remain always with the warden or confrater for the time being, and the other with one of the more discreet of the poor men to be elected by the same poor.

---

[332] i.e. payment for subsistence

[333] the warden's stipend was to be £6 13s 4d; the confrater's stipend was to be £5 6s 8d

XXVI The moiety of goods

.. that every warden, confrater and twelve poor for the time being, at their departure by death, leave for the benefit of their souls one half of all their goods for the repairing and supporting of the almshouse and for defraying other charges belonging to it, the which half or the true and just value of the same, I will that it be always kept in the chest under three locks with three separate keys, until there shall be need of it to meet the necessary charges of the almshouse.

XXVII Bread, wine and wax

.. that the warden or the confrater for the time being shall supply and provide out of their own stipend, bread, wine and wax for light for divine services to be celebrated and performed by them, both in the parish church as in their chapel[334].

XXVIII Shutting the gates

.. that every night the great gate of the almshouse and also all other ward gates of the same house be shut and firmly locked, at eight o'clock or soon after from the first day of the month of May to the first day of the month of September, and at seven o'clock at all other times of the year; and that they remain so closed and locked until the break of the day following; and let the keys of the gates every night remain and be in the custody of the warden of the house when he shall be present, and during his absence, in the custody of the confrater.

XXIX Absence

.. that neither the warden nor the confrater, nor any one, male or female, of the twelve poor of the almshouse, be or stay any night in the town of Stamford or elsewhere within a mile of the almshouse without leave asked and obtained of me Thomas Stokk during my life, and after my decease, without the leave of William Elmes my nephew during his life; and after the decease of us both, without permission of the warden for the time being; and the warden himself [shall not be absent] without the leave of the vicar of the parish church of All Saints in the Market for the time being. And if anyone of the twelve poor shall do contrary to this, for the first night let them lose a week's pension, for the second a fortnight's, and for the third a month's pension; and after that, if he or she be found guilty of constant breach of the rule, let him be excluded for ever from the almshouse, which provision I decree is to be inviolably observed for ever.

---

334 Wright adds the following footnote but gives no indication where it came from, perhaps from the warden at the time Wright was writing, 1890: "We begin to burn candle from Michaelmas Day till Candlemas, and have 12 lbs, whereof 9 pound for the l a m [sic]; the rest for the warden and confrater - 4 candles for the pound will serve 18 weeks, i.e. from Michaelmas to Candlemas". The cost of tapers for the chapel was met from the Hospital funds throughout most of the period of these accounts; see 'tapers' in index.

XXX Exchange of lands

.. that it shall not be lawful for the warden and confrater, nor for their successors, in any manner to remit, release, alter, give in exchange or mortgage any of the lands, tenements, meadows, grazing rights, pastures (*pascua, pasturam*), goods and mills with all and singular their appurtenances now held or hereafter to be held, or any part of them, or in any way to alienate them or hereafter to convert them to other uses than are above named, except it shall be by way of exchange which shall turn to the great profit of the house, and even then never without the leave and consent of me Thomas Stokk while I live, and after my death, without the leave and consent of William Elmes my nephew; and after the death of us both, without the leave and consent of the dean and vicar for the time being. And either the warden or confrater or their successors for the time being shall do contrary to the force, form and effect of this last but one statute, I will that then that act shall be null and void, and that forthwith the warden and confrater by that act infringing this same statute, be wholly removed from the almshouse and from all his profit in the same; and in his place let another warden or confrater be appointed in manner and form abovesaid.

XXXI Reading the statutes

I will also and ordain that four times each year, namely, the day after the feast of the Purification of the Blessed Mary, the day after the Ascension of our Lord, the day after the Assumption of the Blessed Mary and the day after the feast of Saint Michael Archangel, in the chapel of the almshouse in the presence of the warden and confrater and also of all the poor of the same almshouse, all and each of the ordinances and statutes of the almshouse be publicly and distinctly read. And also that they be recited and declared in the vulgar tongue to the poor by the warden or the confrater. And that no poor man or poor woman of the almshouse be absent from the reading and rehearsing of these statutes, save some fitting cause prevent them, under the penalty of losing or having his pension kept back for fifteen days.

Wright adds the following statute in English

The following is found at the end of a translation of the statutes in the possession of the Hospital. The original in Latin I have not seen:

XXXII. And I will that these present Rules, ordinances, Constitutions, and statutes thus penned and duly published by me, T. S., to the praise of God and the glory of the Most Blessed Virgin Mary, His Mother, and of All Saints, and to the augmentation of God's worthiness, and to the prosperity of the living and the utility of the lands, and also to the profit of the almshouse, be effectually and perpetually to endure and to obtain unchangeable.

These, therefore, through the grace of God so soundly ordained, I command a religious obedience therein to the warden, confrater, and to all and every one of the poor living in the same. And I commend unto them the league of unity and the bond of perfect charity. Moreover, in the bowels of Christ I exhort all the poor of both kinds that they have mutual love amongst themselves in Christ

Jesus our Lord, that they pray for the souls of the forenamed. And that they so live and commune that, after this life is ended, they may come to the house of the Kingdom of Heaven, which, by the word of the Lord, is promised to the Poore. Amen. Amen.

Reserving to myself, &c. Dated and sealed at Stamford, Oct 9 14[335] Regis Henrici 7. Witnesses: William Ratcliffe Alderman; Robert Hans, M.E.; Henry Sargeant, parson of St John Baptist; T Hickam, parson of St Peters; and Henry Wycks, vicar of All Hallowes.

---

335 October 14 Henry VII would be 1498 by which date Stokes was dead; the date must be after December 1494 (see preamble to the statutes) and before the death of Stokes, 25 October 1495 - i.e. 9 October 11 Henry VII, 1495. William Radcliffe was Alderman from September 1495 to September 1496, which confirms the date as October 1495. The PRO copy SP46/123/59-60 is correctly dated 9 October 1495.

2. CALENDAR OF DEEDS FROM SIR THOMAS DELALAUND TO THE HOSPITAL 1498

(a copy of these deeds survives in the archives of Browne's Hospital, now in Lincolnshire Archives Office, LAO 7/7/10); some names are missing from this copy. I have added to the LAO list details from my own notes and from the transcripts in Wright Domus Dei *pp 55-60, 493-5*).

1. **Lease**: Sir Thomas Dalelaund to John Taillour warden of the almshouse of William Browne in Stamford and William Hawkins confrater of the same Hospital, of a messuage in North Witham with 40[336] acres [of land] and thirty six acres of meadow situated between a tenement of AB on the east and a tenement of CD on the west, abutting on the highway south and the land of EF on the north, which Sir Thomas Delalaund lately had by feoffment from MB knight [Maurice Berkeley of Wymondham, Leics] and which previously belonged to Richard G [German] of North Witham [husbandman]; for 41 years at a rent of one red rose. Warranty clause. Dated North Witham 28 August 14 Henry VII [1498]

2. **Quitclaim** by Sir Thomas Delalaund to the same warden and confrater of the same properties, 20 December 14 Henry VII [1498]. Warranty clause

3. **Memorandum**: In perpetual memory that Thomas Delalaund knt of North Wytham has given to the almshouse called 'Brouneis halmoshouse in Staunford' lands and tenements in North Witham[337] to the value of 18s p.a. for the perpetual use and benefit of the warden of that house and his confrater and their successors and to increase the allowances to the twelve paupers of either sex dwelling there. The warden is to have 4s p.a. added to the stipend provided by statute paid into his own hands; the confrater is to have 3s p.a. paid by the warden; and the twelve paupers are to have what remains divided between them in addition to their weekly alms given by the warden. For this, the warden and

---

[336] LAO list gives 400 acres of meadow and omits the 36 acres; Wright gives MD instead of MB but the correct reading is MB; another deed in the same collection, LAO, BHS 7/7/9 shows Richard German granting properties in North Witham to Berkeley, August 1494. Berkeley was Delalaund's brother-in-law, see below.

[337] A deed in the Hospital archives, now LAO, BHS 7/7/9, shows the property to have been:

a) a messuage with croft in North Witham between a tenement of Thomas Waltham south and the land called Sculthorp Yinge north; extending from the river Witham east to a path leading to Grantham west; with thirty acres of arable and pasture lying together in North Witham;

b) a cottage lying next to the said messuage with three acres of arable, the first lying on the common pasture and abutting on le Temple, the second lying on the same common land, and the third abutting on Bekforlong west

c) a toft with croft adjacent in North Witham lying between a tenement of Thomas Gowen south and a tenement of Thomas Waltham north, abutting on the water [river Witham] east and on two selions called Pathe Wey west

taken from LAO list

The account book records: to spek with M delaland for hys devocion of gevyng off iij tenements, *fol 22; it cannot be doubted that these are the three properties.*

his confrater and their successors shall make special memorial of the said Sir Thomas Delalaund and Joan his wife while they live among their prayers for the living with the collect '*Deus qui etc*', and among the prayers for the dead the souls of their parents with the collect '*Absolve, quaesumus, Domine etc*'; and after the death of the said Thomas and Joan, their names shall be inscribed among the names of those benefactors who have died on the list (*scedula*) which stands on the altar. And each of the twelve paupers of either sex shall pray for them weekly with the Salutation of the Virgin for the salvation of the said Thomas and Joan his wife while they live and for the souls of their parents, and after their death for the souls of Thomas and Joan as well as the souls of all the benefactors. The obit of T and N[338], father and mother of Thomas, and also the obit of Thomas and Joan once they have departed (*ab hac luce migraverint*) shall be kept annually with *placebo* and *dirige* by the warden and his confrater in the chapel of the almshouse on 16 May each year, and on that day each of the paupers will say for the souls of the said T and M [sic] and T and J a special psalm of the Virgin in addition to the weekly psalm. The said Thomas also asks that his name and that of Joan his consort, whether living or dead, shall be added to the daily prayers, morning and evening, by one of the senior paupers assigned for this purpose. Thomas wills that if any of the said paupers shall omit any part of this, they shall not benefit [from this donation] and will stand accused before God of perjury. Thomas requests that this memorandum shall be written in the book of statutes, not as a statute but as a note [*quoddam mente notandum*] that shall be read to the paupers after the statutes have been read by the warden and confrater annually. All of these requests the warden and confater and twelve paupers and their successors shall implement, of whom the names are John Taillour warden; William Hawkyns confrater; Thomas Brugge, Thomas Andrew, Thomas Normanton, John Burgoyn, Thomas Bentley, William Bakon, Thomas Reynold, William Hesull, dom George Keele clerk, John Cantyng (men) and Matilda Huntley and Elizabeth Huntley (women)

Dated 14 Henry VII [1498-99]

Note: on that day, the said twelve paupers[339] prayed a special psalm of the Virgin Mary for the souls of Thomas, Joan and his parents and afterwards a weekly psalm.

---

338 Wright gives M; but the list below shows his mother's name was Katerine

339 The prayers of the poor were felt to be especially powerful

Wright adds a list which survived in his day, presumably with the book of statutes:
IHS
Ye shall pray for theis salles in especiall with alle other in generall
King Hen' vij quene Elisabeth his wyeffe with all yer childyr
My lord Sir Lyon Welles and dame Jane hys wyeffe with all yer childyr
Robert Watertone and Sisele hys wyeffe with all yer childyr
John Wykes and Alys hys wyeffe with all yer childyr
Sir William Wykes, dame Margaret hys wyeffe with all yer childyr
William Auwsell and hys wyeffe with all yer childyr
Nicholas of Tye [sic] and Jane hys wyeffe with all yer childyr
Sir John Deveries and hys wyeffe with alle yer childyr
Thomas Delalaund and Margaret hys wyeffe with alle yer childyr
My Lord Sir John Welles and hys doghter
Richard Delalaund and Anne hys wyeffe with all yer childyr
Sir Thomas Delalaund, dame Katerene hys wyeffe with all yer childyr
And ye shall pray specially for the salle of Sir Robert Ratclyffe sometyme Porter of Caleys
Sir Robert Dymmok, dame Jane hys wyeffe and alle yer childyr
And ye shall pray in especiall for the lyffes and salles of me Sir Thomas Delalaund and Dame Janie my wyeffe with our fadyrs and modyres whiche wasse Sir Thomas Delalaund, dame Katerine hys wyeffe, Sir Moses [sic] Berkeley, dame Margere hys wyeffe our bredyr and sisteres, with alle our kyn and good benefactores, that we are moste bounde to pray fore as well as they were reherssed be name, and for all Cristen salles, that God wille have praied fore, beyng in the paynes of purgatorie or in any other place where it plesed God to comaunde them. Amen

3. BOARD OF DONATIONS TO THE HOSPITAL

Wright also prints the following: it would seem that the Donation Board had disappeared by the time Wright was writing, 1890, but that a copy of it was kept among the Hospital archives. Since it contains another account of the foundation and endowment of the Hospital, it is included here. Although it appears to be early seventeenth century in origin, it has new material dating from the late fifteenth century.

At the beginning of the last century a tablet hung in the Audit Room, of which a copy is now given, as it contains some interesting particulars, not only of the foundation and property of the Hospital, but also of the Founder and his family.

MEMORIAE SACRUM.
The Fabrick of this House, with the Chappell annext, was built in the Reign of Edward the 4th by Mr. William Browne, of Stamford, in the County of Lincoln, Marchant of the Staple of Calais, in which he maintained several poor people till the time of Richard the 3rd, from whom he procured Letters Patents to impower him or his Executor to make it an Hospital for the maintenance of two secular priests, the one to be called the Warden, the other the Confrater, of the said House, to celebrate divine service in the Chappell aforesaid, and ten poor men and two poor women unmarried, to cohabit in the said house under the government of the said Warden; to that end he settled lands in trust for the maintenance of the said House, but, dying before he could complete his pious undertaking, left it to his Executor, Mr. Thomas Stokk, Canon of York, Chaplain to ye Lord High Chancellor of England (and brother to Mrs. Mar. Browne, relict of the said William Browne) to finish his charitable work ; who (to his immortal praise) performed his trust with great care. The said Thomas Stokk, at his own charge, procured a new Charter from King Henry the Seaventh, to incorporate the said Hospital and settle the lands left by the Founder to the uses aforesaid. The said Mr. Thomas Stokk made many wholesome constitutions for the well government of the said House, amongst which it is ordained that the House shall be called 'The Hospital of William Browne, of Stamford, in the County of Lincoln.' On the 22nd of December, in the year of Grace 1494, and in the 10th year of the reign of King Henry the Seaventh, by vertue of the Letters Patents the said Mr. Thomas Stokk founded this Hospitall, at which time the Chappell was consecrated to divine service by the Bishop of Lincoln, and solemnly dedicated to the Most Glorious Virgin Mary and all Saints.
The said Mr. Thomas Stokk gave five marks to buy vestments for the Chappell, he gave a common seal of silver[340], a silver chalice, several jewells, and many other utensills for the use of the Warden and Confrater.
Mr. William Elmes, son-in-law to the Founder, gave a stock of 20 marks to the House
Mrs. Margaret Browne, aforesaid, gave, in the time of her widowhood, 65 acres of wood for the use of the Hospital

[340] the seal, now missing, bore the arms of William Elmes, not Thomas Stokes

[341]Afterwards, in the reign of King James, certain covetous minded persons, finding some flaw and invalidity in the Foundation, undertook to subvert it and beg the lands to their own private uses; but that noble and charitable prince was so far from complying with their greedy desires, that out of his own motion and bountiful disposition, new founded the said Hospital, and by his royal charter, bearing date the fourth of May, in the eighth year of his reign over England, &c., settled all the lands given by the most bountiful Founder, and granted ...[342] priviledges and immunities, given by his most noble progenitor, King Henry the Seventh; he confirmed all the Constitutions made by Mr. Thomas Stokk, except those which were repugnant to the Laws of the Kingdom; he ordained that the House should now for ever be called the Hospital of William Browne of the Foundation of King James; he also granted that the Corporation should consist of two Chaplains to celebrate divine service, one to be called the Warden, and the other the Confrater, of the said Hospital, and ten poor men and two poor women, to be maintained in the said House, and to live under the government of the said Warden.
[343]The lands given by the Founder for the maintainance of this Hospitall.

In the County of Lincoln:
Swayfield Mannour ... North Witham Mannour ... South Witham, one farm ....Twiford, one farm ... Woolsthorpe, three cottages and three acres arable ... Colsterworth................Wiltsthorpe, one farm ... Castle Bigtham, one farm, five acres pasture ... Gowathorpe [Counthorpe], severall lands and tenements ... Carlby, one farm ... Gunby, several rents.

In Stamford
In St. Peter's parish ... In All Saints' parish, seven ... In St. Clement's parish ... In St. Michael's parish. ... In St. Marie's parish ... In St. Andrew's Parish ... In St. George's parish ... one ... Yard ... and meadow.

In the County of Northampton:
St. Martin's by Stamford, four tenements ... Burleigh, severall lands ... Worthorpe, four cottages ... Easton, three farms, two cottages ... Barnick, two farms ... Pilsgate ... Walcot, severall lands arable ... Warmington, one farm ... Papley ... lands, arable, and pasture.

In the Counties of Rutland and Leicester:
North Luffenham, one farm ... Sculthorpe, twenty-four acres of pasture ... Stretton, one farm......... ... Stretton Stocking, eighteen acres pasture ... Thistleton, severall lands arable, Seustern, severall chief rents ... Steinby, severall chief rents.

---

[341] there is no evidence if this is a later addition or if the board was written at this time

[342] it is clear that these gaps were illegible on the original

[343] this list is slightly different from the list in Browne's endowment deed and presumably represents changes in the estate between 1488 and 1610

APPENDIX IV: DOCUMENTS FROM THE NATIONAL ARCHIVES RELATING TO THE LAW SUIT BETWEEN THE GILD AND THE HOSPITAL.

All the documents (except the first) are undated, and the sequence is not entirely clear. The case started in the court of Lady Margaret Beaufort at Collyweston but was taken by Christopher Browne into Chancery in May 1506. The warden however took the case to the Court of Requests apparently in parallel with Browne's case.
There may be other documents to be located - these are scattered in the Public Record Office. I am grateful to Dr James Ross, at that time of the Public Records Office, for help with the processes involved.

TNA Early Chancery Proceedings C1/357/15-18

15 Complaint of Christopher Browne Alderman of the Gild of All Saints: *this would seem to be the start of the suit in London after having been determined in the court of Lady Margaret Beaufort at Collyweston*

To the most reverent ffadir yn god Wyllam archebisshope of Caunturbury and Chaunceler of ynglond [William Warham, Chancellor Jan 1504- Dec 1515]

Humbly besecheth yowr gud grace your trew and dayle Oratour Christofer Broun Alderman of the gylde of all hollowez withyn the towne of Staunford yn the Counte of lyncoln and hys bredren of the same gylde: yt wher oon John taillour warden of the almeshowse yn Staunford befor seid borowed and resceyved of oon Wyllam Elmes then alderman of the seid gyld and of hys bredren by the hands of oon s' henr' wykes then vicar of all hallowes yn staunford befor seid xx li of lawfull money of ynglond at severall days yn the xij^th^ yer of the reign of kyng henr the vij^th^ [1496-97[344]] to the use and profytt of the seid almeshowse of the goods and money perteignyng to the seid gylde, and the same to be contented and repayed to the seid gylde at the days and fests appoynted by the seid alderman or hys successours by evyn porcions the seid John tayllour then warden promysed and agreed; And aftur the seid John tayllour converted and employed the seid goods and money to the profytt and weyle of the seid almeshowse as ys well knowen and may be duely proved, and then the seid John tayllour resigned and gaffe over the seid benefice and almeshowse; by reson wherof oon wyllam Sharpe ys elected and chosen warden of the same, and the same nowe occupieth and kepith, and yitt the same money to recontent or satisfie unto the seid nowe alderman and hys bredren utterly refuseth and denyeth contrar' to the law and gud conscien. And forsoe moche as the seid alderman and hys bredren are not a body pollytyke and Incorporate able to sue and to be sued by ordur of the comen lawe, yowr seid oratours are remydyles and yn peryll of losse of ther seid money without yowr grace and favour heryn to

[344] John Coton was warden from Michaelmas 1496 to January 1497; John Taylor was warden from January to Michaelmas 1497. Taylor's copied-up accounts record the sum of £20 as received by Coton; the sum is recorded more than once in the book

them be shewyd. In consideracion wher of please hyt yowr grace to graunt a wrytt of sub pena to be directed unto the seid wyllam Sharpe commandyng hym by the same to apper befor the kyng yn hys chauncer' at a certen day and uppon a certen payn by yowr grace to be lymytte to answer to the premyssez and yowr seid oratour shall dayle pray to god for the prosperous preservacion of yowr gud grace.

Pleg de pros' John White de London Gent and
Wills Smyth de eadem Gent
Endorsed: Coram dno B in Canc' sua in Crastino Ascencionis Anno H sept' xxj *[21 Henry VII; 22 May 1506]*

16: Answer of William Sharpe Warden of the Almshouse in Chancery

Thanswere of William Sherpe Warden of the Almeshouse of Staunford to ye bill of Cristofer Broun Alderman of the Gylde of all halowse

The seid Warden seith that the seid bill is not certen ne sufficient to be answered unto And the mater therin conteigned determinable at ye commen lawe and not in this courte Wherto he praieth to be remitted and thannauntage therof to hym sa[v]ed seith by protestacion not knowing that S' John Taillour predecessour to the nowe Warden borowed the seid summe of money in the seid bill specified, but for answere seith if the seid S' John borowed ony suche sume of money it was to his owen use and not to thuse of the seid almeshowse ne ony parte therof converted to thuse of the seid howse as shall playnly appere by bokes of accomptes therof, and the seid nowe warden seith yt the seid S' John Taillour his late predecessour is yet alyve and a man of good substaunce ageyn whome the seid Alderman may have good remedy by the lawe for the seid dette if ony suche were borowed of the vycar of All halowse in matier and fourme as by the seid bill is supposed, but if it had ber of trouthe as it was not that the seid money had bene converted to thuse of the seid almeshowse, yet the seid nowe Warden cowde make no profyte answere to the seid bill (forasmoche as by the seid bill it is supposed that there was parte of the seid somme belongyng to the seid Gylde *del*) the certente Wherof noo thing apperith withoute that yt the seid nowe Warden denyeth to do ony thing contrary to the lawe or good conscience All whiche maters the seid William is redy to prove and make good As this .courte wyll awarde and prayeth to be dismissed out of this court for his wrongfull vexacion and trouble susteyned in this behalfe

17 Replication of Christopher Browne in Chancery

The Replicacion of Christofor Broune Alderman of the Gilde of all hallowes to thaunsewere of William Sharpe warden of thalmeshous of Stanforth
The said Christofor saith and averyth in every thyng as he hath said in his bill of compleynt and that his said bill is sufficient and certen Wher unto the said

warden ought to make aunsewer and the mater therin conteyned is determinable in this court of Chauncery. And furthermore saith that the said John Taillour warden of the said almeshous borowed of the said William Elmes then Alderman of the said Gild and of his Brethren the som of xx li of the goods of the said Gilde Which goods was converted and imployed by the said John Taillour then warden [to thuse] of the said Almeshous as by the said bill of compleynt is alleged, so that the said Christofor Broune myght have his remedie ayemst the said now warden of the said almeshous and not ayemst the said John Taillour without that that the said John Taillour borowed the said som of xx li unto his owne use onely and not to the use of his said house as by the said bill is specified

18 Rejoinder of William Sharpe Warden in Chancery

The rejoindre of William Sharpe Warden of the Almeshowse of Staunford to the replicacion of Cristofer broun Alderman of the gylde of alhalowes

The seid Wardeyn seith and averith in every thing as he hathe seid in his seid answer, withoute that yt the seid xx li was borowed of the seid Elmes in the seid replicacion specified, or converted imployed to thuse of the seid almeshowse by S' John Tayllour sumtyme Warden of the same, In maner and fourme as by the seid bill is supposed. All whyche maters the seid nowe Warden is redy to prove and make good as this Court wyll award; and praeth as he hath praied

****

TNA Court Requests REQ 2/4/216

The Warden appeals to the Court of Requests against Christopher Browne and the Gild: *the date of this is not known but it appears to be November 1506.*

To the king our soverain lord
Mekely sheweth unto your Excellent highnes your dailly Oratours and contynuell bedmen the Warden and almesmen of ys almshouse of Stawnford within your Countie of lincoln; That wher as the predecessours of your said bedmen peasibly enioyede the said Almeshous with all maner buyldings and other dueties thereunto belonging without any title or claime making of any person to the contrary. Soo it is nowe moost gracious souverain lord that oon Christofre Browne merchaunt of your Countie of Rutland pretendeth title unto the hall (ch *del*) kechyn and pantre of your said Almeshouse for so moche as he is Aldreman of the gild of Alhalowes in Stawnford forsaid contrary to the statuts and deds of your said house. And morover the said Christofre hath put your said besechers to great coosts and chargs as for sut making for the same with the counsaill of your derest lady and moder the countesse of Richemount and Derby by whom the said Christofre was commaunded noo further to entromedle with the said houses, that not with standing he of his further malicious mynde hath sued your said besechers in your comen place for the somme of xx [ti] li whiche was geven unto the predecessour of your said besechers by oon William Elmes gent

towards the mayntenyng and upholding of your said house, and to bee prayed for within the same. And over this the said Christofre demaundeth of your said besechers a certain .. chief Rent of the somme of l s out of the manour of Swayfeld belonging unto your said bedmen Whiche your said Oratours aught not to paye unto hym, as it is evidently knowen both by the countreye ther as also by certain their deds; yit he herewith not satisfiede dailly sueth your said besechers to their expresse wronge and uttre undoing forever oonles your grace moevede with petee be unto theym shewede in this behalf. Wherfor it mayt please your highnesse the premisses tendrely considered and forasmoch as your grace is founder of the same house to see suche ordre and direccion to be had in the said matiers soo as your said besechers have noo cause reasonable to poursue unto your grace for their further remedye in this behalf. And theye shall contynuelly bee your true bedmen during their liffes and specially praye to god for the preservacion of your moost noble and Royall estate long to endure

TNA Court of Requests REQ 2/5/93

Christopher Browne makes a rejoinder: *Browne is replying, not to Sharpe's 'Answer' but to a 'Replicacion'.*

The Reioynder of Christofore Broune to the Replicacion of the warden of thalmeshous of Stanforth

The said Christofor saith and averyth in every thyng as he hath said and averyed in his said aunswer and for as mych as the said warden hath confessed by his said Replicacion that his said predecessour had and borowed the said xx li of money of the said William Elmes towards the charge of the said Almeshous the said Alderman prayth that the said money may be contented and repaid to the Christofore, and over that saith that the said William Broune maid his last will that thaldermen of the said Gilde and ther successour shuld have occupie use and enioye the said hall buttry pantry and kechyn at their pleasur and also that the said warden hylde of the said Christofor by l s a yere as of his maner of Corby of which Rent the said Christofor and they whos astate he hath in the said maner have ben seased by thands of the said warden and his predecessour as by thaunswer of the said Christofor is alleaged, Which he is redy to prove without that that the said William Broune upon the foundacion of the said almeshous gave the said hall buttry pantry and kechyn with all other bildyngs the called Clement now called Brounes Almeshous to the predecessours of the said now warden and to his successours as by the said Replicacion is alleaged and without that that the said Aldermen and their bredren have occupied the said hall buttry pantry and kechyn onely by the sufferaunce of the said Warden and his predecessour but hath occupied the same as in their owne title and right as he hath alleaged.

According to the Account Book, an award was made by the King's Council in December 1506, fol 61.

****

TNA Court of Requests REQ 2/8/114a)
Christopher Browne appeals to the Court of Requests alleging that the Warden has not fulfilled the terms of the Chancery decree; apparently mid-1507.

To the king our soveraigne
Piteously shewith unto your highnes youre Daily Oratour and true liege man Christofer Browne of Staunford Squier that Where alle maters of contraversie bitwene hym and oon sir william Sharpp warden of the Almeshous of Staunford aforsaid were decreed by your moost honorable counseill M doctour Symeon Dean of your most honorabill chappell, M doctour Hatton[345] and M Richard Sutton, the forsaid sir William Sharpe the said decre in no wise will obey and perfourme, Wherfore the said Christofer Browne humbly besechith your highnes to graunt a prevy seall to be directed to the said s William Sharpp commaunding hym by the same to appiere the next terme before your said counsaill there to shew why he shuld not perfourme the decre aforsaid

TNA Court of Requests REQ 2/8/114b
William Sharpe the Warden responds to Christopher Browne's charges

The aunswer of William Sharpe Warden of the almeshows of Stamford to the bill of compleint of Christofer Brown

The same Warden seith that he hath ben all tymes redie and yitt is to performe the commandement and decre of the kyngs most honorable Counceill after the verre true meanyng and entent of the same supposyng that hitt Was never entended by them that the seid Warden ne his successours shuld in eny Wise be charged ne chargeable with the kepyng of eny of the godes of the seid Gild wich mater he referreth to reporte of the seid honorable counceill and also he seith that the seid Christofer deceyveth and wold not delyver to the seid Warden an endenture Wherby he before thys tyme charged the same Warden for the payment of xx^{ti} li notwithstandyng that he hath sett suyrty to the seid Christofer to content and pay the seid some accordyng to the seid decre wich endenture the seid Christofer withholdeth to thentent that he by ..ean therof hereafter myght eftsones troble and charge the same Warden and his successours contrary to (troub *del*) trowth reason and conscience Wherof he praith delyveraunce and the seid Warden on his parte will doo att all tymes as he shalbe commanded by the seid councell as ferr as reason shall requyre and prayeth to be dysmyssed.

[345] probably the Dr Hatfield to whom Sharpe gave wine, fol 59v

APPENDIX V: VISITS TO LONDON BY WILLIAM SHARPE 1506-7

FIRST VISIT TO LONDON 1506 (fol 57v - 61v)

	w/b 1 Nov[346]	travel[347]	meetings noted[348]
Sunday			
Monday			
Tuesday	to Hoggerston[349] and Alconbury		
Wednesday	Baldock Hatfield		
Thursday	London		
Friday	Greenwich	boatmen	
Saturday	Westminster		Archer
	w/b 8 Nov		
Sunday	Greenwich	ferry	
Monday	Greenwich overnight		
Tuesday			
Wednesday	fasting[350]		[Martinmas]
Thursday	Greenwich	ferry	
Friday	Westminster	ferry	
Saturday	Wansbridge[351] overnight	[horse]	
	w/b 15 Nov		
Sunday	[Wansbridge]		dean's servant
Monday			Sir John Hussey
Tuesday	London		
Wednesday	fasting		
Thursday	Westminster		M Bigot
Friday	Westminster	boatmen	
Saturday	Greenwich	ferry	

346 The warden says he left Stamford on Tuesday in All Hallows (1 November) - i.e. 3 November. The places listed are all named in his accounts except for those in square brackets

347 Visits to Greenwich and Westminster by ferry always have a return journey to London which have been omitted here. When no ferry is mentioned, there are sometimes indications that he travelled by horse (e.g. payments for 'horsemeat')

348 These are named individuals when fees, wine or other provision has been given to them; there must have been other meetings

349 Hoggerston is unidentified, but probably Oakington, Cambs, which was an Elmes' manor and sometimes written as Hokyngton

350 On Wednesdays, even when he has travel, he pays for his man's meals but for himself nothing or just a bite in the evening

351 I have been unable to identify Wansbridge; it may be related to the river Wandle south of London. Duncan MacAndrew points out that Bleau's map of Surrey 1648 shows only one bridge on the Wandle with Merton Priory on the west and Tooting Graveney on the east bank.

	w/b 22 Nov		
Sunday			M Breknall
Monday	Richmond overnight	ferry	dean of King's Chapel
Tuesday	back to London	ferry	
Wednesday	fasting		
Thursday	Greenwich	ferry	
Friday			
Saturday			
	w/b 29 Nov		
Sunday			
Monday	[Roger Sharpe sent back to Stamford]		
Tuesday	Greenwich	ferry	dean's servant; Sir John Digby; M Bigot[352]
Wednesday			Richard Sutton; Dr Hatfield
Thursday	Greenwich	ferry	Sir John Hussey
Friday			
Saturday	Westminster	ferry	
	w/b 6 Dec		
Sunday	[Roger Sharpe returns from Stamford]		[St Nicholas]
Monday	Greenwich	ferry	
Tuesday	Westminster	ferry	Archer
Wednesday	Greenwich	ferry	
Thursday	Greenwich	ferry	
Friday	Westminster	ferry	Archer
Saturday	Westminster	ferry	M Bigot's clerk
	w/b/ 13 Dec		
Sunday			
Monday	Greenwich	ferry	
Tuesday	Greenwich	ferry	
Wednesday	Greenwich	ferry	
Thursday	Greenwich	ferry	
Friday	Westminster	ferry	decree of council
Saturday	Hatfield at night		
	w/b 20 Dec		
Sunday	Baldock, Biggleswade , St Ives at night		
Monday	Stilton, Stamford		

[352] almost certainly Pygot

Tuesday			
Wednesday			
Thursday			
Friday			
Saturday			

SECOND VISIT TO LONDON 1507 (fol 62-64)

	w/b 20 June?[353]		
Sunday			
Monday			
Tuesday	Huntingdon, Royston overnight		
Wednesday	Ware, Waltham, London		
Thursday	Greenwich	ferry	
Friday	Westminster	ferry	clerk of signet; entry; copy of decree; dean of king's chapel; M Pigot and M Pigot's servant for writing my answer to the [privy] seal/bill[354] of complaint
Saturday	Richmond overnight	ferry	Sir John Hussey's servant
	w/b 27 June?		
Sunday	Richmond		
Monday	return to London	ferry	
Tuesday	Greenwich	ferry	
Wednesday	Westminster	ferry	my servant sees the Watch
Thursday			Archer
Friday	Greenwich	ferry	
Saturday	Westminster; to Hatfield overnight	ferry	dismissed by king's council and Archer admitted as attorney; clerk of the council;
	w/b 4 July?		
Sunday	Baldock, St Ives overnight		
Monday	Stilton, Peterborough overnight		
Tuesday	Stamford		

353 this date is not certain; it could be a week later. The warden says it took place at 'midsummer'

354 see note to folio 62v

APPENDIX VI: THE DATE OF THE ACCOUNT BOOK

I date the start of this account book to late November/early December 1506. The argument relates to the dispute over the sum of £20 claimed by the gild from the Hospital.

In May 1506, Christopher Browne tabled his bill of complaint concerning the £20 in the chancery and Sharpe (warden) was summoned to London. I am sure that Sharpe consulted John Taylor, his predecessor, before he left; after all Browne had been pursuing the Hospital in the court of Lady Margaret Beaufort for some years. Sharpe left Stamford on 3 November and arrived in London on 5 November. His answer to Christopher's claim was all over the place - that no money had been given; that if it had, it had been given by William Elmes personally and not the gild; that it had been given to Taylor who should answer for it; that it was for Taylor's personal use and not for the Hospital, so it did not implicate Sharpe, etc. Anything but a loan from the gild.

At the same time or shortly after, Sharpe's countersuit in the Court of Requests claimed (among other things) that Browne was troubling the Hospital with an unjustified claim for £20 which Sharpe said had been given by Elmes personally to the Hospital for prayers. We do not have Browne's 'answer' in the Court of Requests, nor Sharpe's replication, but it is clear from Browne's rejoinder that Sharpe changed his claim in his replication and now "*confessed by his said Replicacion that his said predecessour had and borowed the said xx li of money of the said William Elmes*". What made Sharpe change his plea so abruptly?

The only thing I can see is that on 30 November, Sharpe sent his man (Roger Sharpe) back to Stamford. Roger left on Monday and returned by Sunday 6 December. A journey of three days each way (and he may have made a hasty journey in a shorter period) would give him a full day in Stamford. The only purpose for such a journey I can think of was to collect 'the book of accounts' which Sharpe had said in chancery would prove his point: "*as shall playnly appere by bokes of accomptes therof*".

Taylor back in Stamford had (I think) already been at work compiling the *'bokes of accomptes'*. He acquired the quires and wrote the tendentious Narrative, clearly intended to be read in court (note the phrase 'in the second place'). That he was aware that the heart of the issue was the chancery plea for £20 is shown by the fact that the first entry he made, before listing Coton's first account, was to state (fol 2):

Recept'

In primis memorandum that my predecessor forsayd syr John Coton Receyvd off Mastyr Wyllam Elmes forsayd patron off thys almoshows ffor a stoor or a stok afor'hand' to hafe fo to pay in tyme off neede as hytt aperyth in the booke off payments wrytyng in the begynnyng with the hand off the seyd S' John Coton for thys present yer xx li

Summa Recept thys yer bysyde the Rent xx li

He is clearly stating that he (Taylor) did not receive this sum, but that Coton received it from Elmes for the use of the Hospital.

He then copied up all the accounts of Coton and himself from 1495 to 1504. To make sure the document stood up in court, every page of the annual accounts was audited and signed by Henry Wykes vicar of All Saints and patron of the Hospital. But as he copied up the later accounts, he added to the account for October 1503 (very nearly at the end of his copying) an admission that the sum had been a loan from the gild (fol 41):

Item ther was borod off all halo gylde afortyme *xx li.*

This change of statement could not have been written during the very first pleas in both courts, because at that time he and Sharpe were still claiming the money was a gift from Elmes.

This sequence would account for the fact that the first three accounts of William Sharpe (away in London) are missing. There is one other indication that this reconstruction is sound. Taylor has added on a scrap of paper a note about the distraint which Christopher Browne had taken in Swayfield which does not appear in any of the annual accounts - this is now fastened in at folio 38b. It seems clear that Taylor, hearing the news from Roger Sharpe of how the pleadings were going, added this note on a slip of paper to inform the court of the ongoing nature of this second area of dispute. Its writing suggests it was written in haste.

Sharpe then received the book of accounts in London and saw that Taylor had conceded the point and so he changed his plea in his replication in the Court of Requests. I cannot see these accounts and statements being made after 18 December when the king's council issued the decree saying the money should be repaid to the gild, nor before Roger Sharpe had reported to Taylor from London.

I do not think the book of accounts was tabled in court; experience elsewhere suggests that if it had been, it would have been retained either by chancery or in the Court of Requests.

It therefore seems most likely that the first 53 folios were written by Taylor during the month of November or first week of December 1506 while Sharpe was in London. It could not have been earlier, for Sharpe would have taken it with him; it could not have been written in this form after 18 December 1506. Sharpe kept the book; when he returned to Stamford, he did not copy up his earlier accounts but at the end of the year 1506-7 as he was leaving the Hospital, he wrote up his final year's accounts including the costs of his two journeys to London, and subsequent wardens continued to use the book until 1518.

GLOSSARY

This glossary has been compiled jointly by Alan Rogers and Ann Matthews of the Stamford Survey Group. We have drawn on the help of many others, especially Nat Alcock, Chris Currie, Vanessa Doe, David Dymond, Stephen Hart, John Hartley and Nick Hill. Among the sources we have used are

L F Salzman, Building in England down to 1540, *Clarendon 1952; David Yaxley,* A Researcher's Glossary *Larks Press, Norfolk, 2003;* Book of Morton *Northants Record Society 16, 1954; Eric Gee,* A Glossary of Building Terms *Frome 1984; Stephen Alsford,* Medieval English Towns - Glossary *1998;*

Lincolnshire glossary - http.www.cantab.net/users/michael.behrend/repubs/good.glossary/pages/words.html; *Fen-edge encounters* - http://dawnpiper.wordpress.com/land-words; *Osborn: Notes of a lecture entitled 'Collyweston and its Trade', given in 1976 by Bob Osborn of Collyweston, a Master Slater and quarry owner (we have been unable to find if there is any copyright holder of these notes);* Building Accounts of Tattershall Castle 1434-1472, *Lincoln Record Society vol 55.*

We have included a folio number only when there is a special mention of the word.

ı bowth		about
ı for, aforne		before
ı geyn		again
ı geyn		against
ı gret		by agreement, contract
ı lowy(d)		allowed
ı naker		an acre
ı neynd		an end
ı nold		an old
ı Noyffin	76	*probably* an oven
ı peyr		appear
ı yis syd		at this side of
ıbatements		deductions
ıckers, akyrs		acres
ıid (king's)		an occasional imposition made by the king for specific purposes
ıll halos		All Saints (parish, church, gild)
ılloyd		allowed
ılmysse		alms[house]
ılyas capias	85v	writ to seize possessions pending trial
ımeld [jewelry]	61v	*perhaps* enamelled
ın noon		now, currently, at present
Aº R' R'		*anno regni regis*; in the year of the reign of king [Henry]

asch, aschese, aschys, ascys, assys, asse		ash tree(s)
assize, rents of assize		customary manorial dues from tenants as distinct from 'farms' (agreed rents)
assuyng		suing
asynyd		assigned [a court decision]
awght		owed
awtar		altar
ayl		ale
balks	44	baulks, tie beams
balys		bailiffs
bands, door bands of iron; window bands	10v	metal bands reinforcing doors; maybe hinges on metal plates
bargyn		contract
baros		(wheel)barrows
baryn		barn
basterd stone	118v	a hard stone broken up[355]
baston, bastyn roppe		rope made of bast fibre, Salzman
batyng		deducting
be		by
bedgat		retiring [to bed]
bench [made by masons]		either long seating or work top
betyng		beating [plaster]
betyng		'baiting', i.e. eating a meal
bey		bay [of building like a barn]
beyldyd		builded, built
blind chimney		*presumably* disused/blocked chimney
bol(l), bollys		bowl(s)
bonche [of laths etc]		bunch
bords		boards of various sizes and dimensions
born, bornyd		burn, burned [lime, plaster] - *see* bren
borosokn		duty of attending court of soke of Peterborough
boschell [of peas]		bushel
bot		but, only
botras		buttress
bowht, bohte, boyhte, bowghyt, bowte, boyghte, boyht		bought
bowndyng [our land]	53v	*either* hedging our land *or* measuring our land
boyr - dwelled at ye boyr in Stretton	95v	*presumably a placename in Stretton ?* bower?

[355] "There is a layer of blue rag, a very hard stone known in the trade as bastard, and the only use for that is to break it up and build pillars to hold up the ceiling". (Osborn). This, I think, is the meaning here rather than the softer brown ironstone used widely for building in north Northamptonshire which is also known as bastard stone (D S Sutherland, *Northamptonshire Stone* Dovecote Press, 2003, pp 46-49) since it only appears once in these accounts and in a small quantity. See also Salzman 233 for bastard slate.

boythe		both
brasys; brase loggys	44	braces (timber); brace spars
bredcroft, bradcroft		Bradcroft, small settlement forming western suburb of Stamford lying in Rutland [buildings]
bren, brent		burn, burned
breyg		bridge
brode ston	52	*while many equate this with* freestone, Salzman 233 suggests large slates used for wall infilling instead of wattle and plaster
brykk		brick
bwlkes		*see* balks
bye		buy
bynwark		parish and church of St Mary Bynwark in western corner of town
calyd		called
carwar		carver
caryeg		carriage
catt of iron		*probably* gad of iron, weight Salzman 287; Tattershall 42
cayle	5	*here most likely* stone used for flooring, *see* Osborn[356]
chales		chalice
chef		chief rent
cheryf		sheriff
cherys		cherries
cheyneys		chains
chief rent		annual payment to landlord, ground rent
chyrch revys		churchwardens
clasp, claspe [of iron] for gate	44v	iron bracket [to mend ladder rung]; bracket for gate; door fastening
cleymowntt		Claymont, market place of Stamford, now Broad Street
clossys, clossis		closes, enclosed plots
clowt nayle		clout nails, flat-headed
coffer		chest
collys		coals
cope		copy; *also* coping stone
copwll copull		pair of rafters
corby; two corbys for lead	5	*unidentified*
corn schawmbyr		*either* corn chamber *or* corner chamber
corrections		fines on bedesmen for infringement of Hospital rules
cottears, cotyard		cottagers
countyng hows		store room for accounts; office
couples		*see* cowples

356 "There's only roughly about ten inches of soil, and then you get four or five feet of crash or kale as we call it ... in the olden days it was used for roadmaking" (Osborn). The *Lincolnshire glossary* says: "keal, kale: pieces of stone in very small masses, and uncertain and irregular shape; ... "Whether they are pieces or shreds of the limestone, of the ragg, or of our ordinary sandstone, they have all the name of *keale*"; in some parts of the county it is more especially applied to the scalings or fragments of the sandstone, as *craach*, or *crash*, is to the limestone; cf. Anglo-Saxon *scylan*, French *chaille*, 'a rocky earth'".

cowchyng	13, 34v	bedding down; stacking, storing
cownand, covande		covenanted, agreed, contracted with
cownte		account
cowple sparrs, cowpwlls	44	pair of rafters
coyn of long wall, coynys [of shop windows]	52, 39v	? quoins
crahcs	73	cracche, crib or rack for animal fodder, Yaxley
crest		ridge tile of stone or sometimes clay[357]
cross house in the yard	28v	*uncertain; it may be* a building at back of yard crossing between the two wings
crowper [saddle]		crupper [harness]
croys	82	*perhaps* crows
crystonmes		christmas
cumin		spice
cuthbert court		court of St Leonard's priory, Stamford
cycientes	62	[legal] sessions
dabyng		plastering, rendering - *see* dawbyng
daleland		Delalaund
darnys, dornys [pair of door durns]; dornis, dornys, dwrnes for a barn door	51v	door posts, frames
dawbyng		plastering, rendering, laying earth for the floor, *or* whitewashing - *both meanings appear in these accounts*
dells		dwells
denerse		dinners
det		debt
dewete		duty
dey		day
deyd		did
di', di[m]		half
dofcote, dowfhows, dowfhos, duffcot, dwff cott, dwfcote		dovecote
doon, doyne		done
dornis		*see* darnys
dorr, dur, dwr		door
dos'		dozen
draw in spars; drawyng a balk, timbers, floor joists;		set in place, insert? laying floor timbers? assembling?
draw, draw thatch, draw in thatch, drawer of thatch	50	combing to make straws parallel, preparing straw for thatching, Salzman 224; Morton

357 "a stone ridging ... that used to come from Weldon, ... and it was sawn, another job that used to be done in the wintertime. And also they used to make clay ridge tiles at Peterborough, Whittlesea, even at Stamford, which more or less matched the colour of the slating" (Osborn).

drawgt (sege)	4v	privy [probably inside room]
drawyng in [a house]; drawyng ye hows, dray		constructing a building or a room (Morton)
drawys (expenses this year draws £...), **drays**		amounts to
dray, drayng,	82v	*see* draw
drye ston wall	32v	dry stone wall
dryve, dryff [a floor]		? laying a floor, probably of earth
dur bands		Salzman 208 *equates these with* 'vertivals' or plate hinges, *but I think they occur too frequently for this to be true every time; they may be* metal bands to reinforce wooden doors; *see* bands
durnys		*see* darnys
dwtey		duty
dyghtyng, dythtyng, dyhttyng	61v	preparing [food], washing, cleaning [clothes], grooming [horse]
dyryge		memorial service for the dead, requiem; book of the service
dystreyne		seizure of cattle or goods in recompense for non-payment of rent or other charge; *see* stresse
edyryng [felling of stakes and edyryng]	17v	? ordering, i.e. stacking?
end		end of a wall, *perhaps sometimes* a gable end
enke	56v	ink
entertes [making of an]		tiebeam, Salzman 212
entrese		*perhaps* entry [into court, entering a plea]
erabyll		arable
ernyst, ernese		initial or down payment for contract
erthe, yorthe		earth, mainly clay, used for flooring, Salzman 147
esseyng		essoining
essoin, essoyn		excuse for absence or other fault in court
est stone - eft stone	118	*unknown*
evyn		evening
evys, evys boord, evys slates		eaves, eaves boards, eaves slates
eyd(e)		aid
eynd		end
eyrn, eyryn		iron
eys, eywys		eaves
falo		fallow
fardest, farryst, ferryst		furthest [the furthest house]
fawgts, fawyt		faults
feld		field
fen thak		reeds for thatching
fen, feyn		fain; must
ferm		an agreed rent for leases, usually an annual charge for a period of years and then re-negotiated; frequently with substantial entry payment and smaller annual payment
ferm, feyrm		farmstead

fewyng a gwtter, ffeyng, fewyng [a privy, a mess]		cleaning, clearing up
fagoattys		faggots for fuel
falloys		fallows
feiffers		feoffees, trustees
fled [a chamber that was fled]	88v	*apparently* falling down *or* fallen
florth, floryht		floor
foder, foodyr		load or weight of lead, Salzman 122
folowehte		follows
fornas		furnace, oven, kiln
frank post		*uncertain*
frett of ladder	44v	ladder rung
fro		from
fur, furryng up gables		nailing extra pieces of timber to make surfaces even or for protection, Salzman 305; Yaxley
fyllyng, bem fyllyng bytwene the trasyngs	19, 39v	filling in between the [floor or wall] beams or joists with lath and plaster, wattling (and plaster), stone or occasionally brick
gaderyng, gederyng, gethurryng		gathering, collection [of rents]
game - making game a wall	100v	repairing?
garner		corn store
garrett gate	47v	*perhaps* entry with tower, Yaxley
gawme for windows **geamaws pair of; geawmbb [in stone]; geanows** pair of, for the shop windows	68, 44, 114; 39	? jambs or hinges, Yaxley
geyl spenc	98	*this may be* 'gild larder/pantry' ('spence' is a larder, Salzman 484) *or it may be* 'gild expenses'
geyt		get
golf, golve		*see* gowel
goter, gwter		gutter
goth with		goeth, goes with, has been joined to
gowel, govel,		gable[358]
gowyll, golve		gavel, rent payment
granse - bran and granse for the horse		grains
grese, gresyng, greys		steps, stairs
gret leet		king's leet court in Stamford
gret water		flood
grete		agreement, contract work
greyte yaat		great gate

[358] The 'govel, golve' in Easton payable to the gildhouse of Our Lady may be either an annual customary rent due to the gild of St Mary in Easton or a payment due to the connection of the tenant's house to the gable of the gildhouse - it is not possible to determine which this is.

ȝrondsell, growndsole		groundsill; can be foundation course of stone or timber
ȝrynd, grynde of iron [of the barn door]	6v, 18, 39v	?door fitting?
ȝwd		good
ȝwttar		gutter
ȝy hows in the yard	47	*perhaps* privy
ȝy(e)		Guy
ȝyffyng		giving
ȝyle of corpus Xti		gild of corpus christi
ȝyle, gyll, gild howse		*either* house used by gild for meetings *or* house which belonged to and paid rent to a gild [gild of St Mary in Easton; or house next to All Saints vicarage which was used by or paid rent to the gild of All Saints, Stamford]
ȝymmos, gymmoys, gymms - pair of		*probably* hinges Yaxley; *but see* geamaws *above*
ıach		hatch
ıaf		have
ıaf		half
ıal		hall
ıaloyng, halow		hallowing, consecrating
ıalylofe, haly lof		payment (of 1d, 2d or 3d) to the parish due on different dates from some properties (by rota) in both rural and urban contexts, presumably for exemption on this occasion from providing the parish holy loaf; normally paid by the tenant. See E. Duffy, *Stripping of the Altars* pp 125-7.
ıart lath		laths from inner wood
ıeche, heggs		hedge, hedges
ıecter?		hectare?
ıelmys		Elmes
ıeng lok [for a door], henglok	13v, 44	*probably* padlock (Yaxley)
ıengels, henghelis [usually with hooks]	12v	*most likely* hinges (simple pin hinge); *unlikely here to be* hangells, hooks which form part of the equipment of an open fire for cooking (Yaxley)
ıenges		hinges
ıengyng [hengyng the house]	89	*uncertain; may be related to* hinges; *or* hanging windows and doors etc
ıenkylls		*probably* hengels
ıent nown		before noon?
ıer		their
ıerdylls, hyrdels		hurdles
ıespys		hasps
ıey, hey hows		hay, hay barn
ıeyd plac		manor house
ıeyng		hang
ıeyr		here, her, their
ıogstyes		pigstyes
ıole, holl		whole
ıolys		holes

ıoopyng of soo, hopyng, hoopyng of bowls		*probably* providing iron hoops around the bowls or buckets
ıoopys off yrn		iron hoops
ıoose, hws, hos, hose, howsse, howsys		house, houses - *frequently used to mean* a room in a house, a chamber; *but* 'hus' *can also mean* a door, Salzman
ıord bred		fodder
ıotts		oats
ıowk		hook [for door], latch
ıowm		home
ıowte		owed
ıoyle, hollyd, holly		whole, wholly
ıus, hws		us; *see* hoose
ıwe		Hugh
ıwks		hooks
ıye		high
ıyeryng, hyard		hiring [horses, guide, messenger]; hired [land]
ıyllyng		covering (books) , roofing (buildings)
ıyr		here
ıyr		hire
ıyt		it
lhs est amor meus		Jesus is my devotion
nsett house	24	*described by Yaxley as a puzzling term, its meaning here is uncertain, perhaps* an interior room (*see* hoose) or farm building for animals
agge [of straw]	112v	small cart-load, OED
ame [mendyng a jame] **jeawmys -** carpenters making divers jeawmys and undersetting the walls	81v	? jamb? *but see* jeamys, geamaws
ealmys - paid a mason to mend	49	*perhaps* hinges set in stone, the iron pintle hinges set into masonry jambs to receive iron strap hinges
eamys of the hall **eamaws for a door;** **eawnys, jemos**	11, 40v 45 23v, 74	?hinges Yaxley (gemel)
oyst tree	114	joist
ĸaryag		carriage
ĸebull, bord kebull, kebbyll, kebwl	44	*almost certainly* 'couple'
ĸechyn		kitchen
ĸerver		carver
ĸing's eyd		tax at will of king, *see* aid
ĸnafe nykkol - Item for to help to tak down ye sclats to a knafe nykkol iijd	94	*is it possible that* 'knafe nykkol' *is a personal name? Rafe Nyccol?*
ĸoyns of freestone, hewyng of	13v	hewing quoins
ĸybulls [wooden]	31v	*probably* couples [q.v.]
ĸydds		faggots of wood for fuel

kyllyng, kylyn		kiln *[probably for malt]*
kyngs xv	18	king's tax of one fifteenth; *in towns like Stamford, paid at one tenth of rateable value but still called a fifteenth*
kynkys		king's
ade		lady
adys rent		*see* gyle, gild house *above*
app of iron	39	*perhaps* a measure of iron; *or is it possible that this is* a flap of iron to cover a keyhole? Salzman 302
aryfax		*perhaps* caryfax? *the placename is otherwise unknown in Stamford*
aterynd		latter end
aton		bell metal used from memorial brasses
atts		laths
eads, leds		lead framing in window glass in chapel
eche		doctor
eddyr		ladder
edyng [of stone, mortar etc]		carting [stone, mortar etc]
egbys	52	leghys?
eghys, ledghys, leyg, legths, legyhys, legys to a door, leyge, legge	23, 44, 33v	ledges [e.g. window ledges], square-sectioned braces on doors, windows etc; a term still used for the horizontal board to which the vertical boards are nailed in a boarded door
eyd		lead *for roofing or gutters*
eyd to		joined with
eyng		laying
eyn'hte	82v	*probably here* length
eytt		leet court
oggs		sawn timber; posts and spars[359] etc
ongs, longyn		belongs, belonging
ovar, lower	31v	louvre; wooden slatted tower in roof as a smoke vent
oyd, loydyd		loads
ycens		licence
yflode		*the best translation is* 'estate'
yg over		lie over
yttar	32, 52	*perhaps* litter, rubbish
naad		made
naner		manor
nanteltre	32, 52v	mantelpiece above fireplace
narbuler		metal engraver
naschfatt	46v	mash vat - large wooden tub containing the mash for brewing - Yaxley
nasyn		mason
nawnger		manger
nedo		meadow
nercyments		fines in court

[359] These are clearly timbers here rather than the 'logs' of stone ('pillars') which Osborn refers to in Collyweston

nersyed		amerced, fined in court
net, mete, meyte		meat, food
neyt, met, mett	10v	measure, measured
nichelys, myhel, myhelemes		michael, Michaelmas
no, moo		more
noren		morn[ing]
noyng		mowing [hay]
nwdwall		mud wall
nwst		must
nydow		meadow
nyllyn, mylner howse		mill, mill house, miller
ıell, neylys,		nails
ıete gate [in field]	49v	?cattle gate, cattle grid?
ıett - for mending a nett [?mett?] [in items in store]	125v	*uncertain reading and meaning*
ıett - long nett hows	52	?cattle shed?
ıohte ar		are not there
ıonnys		nuns
ıoo		no
ıoo		now
ıoyffyn		*probably* an oven
ıyht		night
ɔder		other
ɔn hole yeyre		one whole year
ɔn, oon		one
ɔnys		once
ɔppynynyg		opening
ɔr		ere, before
ɔs		as
ɔstyy wall - in the Angel Inn	11	*unknown; it may be the wall of the hostellry*
ɔwen		oven
ɔwen		own
ɔwer		over
ɔwt		ought, out
ɔyer		other
ɔyn		own
ɔak thred		pack thread for thatching
ɔale		fence
ɔalle [carpenter mends a palle]	118	*probably* fence or stake
ɔanys in the govel		*perhaps* panels in the gable
ɔar of, pare		pair of, pair
ɔargetting		plaster work to walls and gables, often ornamental
ɔauper		paper
ɔayngtyng		painting

payth, peyth		pays
pec, peec, pese, peys		piece
pekax		pickaxe
pelor logg	44	pillar spar, upright for doors and windows, *or* supporting post
pentter		painter
pentts, pentys, peyntes	94v	penthouse, pentice, lean-to; *can also be* roof over oven, Yaxley
pepur, pepyr, peyper		pepper
pertener, pertenynyys, perteyngs, ye perteneys yerto		appurtenances, belongings; the appurtenances belonging to some properties
pese		piece
pey, peyd		pay, paid
peynter		painter
peyr		pair
peyse		peas (horse fodder]
pingulfeld		pingle : a small enclosure of low shrubs, or underwood, or gorse; a close, small meadow; a small spinney; pingle close : a small meadow, *Lincolnshire glossary*; here, it is a field name in Stamford
plaschers, plaschyng		hedge cutters, hedging; pleaching, interweaving branches to make a solid hedge to retain cattle.
plats [of iron to lay under the great gate]	39v	plates
platts [timber]		wooden plates, timber beam laid horizontally, Yaxley
playsterer		plasterer
plommar, plwmmer		plumber
plot [mending a]	94v	*perhaps* a patch
poll		measure of length
pond		pound
post fest mychael		after Michaelmas
powlys		[St] Pauls
poyntyng, pwentyng		pointing [of stone work]
prentes		apprentice
prests	9v	charges, payments or levies (*for services etc*)
probatur est per me		[this page] is approved/audited by me
prowand(e)		provender, fodder for horses
pryncypal copull	100	principal rafters
pultre merkett	4v	poultry market
pyk of iron	52	*perhaps* pickaxe, pike
pyns, pynns, pynnes		pins, *especially* slate pins
pytt		quarry
quart' wags		quarter's wages
qwer, qweyr		where
qwest, qwert?		jury in court
qweyt	86v	wheat
rakys		rakes [iron]
ramell		rubbish, spoil heap after building

edyng [bornyng, betyng, syftyng, redyng, schotyng the floor]	44v	reeding, laying reeds in floor; [burning, beating, sifting (the plaster), laying reeds and finishing/smoothing the floor]; Morton suggests it could be colouring the floor with red ochre
ekynd		reckoned
ensak	45, 45v	dig up (old stone) for re-use
ent off a syse		rent of assize, chief rent; customary payments from manorial tenants
esewyd		received
ewyng		*perhaps* renewing
eyd		reed for thatch
eyng - for a reyng to ye leyd	100	*Morton suggests* cleaning (reeing) as with corn; *may be* cleaning lead? *or it could here be* 'arraying' the lead, laying it out, flattening it
eysed		raised
igg, rygg (verb), 'earth and mortar to rygg withall'	12v, 18v, 48v, 49	b) rigg as a verb is always linked with thatching, making the ridges of roofs, a process in which clay and mortar is often used
iggs, ryggs - Crodon Riggs in Swayfield;		a) riggs in Swayfield are no doubt fields, closes, in ridges owned or once owned by someone called Crodon? (*Lincolnshire glossary*); could it be land where turves are cut? Yaxley
od, rode, roode,		rood
oftre, rowftre, rwftre		rooftree
Rokkyng [plastering/rendering and rokkyng]	40, 49	*JSH suggests* raking, combing, *but it may be* inserting stones into the plaster
Rollys		[court] rolls
on a neynd		?run an end?; Yaxley *found* 'run furs', *so this may be* to run furring over an end, i.e. gable
oyd, rode	101	rood [defined as three feet]
oyffe		roof
oys - roys a boun	102	?rows? *unknown*
ygg		*see* riggs
am		same
ap lath		laths from outer sap wood
awer		sawyer
awyn trasyngs	44	sawn joists
chater		slater
chef		chief [rent]
cherefs tern', scheryff geld		annual payment to sheriff for his jurisdiction due from some holdings
chevys		sheaves
chew - paid to schew our lands		?plough, harrow? *or could it be* to measure our lands?
chop bothys		area in Stamford usually named Shobothes
chotyng of lead; schott the floor	17v	*probably* pounding lead before laying it; *also* spreading and watering clay before using it for flooring, Yaxley; *the word survives in* wainscotting *but here refers to flooring*
choyng		shoeing horses
chreddyng of ashes	14v	stripping bark off coppiced ash wands before use in wattling or basket making

sclat, sklatter		slate, slater
sclate pynse		slate pins
scledd	18	horse-drawn sledge for stone
sclottys [for a door]		bolts for doors, Salzman
scole		school
se		see
seage in the high chamber	19v	indoor privy
seam, sem, seem, seyme		packhorse load or cartload (lime, plaster, mortar etc)
seeg, seyge, sege	19	cesspit, privy [in garden with thatched roof]
seiled		sealed
seison		possession, seisin
selar		*probably* cellar
sennyt		week (seven nights)
sere [the sere john henley]	46	*perhaps error for* 'the seyd john henley'
sergeaunt	111	serjeant [at law]
servar, serwar,		labourer, assistant
serwyng		serving [as labourer to craftsman]
serwyng		sewing [thatch]
sessyng	10	assessing
seve		give
sewerte		surety
sewstern		cistern
sewyng, serwyng		sewing [thatch]
seyge		*see* seeg
seyng		seeing, view
shon		shoes [horse]
sigell	62	seal [privy seal writ]
skatyrd		scattered
sklat, sklattar sklaatar		slate, slater
sklatt pynnys		slate pins
skofgate		Scotgate in Stamford
skottyl		scuttle or basket
skowryng		scouring, cleaning (cloth)
slekkyd		slaked [lime]
slhate		slate
slyf		slid down [thatch]
so, soo		water bucket, tub, soe
soder, soderryng, sowder, sowdyr, sowderyng		solder of lead, soldering [leads of chapel window]
some		sum
somertre		*see* summertree
sond		sand
sparr		wall studs
speer at bench end	51	wooden screen, Yaxley, Salzman

Term	Folio	Meaning
spens door		spence, larder door, Salzman
spent		used up
splentyng [a gable], splyntyng		inserting splints in walls and/or laying laths, Yaxley, Salzman, Morton
splintes		nails; or stakes, Salzman
spone		spoon for holy oil
spruse cofer	3	pine chest
spurnes [with staples, for the gate]	123v	*it seems to be* some form of metal fitting for the gate, *probably* the catch to the gate latch
spykyngg		large nails
stabylls		staples
standard, standers of doors		uprights?; *see* Salzman 513
stayng the barn by carpenter		strengthening?
step - for mending stairs [paid] to a wright with a step to the same	124v	?step
stepull	17v	steeple
sterey, straye, strey		straw
stoble, stobull		stubble [straw for thatching]
stodds, stod loggys	44	[wall] studs
stok		cash in hand, reserve funds
stolp, stulpe, stolpys		staple, for gate; *see* stulpes
stor for the lyflode	34v	building materials kept in store in the Hospital to be used for the estate
stres, stresse		distraint
strey		straw
streyts	22	orders of distraint by the court
stryk		strike, measure of wheat, malt, peas, oats, straw, lime etc , related to bushel, Yaxley
studdyng		erecting studs in a wall
stuff, stwf		building materials
stulpes		*probably* staples; *see* stolpes; *to be distinguished from 'stulpes'*, stumps of trees, boundary posts (*Lincolnshire glossary*)
summertre		summer, main cross beam
swm		sum
swte, swuytt, swyt, suet		suit
swyncote, swynkott		pigstyes
swynhaw		Swinehaw wood in North Witham
syd		side
syd tre, syddetre		sidetree timber
syf, syff		sieve, sift
sygt		sight
synet	62v	signet [clerk of the royal signet]
synke		drain
sysse		session of court
syuyng, swuyng		suing

apurys		tapers, altar candles
aylefete, telfett	47, 100	tailfeet [timber structure, *probably* part of roof] *may be related to* tailtree, short timber with one end tied into a frame, Yaxley; Morton *suggests* short pieces of wood attached to feet of rafters
elyor, telyer		tailor
emper, tempering		mixing earth (clay) with straw and stubble
eryng of floor; laths for teryng **floor**		laying earth on the floor, Salzman
habbay		the abbey, the abbot
hak, thakkar, thak rope		thatch, thatcher, thatch rope
herle		the earl
hoo		those
horo		through
housand (slates, nails or kydds etc)		a heap or collection , not a numerical term[360]
hydur		thither
hyng - 'Eltham thyng' in Carlby		small holding, sometime belonging to Eltham? Morton 176
on		the one (*before* tother, the other]
otalis oneris, onoris		total charges
rasyngs, trasons		joists
well mond'		twelve months
ymys		times
ndyrsett		provide support to, strengthening foundations before building work starts or driving in wedges to help timber-framed building to settle, Salzman 202
art nayls	49	hinge nails
ertvales, vertwall		metal fittings to doors or gates, Salzman
idua		widow
ache		the watch, London police
alor		value
alplat		wallplate, base timber to wall
and		wattling and roofing wands, probably of ash or willow
ark		work
attel, wattlyng		wattle for wall
ebbys of lead	17v	sheets of lead
edder		whether
edhys of iron	38v	iron wedges to split timbers and stone
effare, wefer, weffer, wefar, wever, weyvar, wewer		weaver [tenant in St Martin's, Stamford]

[360] thousand of slates: "when you get your slates holed they're set up in heaps, and a heap is a slater's thousand, which is like a baker's dozen. It isn't very accurate, there isn't a 1000 slates in it but it's known as a 1000. There's so many cases of slates and a case of slates is three, and you put in so many case to a heap, and a heap is supposed to cover roughly two square. A square in slater's measurement is ten feet by ten feet... a hundred square feet" - a thousand in this reckoning is enough slates of varying sizes to cover two hundred square feet; Osborn

welow		willow
weyht		weight
weyr		were
whe		we
whete strey		wheat straw for thatching
whyll		while
withdrawgt, withdrawgt in the high chamber	11, 33v, 45	*I think it is* a privy inside a chamber; *it is less likely to be* a private withdrawing room inside a chamber.
wollyng rope for scaffolding	13	strong cord for scaffolding, *see* Yaxley 'wolding line'
wootys		oats
wpp		up
writh		wright
wrohte		wrought
wrygt		write
wryte, wryyt, wrygt		wright, carpenter or smith
wyccareghe		vicarage
wymbell	86	gimlet to bore stone etc
wyndull (Item j grete wyndull to putt in naylys)	44	basket, skep, Yaxley
wyne rynyche		Rhenish wine
wyrte		writ
yat		that
yaytts, yat, yate, yaytt		gates
ye		the, they, their
yem		them
yen		then
yer		their, there, year
yer os [yer os laxton dwelt]		there as, i.e. where laxton dwelled
yerfor		therefore
yern		iron
yeroff		thereof
yerto		thereto
yether		thither
yeyre; yis yyer		year; this year
yis		this
yorthe		earth
yrn, yern		iron

INDEX

The numbers are folio numbers, not page numbers. The words and numbers in italics refer to pages of the Introduction and Appendices.

There will often be more than one reference on each folio. I have given the first mention of personal and placenames in this index a capital letter, but I have left many names without a capital letter as in the original to assist searching.

The counties are the pre-1974 counties

Lightning Source UK Ltd.
Milton Keynes UK
UKOW02f2322240214

227055UK00001B/9/P

9 781845 495992

THE WARDENS: MANAGING A LATE MEDIEVAL HOSPITAL

On behalf of the Stamford Survey Group and the publishers, we apologise for the faulty printing of the glossary. A copy of the glossary is provided separately.

GLOSSARY

This glossary has been compiled jointly by Alan Rogers and Ann Matthews of the Stamford Survey Group. We have drawn on the help of many others, especially Nat Alcock, Chris Currie, Vanessa Doe, David Dymond, Stephen Hart, John Hartley and Nick Hill. Among the sources we have used are

L F Salzman, Building in England down to 1540, *Clarendon 1952; David Yaxley,* A Researcher's Glossary *Larks Press, Norfolk, 2003;* Book of Morton *Northants Record Society 16, 1954; Eric Gee,* A Glossary of Building Terms *Frome 1984; Stephen Alsford,* Medieval English Towns - Glossary *1998;*

Lincolnshire glossary - http.www.cantab.net/users/michael.behrend/repubs/good.glossary/pages/words.html; *Fen-edge encounters -* http://dawnpiper.wordpress.com/land-words; *Osborn: Notes of a lecture entitled 'Collyweston and its Trade', given in 1976 by Bob Osborn of Collyweston, a Master Slater and quarry owner (we have been unable to find if there is any copyright holder of these notes);* Building Accounts of Tattershall Castle 1434-1472, *Lincoln Record Society vol 55.*

We have included a folio number only when there is a special mention of the word.

a bowth		about
a for, aforne		before
a geyn		again
a geyn		against
a gret		by agreement, contract
a lowy(d)		allowed
a naker		an acre
a neynd		an end
a nold		an old
a Noyffin	76	*probably* an oven
a peyr		appear
a yis syd		at this side of
abatements		deductions
ackers, akyrs		acres
aid (king's)		an occasional imposition made by the king for specific purposes
all halos		All Saints (parish, church, gild)
alloyd		allowed
almysse		alms[house]
alyas capias	85v	writ to seize possessions pending trial
ameld [jewelry]	61v	*perhaps* enamelled
an noon		now, currently, at present
A° R' R'		*anno regni regis*; in the year of the reign of king [Henry]

asch, aschese, aschys, ascys, assys, asse		ash tree(s)
assize, rents of assize		customary manorial dues from tenants as distinct from 'farms' (agreed rents)
assuyng		suing
asynyd		assigned [a court decision]
awght		owed
awtar		altar
ayl		ale
balks	44	baulks, tie beams
balys		bailiffs
bands, door bands of iron; window bands	10v	metal bands reinforcing doors; maybe hinges on metal plates
bargyn		contract
baros		(wheel)barrows
baryn		barn
basterd stone	118v	a hard stone broken up[355]
baston, bastyn roppe		rope made of bast fibre, Salzman
batyng		deducting
be		by
bedgat		retiring [to bed]
bench [made by masons]		either long seating or work top
betyng		beating [plaster]
betyng		'baiting', i.e. eating a meal
bey		bay [of building like a barn]
beyldyd		builded, built
blind chimney		*presumably* disused/blocked chimney
bol(l), bollys		bowl(s)
bonche [of laths etc]		bunch
bords		boards of various sizes and dimensions
born, bornyd		burn, burned [lime, plaster] - *see* bren
borosokn		duty of attending court of soke of Peterborough
boschell [of peas]		bushel
bot		but, only
botras		buttress
bowht, bohte, boyhte, bowghyt, bowte, boyghte, boyht		bought
bowndyng [our land]	53v	*either* hedging our land *or* measuring our land
boyr - dwelled at ye boyr in Stretton	95v	*presumably a placename in Stretton ?* bower?

355 "There is a layer of blue rag, a very hard stone known in the trade as bastard, and the only use for that is to break it up and build pillars to hold up the ceiling". (Osborn). This, I think, is the meaning here rather than the softer brown ironstone used widely for building in north Northamptonshire which is also known as bastard stone (D S Sutherland, *Northamptonshire Stone* Dovecote Press, 2003, pp 46-49) since it only appears once in these accounts and in a small quantity. See also Salzman 233 for bastard slate.

boythe		both
brasys; brase loggys	44	braces (timber); brace spars
bredcroft, bradcroft		Bradcroft, small settlement forming western suburb of Stamford lying in Rutland [buildings]
bren, brent		burn, burned
breyg		bridge
brode ston	52	*while many equate this with* freestone, Salzman 233 suggests large slates used for wall infilling instead of wattle and plaster
brykk		brick
bwlkes		*see* balks
bye		buy
bynwark		parish and church of St Mary Bynwark in western corner of town
calyd		called
carwar		carver
caryeg		carriage
catt of iron		*probably* gad of iron, weight Salzman 287; Tattershall 42
cayle	5	*here most likely* stone used for flooring, *see* Osborn[356]
chales		chalice
chef		chief rent
cheryf		sheriff
cherys		cherries
cheyneys		chains
chief rent		annual payment to landlord, ground rent
chyrch revys		churchwardens
clasp, claspe [of iron] for gate	44v	iron bracket [to mend ladder rung]; bracket for gate; door fastening
cleymowntt		Claymont, market place of Stamford, now Broad Street
clossys, clossis		closes, enclosed plots
clowt nayle		clout nails, flat-headed
coffer		chest
collys		coals
cope		copy; *also* coping stone
copwll copull		pair of rafters
corby; two corbys for lead	5	*unidentified*
corn schawmbyr		*either* corn chamber *or* corner chamber
corrections		fines on bedesmen for infringement of Hospital rules
cottears, cotyard		cottagers
countyng hows		store room for accounts; office
couples		*see* cowples

---

356 "There's only roughly about ten inches of soil, and then you get four or five feet of crash or kale as we call it ... in the olden days it was used for roadmaking" (Osborn). The *Lincolnshire glossary* says: "keal, kale: pieces of stone in very small masses, and uncertain and irregular shape; ... "Whether they are pieces or shreds of the limestone, of the ragg, or of our ordinary sandstone, they have all the name of *keale*"; in some parts of the county it is more especially applied to the scalings or fragments of the sandstone, as *creach,* or *crash,* is to the limestone; cf. Anglo-Saxon *scylan,* French *chaille,* 'a rocky earth'".

cowchyng	13, 34v	bedding down; stacking, storing
cownand, covande		covenanted, agreed, contracted with
cownte		account
cowple sparrs, cowpwlls	44	pair of rafters
coyn of long wall, coynys [of shop windows]	52, 39v	? quoins
crahcs	73	cracche, crib or rack for animal fodder, Yaxley
crest		ridge tile of stone or sometimes clay[357]
cross house in the yard	28v	*uncertain; it may be* a building at back of yard crossing between the two wings
crowper [saddle]		crupper [harness]
croys	82	*perhaps* crows
crystonmes		christmas
cumin		spice
cuthbert court		court of St Leonard's priory, Stamford
cycientes	62	[legal] sessions
dabyng		plastering, rendering - *see* dawbyng
daleland		Delalaund
darnys, dornys [pair of door durns]; dornis, dornys, dwrnes for a barn door	51v	door posts, frames
dawbyng		plastering, rendering, laying earth for the floor, *or* whitewashing - *both meanings appear in these accounts*
dells		dwells
denerse		dinners
det		debt
dewete		duty
dey		day
deyd		did
di', di[m]		half
dofcote, dowfhows, dowfhos, duffcot, dwff cott, dwfcote		dovecote
doon, doyne		done
dornis		*see* darnys
dorr, dur, dwr		door
dos'		dozen
draw in spars; drawyng a balk, timbers, floor joists;		set in place, insert? laying floor timbers? assembling?

357 "a stone ridging ... that used to come from Weldon, ... and it was sawn, another job that used to be done in the wintertime. And also they used to make clay ridge tiles at Peterborough, Whittlesea, even at Stamford, which more or less matched the colour of the slating" (Osborn).

draw, draw thatch, draw in thatch, drawer of thatch	50	combing to make straws parallel, preparing straw for thatching, Salzman 224; Morton
drawgt (sege)	4v	privy [probably inside room]
drawyng in [a house]; drawyng ye hows, dray		constructing a building or a room (Morton)
drawys (expenses this year draws £...), **drays**		amounts to
dray, drayng,	82v	*see* draw
drye ston wall	32v	dry stone wall
dryve, dryff [a floor]		? laying a floor, probably of earth
dur bands		Salzman 208 *equates these with* 'vertivals' or plate hinges, *but I think they occur too frequently for this to be true every time; they may be* metal bands to reinforce wooden doors; *see* bands
durnys		*see* darnys
dwtey		duty
dyghtyng, dythtyng, dyhttyng	61v	preparing [food], washing, cleaning [clothes], grooming [horse]
dyryge		memorial service for the dead, requiem; book of the service
dystreyne		seizure of cattle or goods in recompense for non-payment of rent or other charge; *see* stresse
edyryng [felling of stakes and edyryng]	17v	? ordering, i.e. stacking?
end		end of a wall, *perhaps sometimes* a gable end
enke	56v	ink
entertes [making of an]		tiebeam, Salzman 212
entrese		*perhaps* entry [into court, entering a plea]
erabyll		arable
ernyst, ernese		initial or down payment for contract
erthe, yorthe		earth, mainly clay, used for flooring, Salzman 147
esseyng		essoining
essoin, essoyn		excuse for absence or other fault in court
est stone - eft stone	118	*unknown*
evyn		evening
evys, evys boord, evys slates		eaves, eaves boards, eaves slates
eyd(e)		aid
eynd		end
eyrn, eyryn		iron
eys, eywys		eaves
falo		fallow
fardest, farryst, ferryst		furthest [the furthest house]
fawgts, fawyt		faults
feld		field
fen thak		reeds for thatching
fen, feyn		fain; must

ferm		an agreed rent for leases, usually an annual charge for a period of years and then re-negotiated; frequently with substantial entry payment and smaller annual payment
ferm, feyrm		farmstead
fewyng a gwtter, ffeyng, fewyng [a privy, a mess]		cleaning, clearing up
ffagoattys		faggots for fuel
ffalloys		fallows
ffeiffers		feoffees, trustees
fled [a chamber that was fled]	88v	*apparently* falling down *or* fallen
florth, floryht		floor
foder, foodyr		load or weight of lead, Salzman 122
folowehte		follows
fornas		furnace, oven, kiln
frank post		*uncertain*
frett of ladder	44v	ladder rung
fro		from
fur, furryng up gables		nailing extra pieces of timber to make surfaces even or for protection, Salzman 305; Yaxley
fyllyng, bem fyllyng bytwene the trasyngs	19, 39v	filling in between the [floor or wall] beams or joists with lath and plaster, wattling (and plaster), stone or occasionally brick
gaderyng, gederyng, gethurryng		gathering, collection [of rents]
game - making game a wall	100v	repairing?
garner		corn store
garrett gate	47v	*perhaps* entry with tower, Yaxley
gawme for windows **geamaws pair of; geawmbb [in stone]; geanows** pair of, for the shop windows	68, 44, 114; 39	? jambs or hinges, Yaxley
geyl spenc	98	*this may be* 'gild larder/pantry' ('spence' is a larder, Salzman 484) *or it may be* 'gild expenses'
geyt		get
golf, golve		*see* gowel
goter, gwter		gutter
goth with		goeth, goes with, has been joined to
gowel, govel,		gable[358]
gowyll, golve		gavel, rent payment
granse - bran and granse for the horse		grains
grese, gresyng, greys		steps, stairs
gret leet		king's leet court in Stamford

358 The 'govel, golve' in Easton payable to the gildhouse of Our Lady may be either an annual customary rent due to the gild of St Mary in Easton or a payment due to the connection of the tenant's house to the gable of the gildhouse - it is not possible to determine which this is.

gret water		flood
grete		agreement, contract work
greyte yaat		great gate
grondsell, growndsole		groundsill; can be foundation course of stone or timber
grynd, grynde of iron [of the barn door]	6v, 18, 39v	?door fitting?
gwd		good
gwttar		gutter
gy hows in the yard	47	*perhaps* privy
gy(e)		Guy
gyffyng		giving
gyle of corpus Xti		gild of corpus christi
gyle, gyll, gild howse		*either* house used by gild for meetings *or* house which belonged to and paid rent to a gild [gild of St Mary in Easton; or house next to All Saints vicarage which was used by or paid rent to the gild of All Saints, Stamford]
gymmos, gymmoys, gymms - pair of		*probably* hinges Yaxley; *but see* geamaws *above*
hach		hatch
haf		have
haf		half
hal		hall
haloyng, halow		hallowing, consecrating
halylofe, haly lof		payment (of 1d, 2d or 3d) to the parish due on different dates from some properties (by rota) in both rural and urban contexts, presumably for exemption on this occasion from providing the parish holy loaf; normally paid by the tenant. See E. Duffy, *Stripping of the Altars* pp 125-7.
hart lath		laths from inner wood
heche, heggs		hedge, hedges
hecter?		hectare?
helmys		Elmes
heng lok [for a door], henglok	13v, 44	*probably* padlock (Yaxley)
hengels, henghelis [usually with hooks]	12v	*most likely* hinges (simple pin hinge); *unlikely here to be* hangells, hooks which form part of the equipment of an open fire for cooking (Yaxley)
henges		hinges
hengyng [hengyng the house]	89	*uncertain; may be related to* hinges; *or* hanging windows and doors etc
henkylls		*probably* hengels
hent nown		before noon?
her		their
herdylls, hyrdels		hurdles
hespys		hasps
hey, hey hows		hay, hay barn
heyd plac		manor house
heyng		hang
heyr		here, her, their
hogstyes		pigstyes

hole, holl		whole
holys		holes
hoopyng of soo, hopyng, hoopyng of bowls		*probably* providing iron hoops around the bowls or buckets
hoopys off yrn		iron hoops
hoose, hws, hos, hose, howsse, howsys		house, houses - *frequently used to mean* a room in a house, a chamber; *but* 'hus' *can also mean* a door, Salzman
hord bred		fodder
hotts		oats
howk		hook [for door], latch
howm		home
howte		owed
hoyle, hollyd, holly		whole, wholly
hus, hws		us; *see* hoose
hwe		Hugh
hwks		hooks
hye		high
hyeryng, hyard		hiring [horses, guide, messenger]; hired [land]
hyllyng		covering (books) , roofing (buildings)
hyr		here
hyr		hire
hyt		it
Ihs est amor meus		Jesus is my devotion
insett house	24	*described by Yaxley as a puzzling term, its meaning here is uncertain, perhaps* an interior room (*see* hoose) or farm building for animals
jagge [of straw]	112v	small cart-load, OED
jame [mendyng a jame] **jeawmys -** carpenters making divers jeawmys and undersetting the walls	81v	? jamb? *but see* jeamys, geamaws
jealmys - paid a mason to mend	49	*perhaps* hinges set in stone, the iron pintle hinges set into masonry jambs to receive iron strap hinges
jeamys of the hall jeamaws for a door; jeawnys, jemos	11, 40v 45 23v, 74	?hinges Yaxley (gemel)
joyst tree	114	joist
karyag		carriage
kebull, bord kebull, kebbyll, kebwl	44	*almost certainly* 'couple'
kechyn		kitchen
kerver		carver
king's eyd		tax at will of king, *see* aid
knafe nykkol - Item for to help to tak down ye sclats to a knafe nykkol iijd	94	*is it possible that* 'knafe nykkol' *is a personal name? Rafe Nyccol?*

koyns of freestone, hewyng of	13v	hewing quoins
kybulls [wooden]	31v	*probably* couples [q.v.]
kydds		faggots of wood for fuel
kyllyng, kylyn		kiln *[probably for malt]*
kyngs xv	18	king's tax of one fifteenth; *in towns like Stamford, paid at one tenth of rateable value but still called a fifteenth*
kynkys		king's
lade		lady
ladys rent		*see* gyle, gild house *above*
lapp of iron	39	*perhaps* a measure of iron; *or is it possible that this is* a flap of iron to cover a keyhole? Salzman 302
laryfax		*perhaps* caryfax? *the placename is otherwise unknown in Stamford*
laterynd		latter end
laton		bell metal used from memorial brasses
latts		laths
leads, leds		lead framing in window glass in chapel
leche		doctor
leddyr		ladder
ledyng [of stone, mortar etc]		carting [stone, mortar etc]
legbys	52	leghys?
leghys, ledghys, leyg, legths, legyhys, legys to a door, leyge, legge	23, 44, 33v	ledges [e.g. window ledges], square-sectioned braces on doors, windows etc; a term still used for the horizontal board to which the vertical boards are nailed in a boarded door
leyd		lead *for roofing or gutters*
leyd to		joined with
leyng		laying
leyn'hte	82v	*probably here* length
leytt		leet court
loggs		sawn timber; posts and spars[359] etc
longs, longyn		belongs, belonging
lovar, lower	31v	louvre; wooden slatted tower in roof as a smoke vent
loyd, loydyd		loads
lycens		licence
lyflode		*the best translation is* 'estate'
lyg over		lie over
lyttar	32, 52	*perhaps* litter, rubbish
maad		made
maner		manor
manteltre	32, 52v	mantelpiece above fireplace
marbuler		metal engraver
maschfatt	46v	mash vat - large wooden tub containing the mash for brewing - Yaxley

[359] These are clearly timbers here rather than the 'logs' of stone ('pillars') which Osborn refers to in Collyweston

masyn		mason
mawnger		manger
medo		meadow
mercyments		fines in court
mersyed		amerced, fined in court
met, mete, meyte		meat, food
meyt, met, mett	10v	measure, measured
michelys, myhel, myhelemes		michael, Michaelmas
mo, moo		more
moren		morn[ing]
moyng		mowing [hay]
mwdwall		mud wall
mwst		must
mydow		meadow
myllyn, mylner howse		mill, mill house, miller
nell, neylys,		nails
nete gate [in field]	49v	?cattle gate, cattle grid?
nett - for mending a nett [?mett?] [in items in store]	125v	*uncertain reading and meaning*
nett - long nett hows	52	?cattle shed?
nohte ar		are not there
nonnys		nuns
noo		no
noo		now
noyffyn		*probably* an oven
nyht		night
oder		other
on hole yeyre		one whole year
on, oon		one
onys		once
oppynynyg		opening
or		ere, before
os		as
ostyy wall - in the Angel Inn	11	*unknown; it may be the wall of the hostellry*
owen		oven
owen		own
ower		over
owt		ought, out
oyer		other
oyn		own
pak thred		pack thread for thatching
pale		fence
palle [carpenter mends a palle]	118	*probably* fence or stake
panys in the govel		*perhaps* panels in the gable

par of, pare		pair of, pair
pargetting		plaster work to walls and gables, often ornamental
pauper		paper
payngtyng		painting
payth, peyth		pays
pec, peec, pese, peys		piece
pekax		pickaxe
pelor logg	44	pillar spar, upright for doors and windows, *or* supporting post
pentter		painter
pentts, pentys, peyntes	94v	penthouse, pentice, lean-to; *can also be* roof over oven, Yaxley
pepur, pepyr, peyper		pepper
pertener, pertenynyys, perteyngs, ye perteneys yerto		appurtenances, belongings; the appurtenances belonging to some properties
pese		piece
pey, peyd		pay, paid
peynter		painter
peyr		pair
peyse		peas (horse fodder]
pingulfeld		pingle : a small enclosure of low shrubs, or underwood, or gorse; a close, small meadow; a small spinney; pingle close : a small meadow, *Lincolnshire glossary*; here, it is a field name in Stamford
plaschers, plaschyng		hedge cutters, hedging; pleaching, interweaving branches to make a solid hedge to retain cattle.
plats [of iron to lay under the great gate]	39v	plates
platts [timber]		wooden plates, timber beam laid horizontally, Yaxley
playsterer		plasterer
plommar, plwmmer		plumber
plot [mending a]	94v	*perhaps* a patch
poll		measure of length
pond		pound
post fest mychael		after Michaelmas
powlys		[St] Pauls
poyntyng, pwentyng		pointing [of stone work]
prentes		apprentice
prests	9v	charges, payments or levies (*for services etc*)
probatur est per me		[this page] is approved/audited by me
prowand(e)		provender, fodder for horses
pryncypal copull	100	principal rafters
pultre merkett	4v	poultry market
pyk of iron	52	*perhaps* pickaxe, pike
pyns, pynns, pynnes		pins, *especially* slate pins
pytt		quarry
quart' wags		quarter's wages
qwer, qweyr		where

qwest, qwert?		jury in court
qweyt	86v	wheat
rakys		rakes [iron]
ramell		rubbish, spoil heap after building
redyng [bornyng, betyng, syftyng, redyng, schotyng the floor]	44v	reeding, laying reeds in floor; [burning, beating, sifting (the plaster), laying reeds and finishing/smoothing the floor]; Morton suggests it could be colouring the floor with red ochre
rekynd		reckoned
rensak	45, 45v	dig up (old stone) for re-use
rent off a syse		rent of assize, chief rent; customary payments from manorial tenants
resewyd		received
rewyng		*perhaps* renewing
reyd		reed for thatch
reyng - for a reyng to ye leyd	100	*Morton suggests* cleaning (reeing) as with corn; *may be* cleaning lead? *or it could here be* 'arraying' the lead, laying it out, flattening it
reysed		raised
rigg, rygg (verb), 'earth and mortar to rygg withall'	12v, 18v, 48v, 49	b) rigg as a verb is always linked with thatching, making the ridges of roofs, a process in which clay and mortar is often used
riggs, ryggs - Crodon Riggs in Swayfield;		a) riggs in Swayfield are no doubt fields, closes, in ridges owned or once owned by someone called Crodon? (*Lincolnshire glossary*); could it be land where turves are cut? Yaxley
rod, rode, roode,		rood
roftre, rowftre, rwftre		rooftree
Rokkyng [plastering/renderin g and rokkyng]	40, 49	*JSH suggests* raking, combing, *but it may be* inserting stones into the plaster
Rollys		[court] rolls
ron a neynd		?run an end?; Yaxley *found* 'run furs', *so this may be* to run furring over an end, i.e. gable
royd, rode	101	rood [defined as three feet]
royffe		roof
roys - roys a boun	102	?rows? *unknown*
rygg		*see* riggs
sam		same
sap lath		laths from outer sap wood
sawer		sawyer
sawyn trasyngs	44	sawn joists
schater		slater
schef		chief [rent]
scherefs tern', scheryff geld		annual payment to sheriff for his jurisdiction due from some holdings
schevys		sheaves
schew - paid to schew our lands		?plough, harrow? *or could it be* to measure our lands?
schop bothys		area in Stamford usually named Shobothes

schotyng of lead; schott the floor	17v	*probably* pounding lead before laying it; *also* spreading and watering clay before using it for flooring, Yaxley; *the word survives in* wainscotting *but here refers to flooring*
schoyng		shoeing horses
schreddyng of ashes	14v	stripping bark off coppiced ash wands before use in wattling or basket making
sclat, sklatter		slate, slater
sclate pynse		slate pins
scledd	18	horse-drawn sledge for stone
sclottys [for a door]		bolts for doors, Salzman
scole		school
se		see
seage in the high chamber	19v	indoor privy
seam, sem, seem, seyme		packhorse load or cartload (lime, plaster, mortar etc)
seeg, seyge, sege	19	cesspit, privy [in garden with thatched roof]
seiled		sealed
seison		possession, seisin
selar		*probably* cellar
sennyt		week (seven nights)
sere [the sere john henley]	46	*perhaps error for* 'the seyd john henley'
sergeaunt	111	serjeant [at law]
servar, serwar,		labourer, assistant
serwyng		serving [as labourer to craftsman]
serwyng		sewing [thatch]
sessyng	10	assessing
seve		give
sewerte		surety
sewstern		cistern
sewyng, serwyng		sewing [thatch]
seyge		*see* seeg
seyng		seeing, view
shon		shoes [horse]
sigell	62	seal [privy seal writ]
skatyrd		scattered
sklat, sklattar sklaatar		slate, slater
sklatt pynnys		slate pins
skofgate		Scotgate in Stamford
skottyl		scuttle or basket
skowryng		scouring, cleaning (cloth)
slekkyd		slaked [lime]
slhate		slate
slyf		slid down [thatch]
so, soo		water bucket, tub, soe
soder, soderryng, sowder, sowdyr, sowderyng		solder of lead, soldering [leads of chapel window]

some		sum
somertre		*see* summertree
sond		sand
sparr		wall studs
speer at bench end	51	wooden screen, Yaxley, Salzman
spens door		spence, larder door, Salzman
spent		used up
splentyng [a gable], splyntyng		inserting splints in walls and/or laying laths, Yaxley, Salzman, Morton
splintes		nails; or stakes, Salzman
spone		spoon for holy oil
spruse cofer	3	pine chest
spurnes [with staples, for the gate]	123v	*it seems to be* some form of metal fitting for the gate, *probably* the catch to the gate latch
spykyngg		large nails
stabylls		staples
standard, standers of doors		uprights?; *see* Salzman 513
stayng the barn by carpenter		strengthening?
step - for mending stairs [paid] to a wright with a step to the same	124v	?step
stepull	17v	steeple
sterey, straye, strey		straw
stoble, stobull		stubble [straw for thatching]
stodds, stod loggys	44	[wall] studs
stok		cash in hand, reserve funds
stolp, stulpe, stolpys		staple, for gate; *see* stulpes
stor for the lyflode	34v	building materials kept in store in the Hospital to be used for the estate
stres, stresse		distraint
strey		straw
streyts	22	orders of distraint by the court
stryk		strike, measure of wheat, malt, peas, oats, straw, lime etc , related to bushel, Yaxley
studdyng		erecting studs in a wall
stuff, stwf		building materials
stulpes		*probably* staples; *see* stolpes; *to be distinguished from 'stulpes'*, stumps of trees, boundary posts (*Lincolnshire glossary*)
summertre		summer, main cross beam
swm		sum
swte, swuytt, swyt, suet		suit
swyncote, swynkott		pigstyes
swynhaw		Swinehaw wood in North Witham
syd		side
syd tre, syddetre		sidetree timber
syf, syff		sieve, sift

sygt		sight
synet	62v	signet [clerk of the royal signet]
synke		drain
sysse		session of court
syuyng, swuyng		suing
tapurys		tapers, altar candles
taylefete, telfett	47, 100	tailfeet [timber structure, *probably* part of roof] *may be related to* tailtree, short timber with one end tied into a frame, Yaxley; Morton *suggests* short pieces of wood attached to feet of rafters
telyor, telyer		tailor
temper, tempering		mixing earth (clay) with straw and stubble
teryng of floor; laths for teryng **floor**		laying earth on the floor, Salzman
thabbay		the abbey, the abbot
thak, thakkar, thak rope		thatch, thatcher, thatch rope
therle		the earl
thoo		those
thoro		through
thousand (slates, nails or kydds etc)		a heap or collection , not a numerical term[360]
thydur		thither
thyng - 'Eltham thyng' in Carlby		small holding, sometime belonging to Eltham? Morton 176
ton		the one (*before* tother, the other]
totalis oneris, onoris		total charges
trasyngs, trasons		joists
twell mond'		twelve months
tymys		times
undyrsett		provide support to, strengthening foundations before building work starts or driving in wedges to help timber-framed building to settle, Salzman 202
vart nayls	49	hinge nails
vertvales, vertwall		metal fittings to doors or gates, Salzman
vidua		widow
wache		the watch, London police
walor		value
walplat		wallplate, base timber to wall
wand		wattling and roofing wands, probably of ash or willow
wark		work
wattel, wattlyng		wattle for wall
webbys of lead	17v	sheets of lead

[360] thousand of slates: "when you get your slates holed they're set up in heaps, and a heap is a slater's thousand, which is like a baker's dozen. It isn't very accurate, there isn't a 1000 slates in it but it's known as a 1000. There's so many cases of slates and a case of slates is three, and you put in so many case to a heap, and a heap is supposed to cover roughly two square. A square in slater's measurement is ten feet by ten feet... a hundred square feet" - a thousand in this reckoning is enough slates of varying sizes to cover two hundred square feet; Osborn

wedder		whether
wedhys of iron	38v	iron wedges to split timbers and stone
weffare, wefer, weffer, wefar, wever, weyvar, wewer		weaver [tenant in St Martin's, Stamford]
welow		willow
weyht		weight
weyr		were
whe		we
whete strey		wheat straw for thatching
whyll		while
withdrawgt, withdrawgt in the high chamber	11, 33v, 45	*I think it is* a privy inside a chamber; *it is less likely to be* a private withdrawing room inside a chamber.
wollyng rope for scaffolding	13	strong cord for scaffolding, *see* Yaxley 'wolding line'
wootys		oats
wpp		up
writh		wright
wrohte		wrought
wrygt		write
wryte, wryyt, wrygt		wright, carpenter or smith
wyccareghe		vicarage
wymbell	86	gimlet to bore stone etc
wyndull (Item j grete wyndull to putt in naylys)	44	basket, skep, Yaxley
wyne rynyche		Rhenish wine
wyrte		writ
yat		that
yaytts, yat, yate, yaytt		gates
ye		the, they, their
yem		them
yen		then
yer		their, there, year
yer os [yer os laxton dwelt]		there as, i.e. where laxton dwelled
yerfor		therefore
yern		iron
yeroff		thereof
yerto		thereto
yether		thither
yeyre; yis yyer		year; this year
yis		this
yorthe		earth
yrn, yern		iron